Dual Source CT Imaging

Peter R. Seidensticker, MD

Lars K. Hofmann, MD

With 209 Figures and 52 Tables

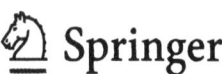

ISBN 978-3-540-77601-7
Springer Medizin Verlag Heidelberg

Bibliografische Information der Deutschen Bibliothek
The Deutsche Bibliothek lists this publication in Deutsche
Nationalbibliographie; detailed bibliographic data is available
in the internet at http://dnb.ddb.de.

Springer Medizin Verlag
springer.com
© Springer Medizin Verlag Heidelberg 2008

SPIN 11770107
Design and Typesetting:
A.UND.W – Agentur für Kommunikation, Berlin
Printing: Grosch! Druckzentrum GmbH, Heidelberg

18/5135 – 5 4 3 2 1 0

Content

Dear Colleagues

The introduction of Dual Source Computed Tomography (DSCT) in 2005 represented a giant leap in the evolution of sectional imaging comparable to the introduction of spiral and later multi-detector CT. The scientific community has responded with great interest and DSCT has opened entirely new clinical fields to CT applications. Equipped with two x-ray sources and detectors mounted in one gantry, DSCT enables many new applications ranging from heart rate independent coronary CT angiography examinations to complete chest pain evaluation in one single scan. Because it is able to run both x-ray sources simultaneously at different energy settings, DSCT is also the first scanner generation to enable routine spiral dual energy imaging.

As today's scanners become faster and more robust, contrast media delivery has become an increasingly critical element of the contrast enhanced CT procedure. It has been necessary over the years to significantly adapt injection protocols with each new scanner generation. This is particularly relevant in the case of DSCT.

Siemens AG and Bayer Schering Pharma joined forces in early 2006 to provide you with a comprehensive overview of DSCT's capabilities together with reliable protocol recommendations for scanner use and optimized contrast media injection parameters.

Based on their extensive experience in CT imaging, physicians from 12 global luminary sites were selected to form the Dual Source CT Expert Panel. Over the course of 18 months and four panel meetings, 25 clinical scan and contrast media injection protocols were developed. All protocols were based on intense discussions among the panel members. To ensure the highest quality, the selected protocols were tested by numerous sites, individually adapted and finally approved during a panel consensus meeting.

This book will provide an introduction into DSCT technology as well as into the basics of contrast media administration. You will find consensus protocols as well as individual considerations, such as tricks and pitfalls, complemented by clinical examples from several of the world's best radiologists and cardiologists. We are confident it can help you to achieve consistently high image quality, optimal patient care, and perhaps a solid starting point for the development of your own unique protocols.

Peter R. Seidensticker, MD

Berlin / Germany

Lars K. Hofmann, MD

Erlangen / Germany

The Dual Source CT Expert Panel

Stephan Achenbach, MD, FESC, FACC

Professor of Cardiology

University of Erlangen-Nuremberg

Departments of Cardiology and Radiology

Ulmenweg 18

91054 Erlangen, Germany

Hatem Alkadhi, MD

University Hospital Zurich

Institute of Diagnostic Radiology

Raemistr. 100

8091 Zurich, Switzerland

Christoph R. Becker, MD

Associate Professor

University of Munich-Grosshadern

Department of Clinical Radiology

Marchioninistr. 15

81377 Munich, Germany

Harald Brodoefel, MD

Eberhard Karls-University Tühingen

Department of Diagnostic and

Interventional Radiology

Hoppe-Seyler-Str. 3

72076 Tübingen, Germany

Roman Fischbach, MD

Associate Professor of Radiology

University of Münster

Department of Clinical Radiology

Albert-Schweitzer-Str. 33

48149 Münster, Germany

Martin Heuschmid, MD

Associate Professor

Eberhard-Karls-University Tübingen

Department of Diagnostic and

Interventional Radiology

Hoppe-Seyler-Str. 3

72076 Tübingen, Germany

Thorsten R. C. Johnson, MD

University of Munich-Grosshadern

Department of Clinical Radiology

Marchioninistr. 15

81377 Munich, Germany

Kai Uwe Juergens, MD

Assistant Professor

University of Münster

Department of Clinical Radiology

Albert-Schweitzer-Str. 33

48149 Münster, Germany

Andreas F. Kopp, MD
Professor of Radiology
Eberhard-Karls-University Tübingen
Department of Diagnostic and
Interventional Radiology
Hoppe-Seyler-Str. 3
72076 Tübingen, Germany

Axel Kuettner, MD
University of Erlangen-Nuremberg
Department of Radiology
Maximiliansplatz 1
91054 Erlangen, Germany

Andreas H. Mahnken, MD, MBA
University Hospital, RWTH Aachen University
Department of Diagnostic Radiology
Pauwelsstr. 30
52074 Aachen, Germany

Cynthia McCollough, PhD
Mayo Clinic College of Medicine
Department of Radiology
200 First Street SW
Rochester, MN 55905, USA

Nico R. Mollet, MD, PhD
Erasmus Medical Center Rotterdam
Department of Radiology
Room HS-207, Department of Radiology
PO Box 2040
3000 CA Rotterdam, Netherlands

Gilbert L. Raff, MD
William Beaumont Hospital
Department of Cardiology
3601 West Thirteen Mile Road
Royal Oak, MI 48073, USA

Dieter Ropers, MD, FESC
Professor of Cardiology
University of Erlangen-Nuremberg
Departments of Cardiology and Radiology
Ulmenweg 18
91054 Erlangen, Germany

Stephan G. Ruehm, MD, PhD
David Geffen School of Medicine at UCLA
Department of Radiology
Peter V Ueberroth Bldg., Suite 3371
10945 LeConte Avenue
Los Angeles, CA 90095-7206, USA

U. Joseph Schoepf, MD
Medical University of South Carolina
Departments of Radiology and Medicine
169 Ashley Ave., PO Box 250322
29425 Charleston, USA

Harald Seifarth, MD
University of Münster
Department of Clinical Radiology
Albert-Schweitzer-Str. 33
48149 Münster, Germany

Joachim E. Wildberger, MD
RWTH Aachen University
Department of Diagnostic Radiology
Pauwelsstr. 30
52074 Aachen, Germany

Eric Williamson, MD
Mayo Clinic College of Medicine
Department of Radiology
200 First Street SW
Rochester, MN 55905, USA

Authors

Katharina Anders, MD

University of Erlangen-Nuremberg

Department of Radiology

Maximiliansplatz 1

91054 Erlangen, Germany

Cesar Arellano, MD

David Geffen School of Medicine at UCLA

Department of Radiology

Peter V Ueberroth Bldg., Suite 3371

10945 LeConte Avenue

Los Angeles, CA 90095-7206, USA

Matthias Braeutigam

Bayer Schering Pharma AG

TRG Diagnostic Imaging

Müllerstr. 178

13342 Berlin, Germany

Christiane Bredenhoeller, RT

Siemens AG

Medical Solutions

Computed Tomography

Siemensstr. 1

91301 Forchheim, Germany

Filippo Cademartiri, MD, PhD

Erasmus Medical Center Rotterdam

Department of Radiology

Room HS-207, Department of Radiology

PO Box 2040

3000 CA Rotterdam, Netherlands

Kavitha M. Chinnaiyan, MD

Director of Cardiac CT/MRI Education

William Beaumont Hospital

Department of Cardiology

3601 West Thirteen Mile Road

Royal Oak, MI 48073, USA

Marco Das, MD

University Hospital, RWTH Aachen University

Department of Diagnostic Radiology

Pauwelsstr. 30

52074 Aachen, Germany

Christian Fink

University of Munich-Grosshadern

Department of Clinical Radiology

Marchioninistr. 15

81377 Munich, Germany

Tobias Fischer, MD

University of Münster

Department of Clinical Radiology

Albert-Schweitzer-Str. 33

48149 Münster, Germany

Thomas Flohr, PhD

Siemens AG

Medical Solutions

Computed Tomography

Siemensstr. 1

91301 Forchheim, Germany

Ralph Gentry, RT (R)(CT)(MR)
William Beaumont Hospital
Department of Cardiology
3601 West Thirteen Mile Road
Royal Oak, MI 48073, USA

Scott Harris, MD
Mayo Clinic College of Medicine
Department of Radiology
200 First Street SW
Rochester, MN 55905, USA

Robert P. Hartman, MD
Mayo Clinic College of Medicine
Department of Radiology
200 First Street SW
Rochester, MN 55905, USA

Ute Huebner-Steiner
Bayer Schering Pharma AG
TRG Diagnostic Imaging
Müllerstr. 178
13342 Berlin, Germany

Stephan P. Kloska, MD
University of Münster
Department of Clinical Radiology
Albert-Schweitzer-Str. 33
48149 Münster, Germany

Gabriel P. Krestin, MD, PhD
Erasmus Medical Center Rotterdam
Department of Radiology
Room HS-207, Department of Radiology
PO Box 2040
3000 CA Rotterdam, Netherlands

Heon Lee, MD, PhD
Medical University of South Carolina
Department of Radiology
169 Ashley Ave., PO Box 250322
SC 29425 Charleston, USA

Michael Lell, MD
Assistant Professor
University of Erlangen-Nuremberg
Department of Radiology
Maximiliansplatz 1
91054 Erlangen, Germany

Sebastian Leschka, MD
University Hospital Zurich
Institute of Diagnostic Radiology
Raemistr. 100
8091 Zurich, Switzerland

Derek Lohan, MD
David Geffen School of Medicine at UCLA
Department of Radiology
Peter V Ueberroth Bldg., Suite 3371
10945 LeConte Avenue
Los Angeles, CA 90095-7206, USA

Elizabeth McDonald, MD, PhD
Mayo Clinic College of Medicine
Department of Radiology
200 First Street SW
Rochester, MN 55905, USA

Andrew Misselt, MD
Mayo Clinic College of Medicine
Department of Radiology
200 First Street SW
Rochester, MN 55905, USA

Dominik Morhard, MD
University of Munich-Grosshadern
Department of Clinical Radiology
Marchioninistr. 15
81377 Munich, Germany

Konstantin Nikolaou, MD
Associate Professor
University of Munich-Grosshadern
Department of Clinical Radiology
Marchioninistr. 15
81377 Munich, Germany

Christoph Panknin, MS
David Geffen School of Medicine at UCLA
Department of Radiology
Peter V Ueberroth Bldg., Suite 3371
10945 LeConte Avenue
Los Angeles, CA 90095-7206, USA

Hubertus Pietsch, PhD
Bayer Schering Pharma AG
TRG Diagnostic Imaging
Müllerstr. 178
13342 Berlin, Germany

Andrew Primak, PhD
Mayo Clinic College of Medicine
Department of Radiology
200 First Street SW
Rochester, MN 55905, USA

Michael Puesken, MD
University of Münster
Department of Clinical Radiology
Albert-Schweitzer-Str. 33
48149 Münster, Germany

Hans Scheffel, MD
University Hospital Zurich
Institute of Diagnostic Radiology
Raemistr. 100
8091 Zurich, Switzerland

Bernhard Schmidt, PhD
Siemens AG
Medical Solutions
Computed Tomography
Siemensstr. 1
91301 Forchheim, Germany

Ulrich Speck, PhD
Charité, Humboldt University
Department of Radiology
Charitéplatz 1
10098 Berlin, Germany

Paul Stolzmann, MD
University Hospital Zurich
Institute of Diagnostic Radiology
Raemistr. 100
8091 Zurich, Switzerland

Pal Suranyi, MD, PhD
Medical University of South Carolina
Department of Radiology
169 Ashley Ave., PO Box 250322
SC 29425 Charleston, USA

Christian Thilo, MD
Medical University of South Carolina
Departments of Radiology and Medicine
169 Ashley Ave., PO Box 250322
SC 29425 Charleston, USA

Christoph Thomas, MD
Eberhard-Karls-University Tübingen
Department of Diagnostic and
Interventional Radiology
Hoppe-Seyler-Str. 3
72076 Tübingen, Germany

Terri J. Vrtiska, MD
Mayo Clinic College of Medicine
Department of Radiology
200 First Street SW
Rochester, MN 55905, USA

Sabine Weckbach, MD
University of Munich-Grosshadern
Department of Clinical Radiology
Marchioninistr. 15
81377 Munich, Germany

Dual Source CT Technology

Bernhard Schmidt · Christiane Bredenhoeller · Thomas Flohr

The introduction of spiral CT in the early 1990s marked one of the important steps in the evolution of CT-imaging techniques.[1,2] The technology allowed clinicians for the first time to acquire volume data without the risk of miss- or double-registration. It also enabled the reconstruction of images at any position along the patient's length axis as well as reconstructions of overlapping images to improve the longitudinal resolution. Furthermore, spiral acquisition reduced scan times significantly as the patient moved continuously through the gantry rather than step-by-step (step and shoot mode).

Despite these improvements, single-slice spiral CT used in daily clinical routine presented many limitations. Because of the small detector coverage, spiral CT was only able to achieve a desired isotropic resolution (i.e. equal resolution in all three spatial axes) for very limited scan ranges.[3] For longer scans (e.g. chest examinations), the spatial resolution along the patient's length axis had to be significantly compromised. The introduction of multi-detector row computed tomography (MDCT) in 1998 solved some of these issues. Larger anatomical volumes could be acquired with a single acquisition. The first generation of MDCT systems offered simultaneous acquisition of 4 slices at a rotation time of 0.5 s, which provided considerably improved scan speed and longitudinal resolution as well as better utilization of the available x-ray power.[4–6] In addition to significantly reducing acquisition time for a variety of clinical protocols, MDCT also made longer scan ranges with substantially reduced slice width feasible, which is essential, for example, in CT angiography (CTA) of the lower extremities.[7] MDCT also expanded into areas previously considered beyond the scope of 3rd generation CT scanners using mechanical rotation of x-ray tube and detector, such as CT angiography of the coronary arteries with the addition of ECG gating capability.[8,9]

Despite these promising improvements, clinical challenges and limitations remained for 4-slice CT systems. True isotropic resolution for routine applications had not yet been achieved for many applications such as CT angiography of the chest.[7] Stents or severely calcified arteries constituted a diagnostic dilemma for ECG-gated coronary CTA, mainly due to partial volume artifacts resulting from insufficient longitudinal resolution, and limited temporal resolution made reliable imaging of patients with higher heart rates impossible.[10]

The introduction of 16-slice CT scanners finally enabled routine acquisitions with isotropic sub-millimeter spatial resolution.[11,12] This technology also opened up other new possibilities such as the diagnosis of an acute ischemic stroke by assessing the status of the vessels supplying the brain and

Dual Source CT Technology

the location of the intracranial occlusion in the same CTA examination. The higher detector coverage again improved the diagnosis of central and peripheral pulmonary embolisms, even in patients with limited ability to cooperate.[13, 14] ECG-gated cardiac scanning was enhanced by both improved temporal resolution as a result of gantry rotation times as low as 0.375 s and improved spatial resolution.[15, 16]

The generation of 64-slice CT systems was introduced in 2004. This technology relies on new scanner concepts, and two different concepts were launched on the market.

The "volume concept" pursued by GE, Philips and Toshiba aims to further increase the volume coverage speed by using 64 detector rows instead of 16 without changing the physical parameters of the scanner from the 16-slice version.

The "resolution concept" pursued by Siemens uses 32 physical detector rows in combination with "double z-sampling" – a refined z-sampling technique enabled by periodically moving the focal point in the z-direction, to simultaneously acquire 64 overlapping slices. The objective is to increase the longitudinal resolution and reduce spiral artifacts independent of pitch (see also figure 1).[17, 18]

CT angiographic examinations with sub-mm resolution in the pure arterial phase are possible with 64-slice CT systems, even for extended anatomical ranges. The entire thorax (350 mm) can be scanned with sub-mm resolution in about 6 s, facilitating emergency scans, for example, to check for acute pulmonary embolism. A whole-body CTA with 1500 mm scan range takes approximately the same scan time that is required for a 16-slice scanner but with a considerably improved longitudinal resolution. Overall, the improvements in spatial and temporal resolution afforded by 64-slice CT systems lead to better quantification and tracking of disease processes such as relative stenosis, perfusion and pulsatility.[19] The improved temporal resolution that results from gantry rotation times as low as 0.33 s increases the robustness of ECG-gated scanning at higher heart rates. This facilitates the successful integration of CT coronary angiography into routine clinical algorithms, although higher heart rates can still be problematic.[20, 21]

Clinical experience with 64-slice CT systems indicates that many of the issues of previous scanner generations have been solved. Scan time – one of the driving factors in the past to increase CT detector coverage – is no longer an issue in 64-slice CT systems. In fact, the table feed has to be reduced in many cases to avoid outrunning the contrast bolus (e.g. in run offs). Nevertheless, some of the challenges in clinical routine still exist. For example, examining obese patients remains an issue because of the limited tube power. In these cases, the patient can either not be examined at all or dedicated acquisition protocols with compromised scan speed have to be used. In addition, although cardiac CT imaging has become clinical routine, image quality is often compromised by motion artifacts in patients with higher heart rates. But higher temporal resolution would generally reduce blooming artifacts caused by stents or calcifications and residual motion even at lower heart rates. Using refined algorithms such as "multi segment reconstruction" techniques theoretically allow the improvement of temporal resolution. However, the temporal resolution can only be increased as desired at certain heart rates (see figure 2). Some "sweet spots" exist in principle; however, it is impossible in clinical routine to somehow adjust and maintain a patient's heart rate to achieve optimal temporal resolution. Furthermore, multi-segment reconstructions rely on data consistency from two subsequent heart beats. Any inconsistencies will lead to blurred artifacts in the images, as data from two different heart beats are mixed for the reconstruction. Because the use of multi-segment reconstruction techniques shows limited clinical stability, beta blockers are routinely and widely used to decrease the heart rate to overcome the lack of temporal resolution.[22]

To solve the clinical constraints of 64-slice CT systems, Siemens Medical Solutions introduced a Dual Source CT (DSCT) system – the SOMATOM Definition – in 2005. This CT system is equipped with two x-ray tubes and two corresponding detectors. The two acquisition systems are mounted onto a rotating gantry with a 90° angular offset (see figure 3).[23] One detector covers the entire scan field of view (about 50 cm in diameter), while the other is restricted to a smaller, central field of view. Both detectors are capable of acquiring 64 overlapping 0.6 mm slices by means of double z-sampling (z-flying focal point technology). The gantry rotation time is 0.33 s. Each of the two x-ray tubes provides up to 80 kW peak power.

DSCT provides temporal resolutions that are one quarter of the gantry rotation time, independent of the patient's heart rate. DSCT scanners also show promising potential for general radiology applications, such as the use of dose accumulation to examine obese patients, or the use of dual energy acquisitions. The potential applications of Dual Energy CT include tissue characterization, local blood volume quantification in contrast enhanced scans and iodine/calcium separation enabling, for example, the automatic removal of bone from CT angiographic examinations.

Dual Source CT Technology

Cardiac imaging

The key benefit of DSCT for cardiac scanning and coronary CT angiography is the improved temporal resolution. In a DSCT scanner, the half-scan sinogram in parallel geometry needed for an ECG-controlled image reconstruction can be split into two quarter scan sinograms, which are simultaneously acquired by the two acquisition systems in the same relative phase of the patient's cardiac cycle and at the same anatomical level due to the 90° angle between both detectors. With this approach, a constant temporal resolution equivalent to one quarter of the gantry rotation time $t_{rot}/4$ is achieved in a centered region of the scan field of view. For $t_{rot} = 0.33$ s, the temporal resolution is $t_{rot}/4 = 83$ ms, independent of the patient's heart rate (see figure 2). Figure 4 shows a clinical example illustrating the performance of DSCT for ECG-gated coronary CTA. Going from a single-segment reconstruction to a two- or multi-segment reconstruction only slightly improves the quality of the images. However, the temporal resolution

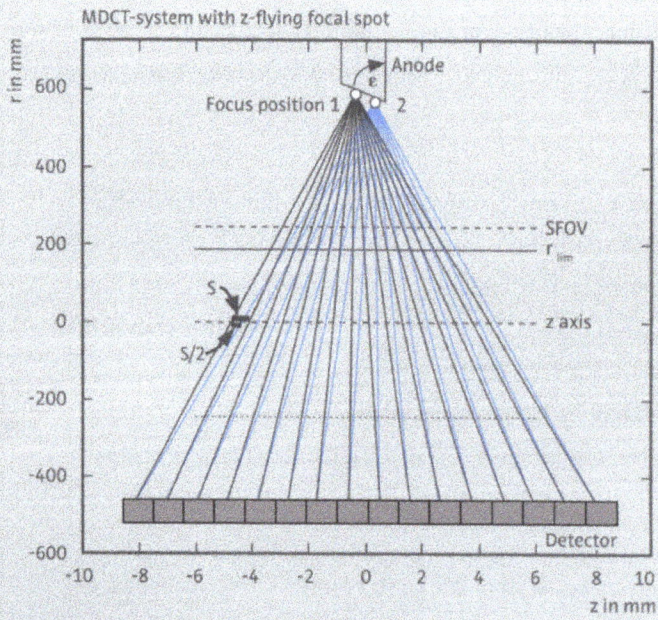

[Figure 1] Schematic illustration of improved z-sampling with the z-flying focal spot technique. Two subsequent M-slice readings are shifted by half a collimated slice-width at iso-center and can be interleaved to one 2M-slice projection. Improved z-sampling is not only achieved at iso-center, but maintained in a wide range of the scan field of view (SFOV).

increase to 83 ms adds significant diagnostic value. Several clinical studies validated this information and have demonstrated that DSCT offers a very robust diagnostic image quality regardless of the heart rate.[24–27] The use of two x-ray tubes for image acquisition immediately brings up the question of patient dose, because one might assume that dose increases by a factor of two. However, the SOMATOM Definition features additional mechanisms and technical improvements that enable you to reduce the dose even below that of Single Source CT (see also figure 5):[28]

· Additional filter: An optimized cardiac bowtie filter – widely used in CT systems – prevents unnecessary exposure outside the central heart region. The cardiac bowtie filter is dedicated and optimized for heart examinations, and it reduces the intensity outside the area of the heart even greater than regular bowtie filters.

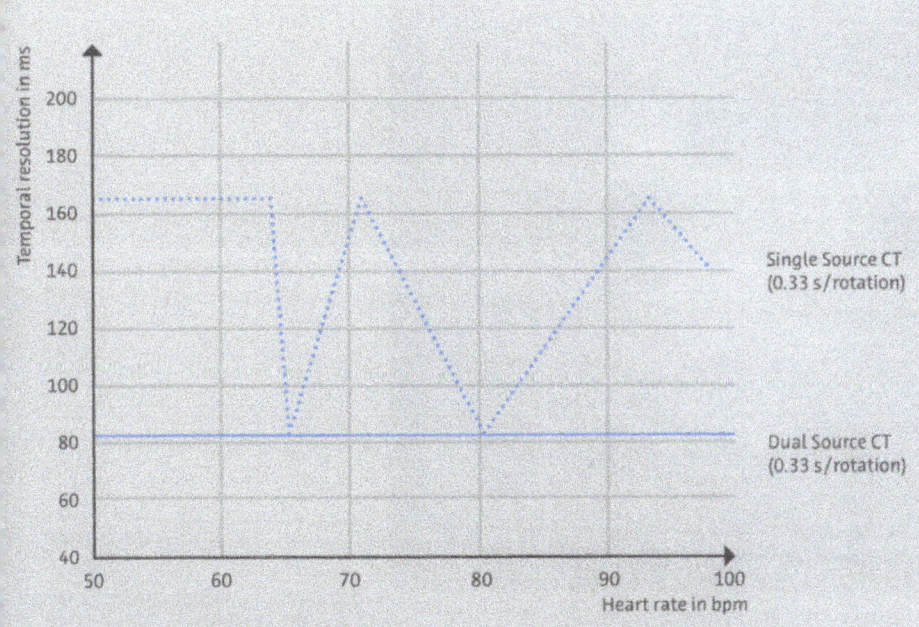

[Figure 2] Comparison of the temporal resolution of single and dual source CT systems: Multi-segment reconstruction technique in the case of the single source systems leads to a strong dependency of the temporal resolution from the heart rate.

Dual Source CT Technology

· Pitch adaptation: Single-segment reconstruction at all heart rates enables efficient adaptation of the table feed: In single source CT, the only way to increase temporal resolution – which is particularly useful for patients with high heart rates – is by using the multi-segment reconstruction technique. Unfortunately, this technique requires the use of a comparatively small pitch during acquisition, resulting in longer scan times and higher radiation exposure. Conversely (and beneficially), the temporal resolution in DSCT is already in the desired range of under 100 ms in single-segment reconstruction, which make multi-segment reconstructions obsolete. Therefore, the scanning pitch can be adapted to the patient's heart rate in DSCT while it cannot in Single Source CT. The pitch increase for higher heart rates significantly reduces patient dose. It is important to note that image noise in cardiac CT is determined by the tube current product per rotation, as about 180 degrees of the complete acquisition is used to generate one image. Assuming the tube current time product (mAs)

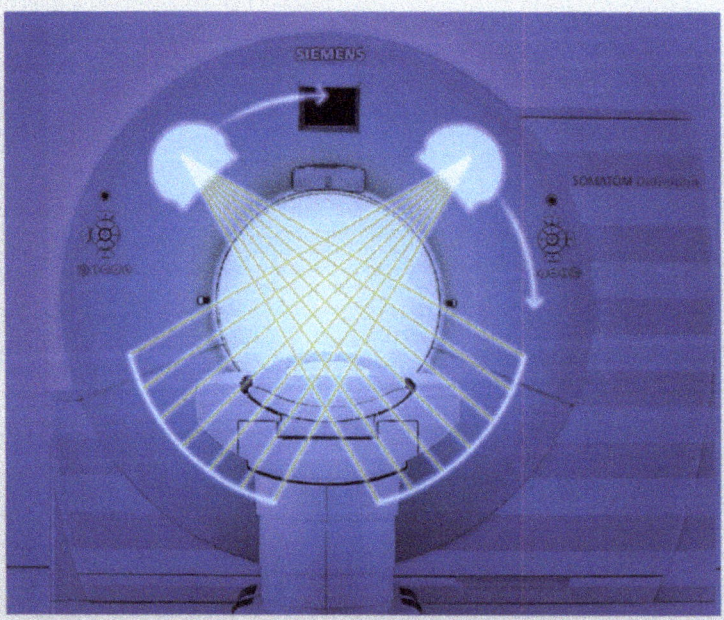

[Figure 3] Schematic illustration of a Dual Source CT (DSCT) system using two tubes and two corresponding detectors offset by 90°. This type of scanner provides temporal resolution equivalent to one quarter of the gantry rotation time for ECG-controlled cardiac CT, independent of the patient's heart rate. Both tubes can also run at different tube voltages for dual energy purposes.

does not change, higher pitch values will not lead to increased noise. This is true for both Single and Dual Source CT systems.

The behavior is different from conventional scanning: image noise changes with the pitch at a given mAs level. Smaller pitch values lead to less image noise than higher pitch values as all data acquired at a certain z-position contribute to the reconstructed image at that z-position.
To avoid this unwanted behavior in conventional scans, the operator specifies the "effective mAs" (mAs/pitch). Because the operator does not increase the pitch for cases of higher heart rates in Single Source cardiac CT examinations, but always uses the same small pitch level independent of the heart rate in order to be capable of multi-segment reconstructions, it was convenient for an operator to enter well-known "effective mAs" values used in regular scan mode.

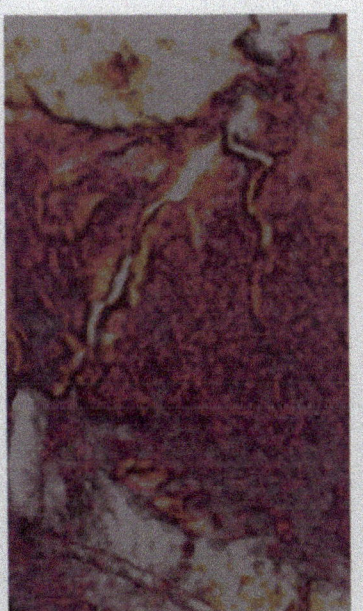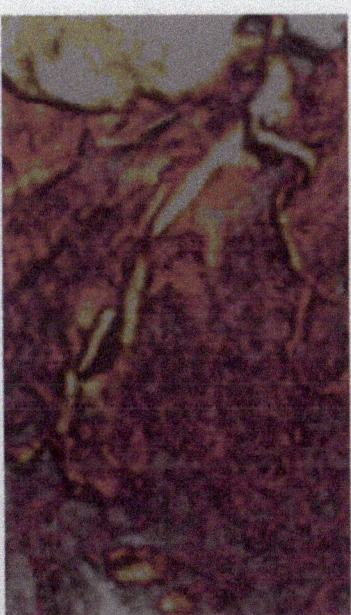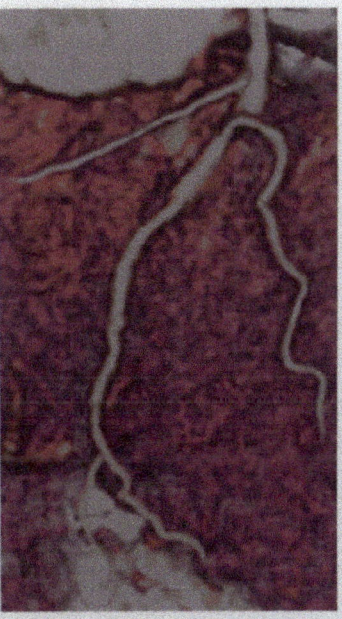

[Figure 4] Various reconstruction technique comparisons of a patient with a heart rate ranging from 86 to 122 bpm. The improvement in temporal resolution from a single- to multi-segment reconstruction only leads to insignificant improvement in image quality. The Dual Source CT reconstruction with a temporal resolution of 83 ms independent of the heart rate leads to a significant improvement in image quality. Courtesy of University Hospital of Munich-Grosshadern/Munich, Germany.

Dual Source CT Technology

The fixed pitch value established a constant relationship between "effective mAs" and the noise determining "mAs/rotation". However, the concept of "effective mAs" is not useful in DSCT systems because the pitch is adapted to the patient's heart rate. Moreover, because of this and how "effective mAs" are defined, the pitch would impact image noise. To eliminate this dependency in DSCT systems, an operator can specify "mAs per rotation". The image quality is then independent of pitch and heart rate. To provide the user control over patient dose, CTDIvol is displayed, which assesses the impact of pitch on patient dose.

· Optimized ECG-pulsing: New ECG-pulsing enables the reduction of exposure even in the presence of arrhythmia. It is one of the most efficient methods for dose reduction in cardiac CT. A high tube current is only used for those phases of the cardiac cycle which are required for morphology. It is

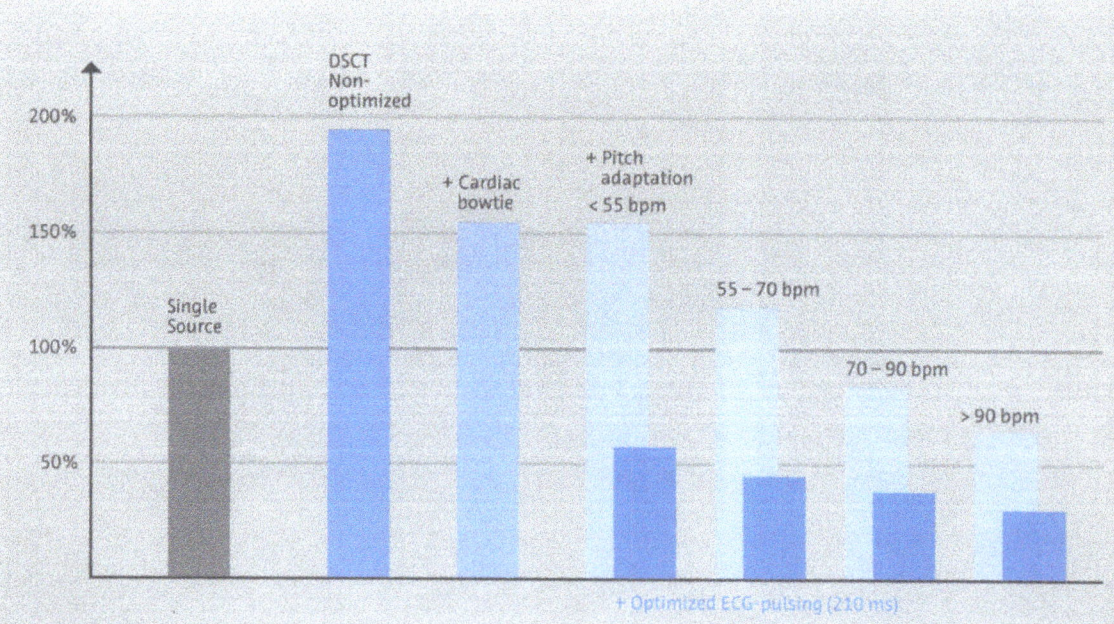

[Figure 5] Several technical improvements help to reduce patient dose in DSCT even below the level of Single Source cardiac CT.[28]

reduced for the rest of the heart cycle. These images are noisier, but they still provide diagnostic information for functional analysis. The minimum window for ECG-pulsing is determined by the time it takes to acquire 180 degrees of data. In Single Source CT, the pulsing window is about half of the rotation time; in Dual Source CT, the desired data is acquired after the gantry rotates 90 degrees. As a result, the pulsing window can be much smaller. Because different heart rates require different reconstruction time points, the plateau of full tube power should be adapted to the patient's heart rate to maximum dose savings but still be able to obtain full image quality in the data needed for a morphological diagnosis (see Table 1).

In addition to the width of the pulsing window, the level of the low dose plateau can also be used for a further dose reduction. Normally, tube current is reduced down to 20% of the nominal tube current

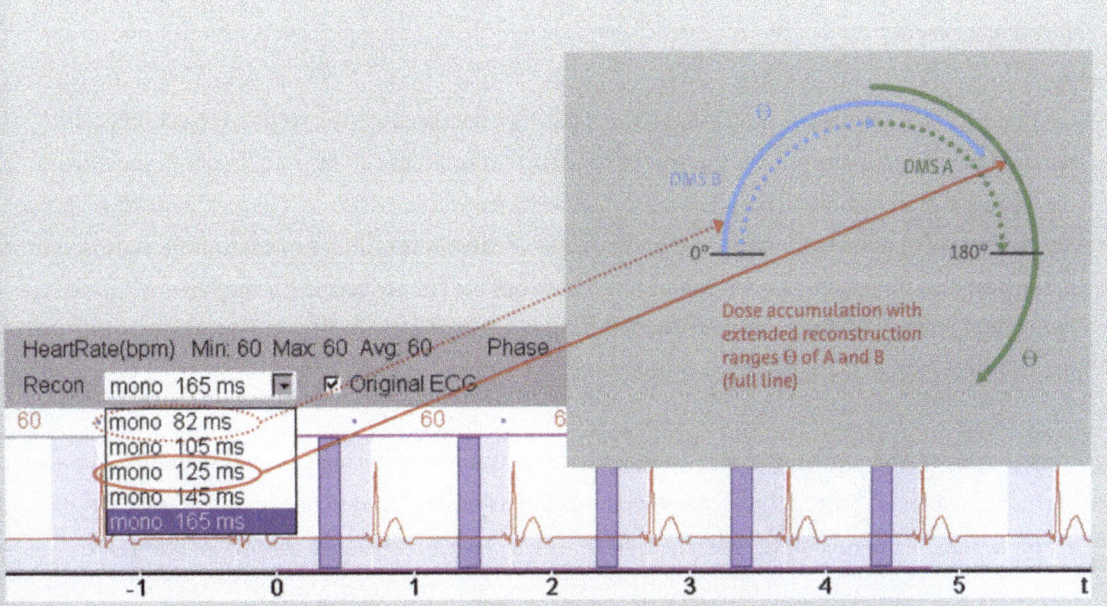

[Figure 6] Cardiac obese scanning: To further reduce image noise in cardiac scanning, temporal resolution of reconstructed images can be lowered in DSCT down to the level of a Single Source CT. Noise reduction up to a factor of $1/\sqrt{2}$ can be achieved.

Dual Source CT Technology

in the low plateau phase. The MinDose™ pulsing mode can be applied to reduce the dose even further, which reduces the dose down to 4% (see figure 3). We must note that this mode does not allow the reconstruction of diagnostic data during the reduced plateau phase.

Obese imaging and cardiac obese imaging

DSCT provides powerful applications for general radiology applications as well. If both acquisition systems are simultaneously used in a standard spiral or sequential acquisition mode, an x-ray peak power of up to 160 kW is available. These power reserves are not only beneficial for the examination of morbidly obese patients, whose number is dramatically growing in western societies, but also to maintain an adequate x-ray photon flux for standard protocols when a high volume coverage speed is necessary. With Single Source CT systems, high mAs-values can only be achieved by reducing the pitch or using a slower rotation time. However, this leads to compromises in scan speed, which is sometimes unwanted or unacceptable, or at least it requires a significant change of the contrast injection protocol.

Compromising scan speed is not necessary in a DSCT system because the second tube simply adds the required power. Furthermore, the enormous tube current reserves can be used for dose reduction in contrast enhanced examinations. The use of a lower tube voltage leads to a higher contrast of iodine. A better signal to noise ratio can be achieved at a lower dose level when a lower tube voltage is used. In the past, lowering of tube voltage was often not possible simply because a single x-ray tube could not provide the required tube current. The limitations of Single Source CT systems are overcome by the ability to double the mAs with a second tube.

Excessive noise when imaging obese patients is not only an issue in conventional scanning, but also in cardiac scanning, especially since reducing the pitch does not lead to less image noise in cardiac examinations. If the tube limit is reached, the only way to reduce noise in cardiac imaging is to compromise temporal resolution and collect more x-ray photons. Single Source CT systems are not

Heart Rate in bpm	Pulsing Window in %
< 60	70−70
60−80	55−80
> 80	40−80

[Table 1] In order to achieve optimal diagnostic results in coronary CTA imaging, the ECG-pulsing window should be adapted to the heart rate of the patient.

capable of this since a temporal resolution of 300 to 400 ms is not acceptable for coronary imaging. Applying the same principle to DSCT, the temporal resolution ends up in the range of about 165 ms (see figure 6), which is still acceptable. In cardiac obese reconstruction, the temporal resolution is equal to a single-segment reconstruction of a Single Source CT. In fact, the SOMATOM Definition leaves it up to the operator to choose the reconstruction type after the examination using the same raw data, which means no additional exposure for the patient. Therefore, he or she can choose whether a regular reconstruction should be performed with a temporal resolution of 83 ms, or a dedicated "cardiac obese" reconstruction, which ends up with a temporal resolution of 165 ms but a noise level reduced by a factor of $1/\sqrt{2}$.

Dual energy imaging

In cardiac and obese examinations, both tubes are operated with the same tube. However, both x-ray tubes can also be operated at different kV- and mAs-settings, allowing the acquisition of dual energy data. While dual energy CT was already evaluated 20 years ago, the technical limitations of the CT scanners at the time prevented the development of routine clinical applications.[29, 30] The biggest constraint was that the dose in the low voltage data was much less than in the high voltage data, since only the tube voltage was switched without adapting the tube current. Therefore, the noise level in the low voltage data was significantly higher, which finally hampered and limited the use of dual energy applications at that time.

With a DSCT system, dual energy data can be acquired nearly simultaneously in spiral mode with sub-second scan times. The ability to overcome data registration problems should prove beneficial to clinicians. Additionally, the limitations of dual energy from the 1980s are overcome by the utilization of two independent tube/detector systems. Noise and dose level can be adjusted independently; therefore, the same noise and dose level in both systems can be achieved by simply using a higher tube current on the low voltage system. Clinical routines have demonstrated that a tube current ratio of about 1:4 for 140kV/80kV is optimal. Depending on the dual energy application and the anatomical area, different collimations can be used for data acquisition similar to conventional scanning. The 64 x 0.6 mm mode is preferred for high coverage and resolution. Thinner or dedicated collimations are indicated for quantitative measurements that demand high-precision CT numbers. One of the biggest concerns is the limited field of view of the B detector (see figure 3) because data are only acquired by the B system inside this area and as a result dual energy can only be performed

Dual Source CT Technology

in this area. Surprisingly, mostly all of the relevant tissue is within this inner field of view. Of course, proper positioning of the patient and the region of interest is a prerequisite. This can be done easily with the use of two topograms prior to scanning: lateral and a p.a.

The use of Dual Energy CT data adds functional information to the morphological information based on x-ray attenuation coefficients that is usually obtained in a CT examination while increasing dose typically by no more than 10–30%. A potential application for Spiral Dual Energy CT is the separation of bones and iodine filled vessels in CT angiographic examinations even in complicated anatomical situations, such as the skull base and the circle of Willis. The bones can be automatically removed, leaving only the vessels in the resultant images. The CT value of iodine increases much greater than bone or calcium with decreasing x-ray tube voltage, which is the basis for iodine-bone separation

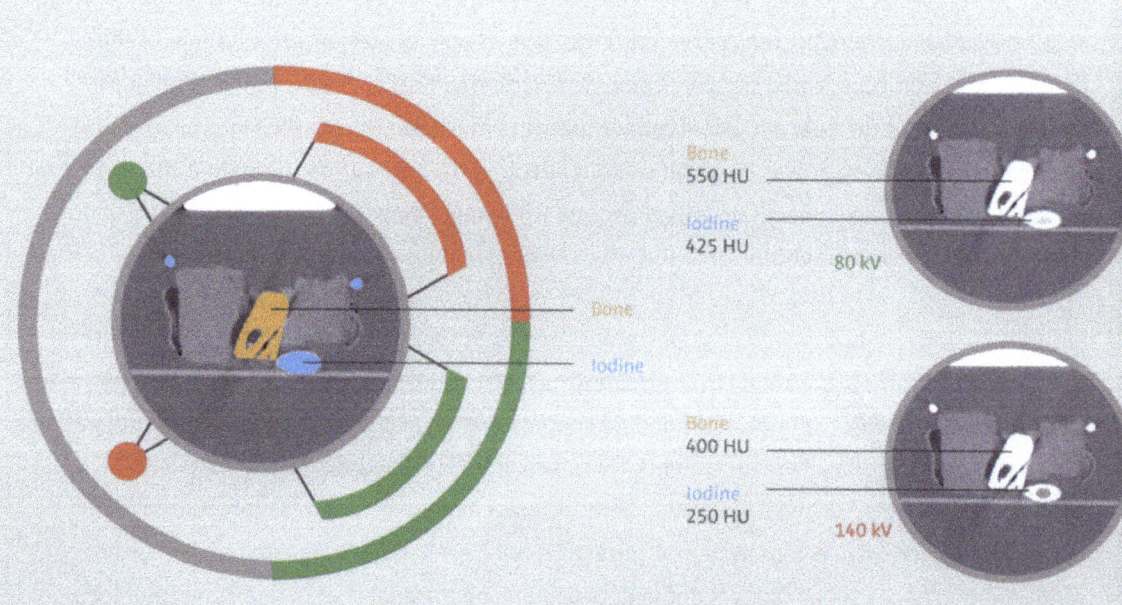

[Figure 7] Schematic illustration of the principle of dual energy imaging with a DSCT system. Although both tube/detector systems are mouthed with an angle of 90 degrees, images at low and high voltage are acquired simultaneously. A specimen with bony structures and tubes filled with iodine are scanned with both energy levels simultaneously. The CT number of iodine increases from high to low voltage by about a factor of 2, whereas the CT number of bone only increases slightly. These differences in CT enhancement are used to distinguish between different chemical compositions.

using Dual Energy CT (see figure 7). The CT values for vessels filled with iodine nearly double when going from 140 kV to 80 kV, whereas bony structures show a significantly less increase in CT values with lower tube voltage.

Another example for tissue separation is the definition of renal stone composition. Uric acid and hydroxyl apatite stones can be differentiated and thus add diagnostic information simply from differences in dual energy behavior. A similar principle applies to the differentiation of a vessel lumen filled with iodinated blood and calcified plaques. In addition to tissue separation, dual energy techniques can also be used to quantify iodine concentration in tissue.[31] This allows, for example, the visualization of perfusion defects in the parenchyma in the case of a pulmonary embolism by displaying the iodine concentration of the different areas of the lungs. Another

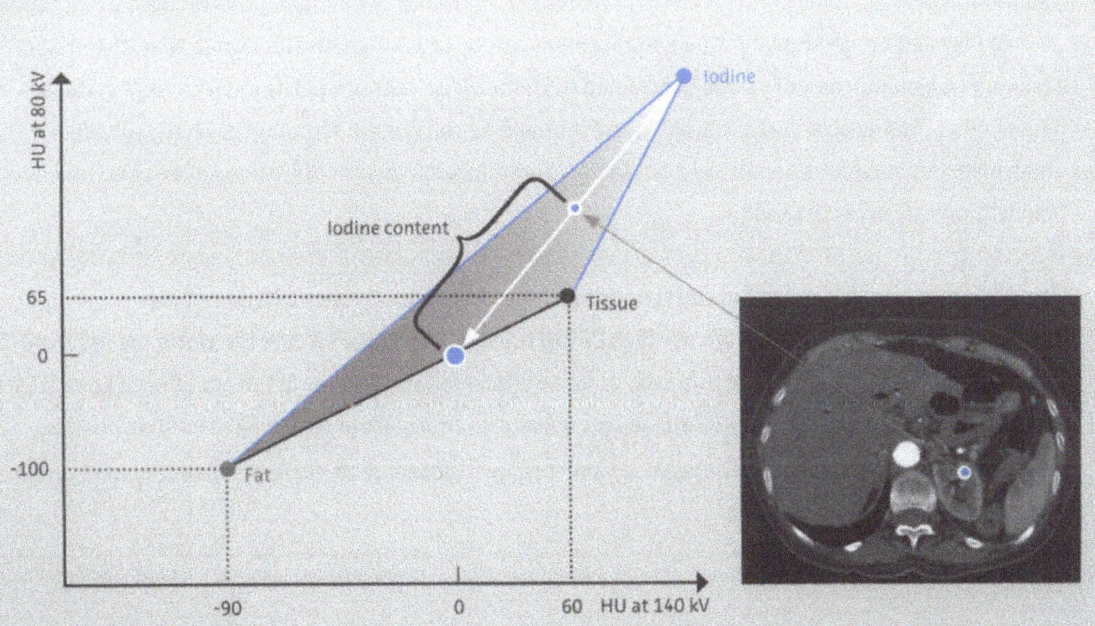

[Figure 8] Three material decomposition: Three appropriate materials are selected depending in the anatomical location. In the case of the liver, this can be, for example, fat, tissue and iodine. After plotting all three materials into an 80kV – 140 kV diagram, a triangle is spanned. To calculate the iodine content of ROI, CT values of this ROI at 80 and the 140 kV are used to determine the position of the ROI within the triangle. After projecting the point down onto the line between fat and tissue, the iodine content is determined.

Dual Source CT Technology

possible application might be the visualization of pure iodine enhancement in abdominal organs such as the kidneys. In this case, additional information about the pure enhancement might be helpful for the differential diagnosis between a hemorrhagic cyst and a renal cell carcinoma. The basic method to determine iodine concentration in tissue – and therefore also to calculate a virtual non-contrast image – is what is known as "three material decomposition".[31] This principle is shown schematically in figure 8. As a first step, three material/tissue types are defined that are of interest and are found in a certain anatomical area. In the liver region, this might be, for example, "soft tissue", "fat" and "iodine". Based on values from literature or clinical experience, these materials are drawn into an 80-140-kV diagram, where they span a triangle.

To evaluate a certain area of interest, the respective CT values in the 80 and 140 kV image are plotted into the existing diagram. Projecting this point onto the line between "fat" and "soft tissue" allows the calculation of true iodine enhancement in the region of interest. By applying this method to the whole field of view, an image showing true enhancement can be calculated. In addition to that, the image showing true enhancement can be subtracted from the weighted sum of the low and high voltage image and by doing so a "virtual" non-contrast image be calculated. Although several dedicated dual energy applications are already available as products, further modifications of existing and new applications are expected soon.

The evolution from sequential to spiral or from single-slice to multi-slice CT systems has revolutionized how CT systems are used in clinical routine. Clinicians all over the world are realizing and experiencing the benefits of this new, innovative technology. Although the era of Dual Source CT has just begun, DSCT systems have already provided proven results in the fields of cardiac imaging, obese imaging and spiral dual energy. Dual Source CT will continue to prove the modality of choice for many other imaging procedures.

References

1 Crawford, C. R., and K. F. King. Computed tomography scanning with simultaneous patient translation. Med Phys 1990; 17; 967-82

2 Kalender, W. A., W. Seissler, E. Klotz, et al. Spiral volumetric CT with single-breath-hold technique, continuous transport, and continuous scanner rotation. Radiology 1990; 176; 181-3

3 Kalender, W. A. Thin-section three-dimensional spiral CT: is isotropic imaging possible? Radiology 1995; 197; 578-80

4 Hu, H., H. D. He, W. D. Foley, et al. Four multidetector-row helical CT: image quality and volume coverage speed. Radiology 2000; 215; 55-62

5 Klingenbeck-Regn, K., S. Schaller, T. Flohr, et al. Subsecond multi-slice computed tomography: basics and applications. Eur J Radiol 1999; 31; 110-24

6 McCollough, C. H., and F. E. Zink. Performance evaluation of a multi-slice CT system. Med Phys 1999; 26; 2223-30

7 Rubin, G. D., A. J. Schmidt, L. J. Logan, et al. Multi-detector row CT angiography of lower extremity arterial inflow and runoff: initial experience. Radiology 2001; 221; 146-58

8 Kachelriess, M., S. Ulzheimer, and W. A. Kalender. ECG-correlated image reconstruction from subsecond multi-slice spiral CT scans of the heart. Med Phys 2000; 27; 1881-902

9 Ohnesorge, B., T. Flohr, C. Becker, et al. Cardiac imaging by means of electrocardiographically gated multisection spiral CT: initial experience. Radiology 2000; 217; 564-71

10 Nieman, K., M. Oudkerk, B. J. Rensing, et al. Coronary angiography with multi-slice computed tomography. Lancet 2001; 357; 599-603

11 Flohr, T., H. Bruder, K. Stierstorfer, et al. New technical developments in multislice CT, part 2: sub-millimeter 16-slice scanning and increased gantry rotation speed for cardiac imaging. Rofo 2002; 174; 1022-7

12 Flohr, T., K. Stierstorfer, H. Bruder, et al. New technical developments in multislice CT--Part 1: Approaching isotropic resolution with sub-millimeter 16-slice scanning. Rofo 2002; 174; 839-45

13 Remy-Jardin, M., I. Tillie-Leblond, D. Szapiro, et al. CT angiography of pulmonary embolism in patients with underlying respiratory disease: impact of multislice CT on image quality and negative predictive value. Eur Radiol 2002; 12; 1971-8

14 Schoepf, U. J., C. R. Becker, L. K. Hofmann, et al. Multislice CT angiography. Eur Radiol 2003; 13; 1946-61

15 Nieman, K., F. Cademartiri, P. A. Lemos, et al. Reliable noninvasive coronary angiography with fast submillimeter multislice spiral computed tomography. Circulation 2002; 106; 2051-4

16 Ropers, D., U. Baum, K. Pohle, et al. Detection of coronary artery stenoses with thin-slice multi-detector row spiral computed tomography and multiplanar reconstruction. Circulation 2003; 107; 664-6

17 Flohr, T., K. Stierstorfer, R. Raupach, et al. Performance evaluation of a 64-slice CT system with z-flying focal spot. Rofo 2004; 176; 1803-10

18 Flohr, T. G., K. Stierstorfer, S. Ulzheimer, et al. Image reconstruction and image quality evaluation for a 64-slice CT scanner with z-flying focal spot. Med Phys 2005; 32; 2536-47

19 Vrtiska, T. J., J. G. Fletcher, and C. H. McCollough. State-of-the-art imaging with 64-channel multidetector CT angiography. Perspect Vasc Surg Endovasc Ther 2005; 17; 3-8

20 Leber, A. W., A. Knez, F. von Ziegler, et al. Quantification of obstructive and nonobstructive coronary lesions by 64-slice computed tomography: a comparative study with quantitative coronary angiography and intravascular ultrasound. J Am Coll Cardiol 2005; 46; 147-54

21 Raff, G. L., M. J. Gallagher, W. W. O'Neill, et al. Diagnostic accuracy of noninvasive coronary angiography using 64-slice spiral computed tomography. J Am Coll Cardiol 2005; 46; 552-7

22 Leschka, S., S. Wildermuth, T. Boehm, et al. Noninvasive coronary angiography with 64-section CT: effect of average heart rate and heart rate variability on image quality. Radiology 2006; 241; 378-85

23 Flohr, T. G., C. H. McCollough, H. Bruder, et al. First performance evaluation of a dual-source CT (DSCT) system. Eur Radiol 2006; 16; 256-68

24 Achenbach, S., D. Ropers, A. Kuettner, et al. Contrast-enhanced coronary artery visualization by dual-source computed tomography--initial experience. Eur J Radiol 2006; 57; 331-5

25 Johnson, T. R., K. Nikolaou, B. J. Wintersperger, et al. Dual-source CT cardiac imaging: initial experience. Eur Radiol 2006

26 Scheffel, H., H. Alkadhi, A. Plass, et al. Accuracy of dual-source CT coronary angiography: First experience in a high pre-test probability population without heart rate control. Eur Radiol 2006; 16; 2739-47

27 Schertler, T., H. Scheffel, T. Frauenfelder, et al. Dual-source computed tomography in patients with acute chest pain: feasibility and image quality. Eur Radiol 2007

28 McCollough, C. H., A. N. Primak, O. Saba, et al. Dose performance of a 64-channel dual-source CT scanner. Radiology 2007; 243; 775-84

29 Vetter JR, Perman WH, Kalender WA, Mazess RB, Holden JE. Evaluation of a prototype dual-energy computed tomographic apparatus. II. Determination of vertebral bone mineral content. Medical Physics, 1986, 13: 340-343

30 Kalender WA, Perman WH, Vetter JR, Klotz E. Evaluation of a prototype dual-energy computed tomographic apparatus. I. Phantom studies. Med. Phys., 1986, 13(3): 334-339

31 Johnson, T. R., B. Krauss, M. Sedlmair, et al. Material differentiation by dual energy CT: initial experience. Eur Radiol 2007; 17; 1510-7

Iodinated Contrast Media: New Perspectives with Dual Source CT

Matthias Braeutigam · Ute Huebner-Steiner · Hubertus Pietsch · Ulrich Speck

Iodinated non-ionic contrast agents (see figure 1) became standard contrast agents in the best sense. They were introduced more than 20 years ago and during these twenty years, millions of patients suffering from every conceivable disease, newborns, pregnant women as well as multimorbid elderly patients, patients with serious conditions such as generalized atherosclerosis, acute brain or cardiac infarctions, advanced cancer, severe cardiac insufficiency, impaired renal or hepatic function and patients of all races and living all over the world received non-ionic contrast agents by any conceivable route of administration.

Low osmolar non-ionic contrast agents – are very well tolerated products which have been administered to critically ill patients at doses for e.g. iopromide or iopamidol of more than 500 ml in adults, which is equivalent to about 150 g iodine.[1, 2, 3] It may be assumed that any risks due to the administration of non-ionic contrast media are known.[4, 5, 6, 7] The properties of this product class have been documented in hundreds of publications and after so many years of experience and use, it is very unlikely that unexpected adverse effects of any of the commonly used products will be observed.

Although all protocols in this book were developed using iopromide formulations, it can be assumed that other contrast media of the same non-ionic low osmolar class (see figure 1) would perform equally effectively when following the respective protocols. The slight differences in the physico-chemical properties of the various contrast media, however, might influence attenuation kinetics and should be the subject of further scientific evaluation.

Imaging technology determines the performance of contrast agents

As with all other x-ray contrast agents, the diagnostic capability of iopromide depends upon the radiological equipment used. Ever since its introduction, CT has again and again drastically changed the use of contrast media (CM). Dual source CT is another major step in this process.

CT changed the efficacy of iodinated CM in several ways (see figure 2a):

· Sensitivity for the detection of iodine in CT depends on the iodine concentration whereas in standard projection x-ray procedures such as angiography the amount of iodine present along the path of the x-ray through the tissue is decisive for its detection.

Iodinated Contrast Media: New Perspectives with Dual Source CT

· CT is much more sensitive to iodine than projection radiography. CT clearly visualizes iodine concentrations of 1 mg/ml in a volume of less than 0.1 ml (see figure 2b). Projection imaging requires at least 20 mg I/ml if an object of 1 cm thickness is visualized. Angiography may serve as an example to illustrate the difference between CT and projection radiography. In spite of high contrast medium doses and very fast injection, intravenous DSA does not reliably yield clinically useful image quality because its sensitivity to iodine is too low. The contrast medium concentration in blood achieved with identical doses is fully sufficient for CT. Conversely, CTA is limited by its spatial and temporal resolution.

A very important feature is speed. The first CT scanners in the seventies took several minutes to acquire the data for a single slice. Short-lasting contrast enhancement was missed.

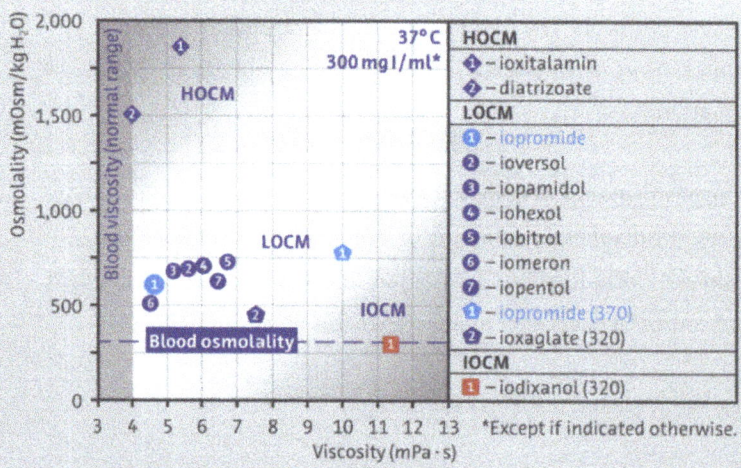

[Figure 1] Iodinated low-osmolar contrast agents.

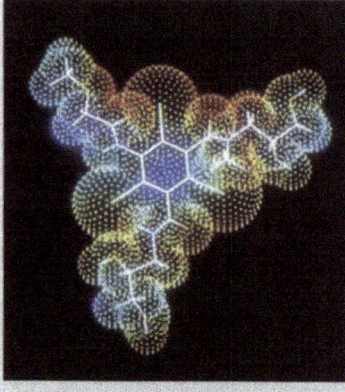

Iopromide
Molecular weight: 791 D
Iodine content: 48%
Size of the molecules: < 1 nm in diameter

Equally important is spatial resolution. If contrast enhancement is restricted to small lesions, it may be missed if low spatial resolution results in the display of average density values over larger volumes. High spatial resolution of moving structures can only be achieved if data acquisition is fast enough to avoid movement artefacts. Movement is critical in organs within or close to the thorax or the heart or in any other organ, tissue or structure in patients who are unable to follow the instructions of radiographers or physicians during image acquisition. The previous chapter points out the dramatic progress in spatial and temporal resolution of modern CT scanners.

CT discovers the multi-talent of non-ionic low osmolar contrast media
Non-invasive angiography and the visualization of perfusion, permeability and interstitial space.

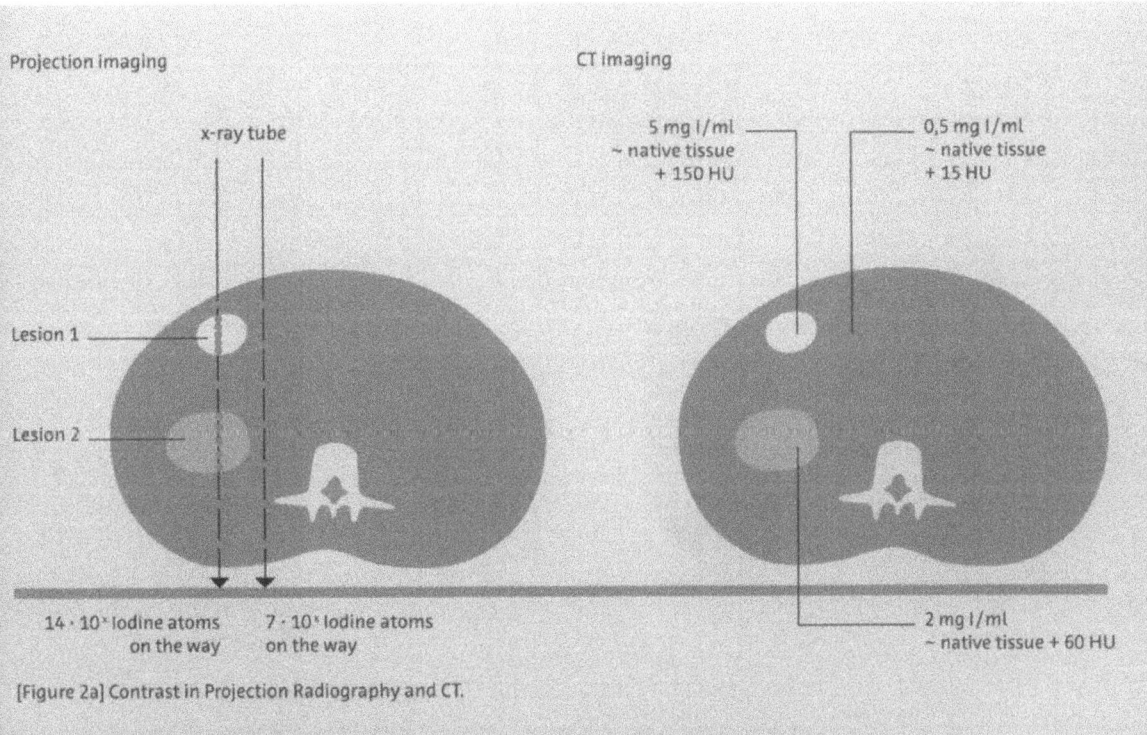

[Figure 2a] Contrast in Projection Radiography and CT.

Iodinated Contrast Media: New Perspectives with Dual Source CT

Non-ionic contrast media are the current end point of a development which begun about 80 years ago with the first intravenous urographic agents. As the name says, these were iodinated contrast media aimed at visualizing the urinary tract following intravenous injection. In addition to urography they were used from the beginning to visualize open and closed body cavities including blood vessels because they mixed with aqueous contents of the cavities, were usually well tolerated and completely excreted within short time. Later on it was realized that compounds belonging to the class of urographic CM did not enter cells or pass biological barriers which in practice means that they are not enterally absorbed nor accumulate in any organs or tissues other than the kidney to a diagnostically useful extent. Because of this property, urographic CM were also called extracellular CM. Before the introduction of modern CT, urographic CM were named nonspecific CM expressing the frustration of their users about the fact that they did not display structures or tissues distant from the site of

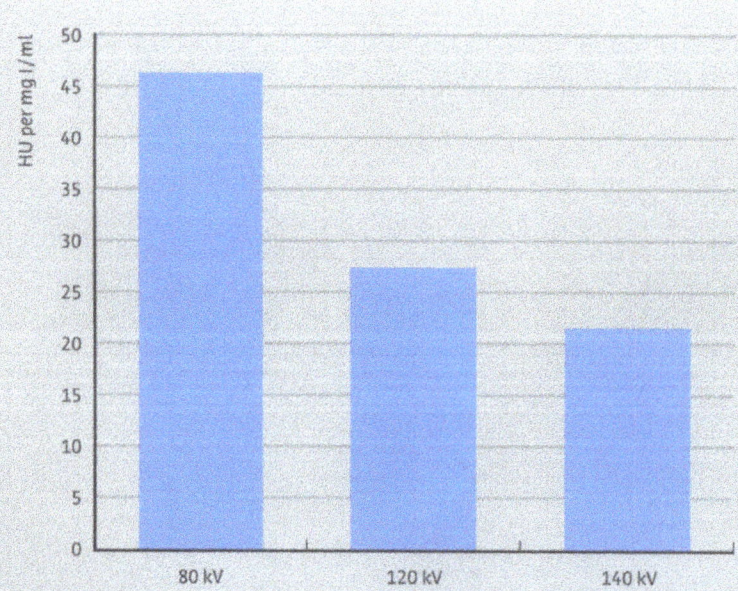

[Figure 2b] Iodine absorption (HU per mg I/ml). Probes of iodine containing solutions were investigated in a human equivalent body phantom. Measurement was performed in a Siemens Sensation 64.

injection and other than the urinary tract although they distribute throughout the body with the exception of the central nervous system to which they have no access due to the blood-brain barrier. The term 'nonspecific' is misleading (see figure 3). It is not the contrast agent which is nonspecific but the way it was used due to the lack of appropriate imaging modalities. The diagnostic benefit of the extracellular CM was only slowly appreciated after the introduction of CT, with the increase in speed of data acquisition and the scanning of large volumes within a few seconds.

Urographic CM are small molecules which are unable to pass cell membranes due to their hydrophilicity. After injection, small extracellular CM molecules ideally do not interact with any body function or constituent. They diffuse through tiny pores wherever the permeability of membranes allows their passage without passing the lipid layer of a cell membrane and are carried by the blood

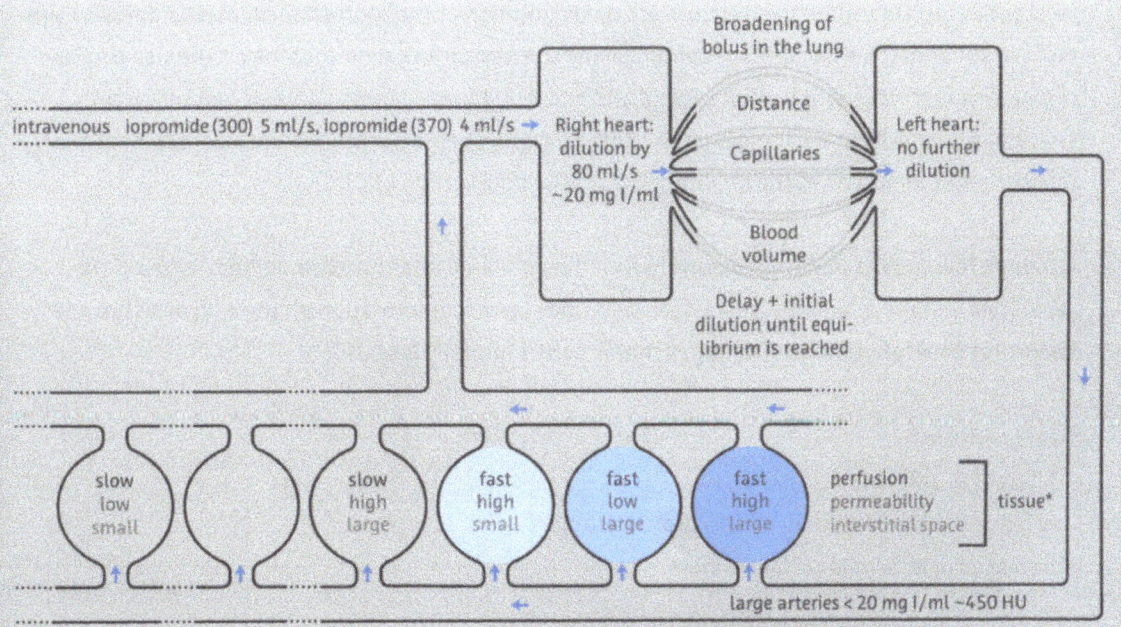

[Figure 3] Dilution and Early Pharmaco-kinetics of Extracellular Contrast Media.

* tissue: interstitial space includes plasma volume (e.g. 5% of tissue volume, contributes about 30 HU) plus interstitial space between cells of solid tissue (e.g. 10% of tissue volume). In brain the interstitial space is not accessible to contrast media due to the blood-brain barrier.

Iodinated Contrast Media: New Perspectives with Dual Source CT

stream to all tissues, exactly reflecting blood perfusion. They are finally filtered by the glomeruli, concentrated in the renal tubules and excreted with the urine. Even if injected behind the blood-brain barrier, e.g. in myelography, elimination from the cerebrospinal fluid follows the same principles: the CM is washed out by the bulk water flow through a valve-like mechanism which allows much larger molecules to pass. Distribution and excretion are completely passive and require no additional energy except possibly concentrating the contrast agent in renal tubules.

If the extracellular CM with standard iodine concentrations of 300–370 mg/ml is intravenously injected at a rate of 3–8 ml/s at a dose of about 1 ml/kg body weight, it is diluted by the cardiac circulation (~ 80 ml/s) and during passage through the lungs to an arterial concentration of 10 to < 20 mg I/ml, providing several hundred Hounsfield units of contrast enhancement in the arterial blood.[8] If scanning is fast enough to follow the arterial contrast agent bolus, even small arteries can be distinguished from adjacent tissue. Only after one recirculation do the dilution of the contrast medium and diffusion into the interstitial space of most tissues diminish the contrast to an extent that makes the visualization of small-caliber arteries impossible. Rapid and precisely timed scanning of large volumes is an essential precondition for CT angiography. Differentiation between calcium and iodine by dual energy capability further improves the quality of diagnostic information of CTA.

Although low osmolar CM float passively with the bulk fluid or diffuse through tiny pores in the capillaries into the interstitial space of tissues, they provide information on the kind of tissue and important pathophysiological changes characteristic of many diseases:

Tissue perfusion
· different in different tissues
· increased in inflammation, rapidly growing tumors
· decreased in ischemia, certain tumors
· absent in cysts, infarcted or necrotic tissue

Capillary permeability
· different in different tissues
· increased in inflammation, angiogenesis, tumors
· detects disturbed blood-brain barrier

Interstitial space (including plasma volume)
· different in blood (about 55%) and tissues (about 5 – 25%)
· increased in inflammation, vascular edema, many tumors
· decreased in cellular edema

The specific distribution is, however, transient; in many cases, it can be observed only for seconds after rapid intravascular injection during the first pass of the contrast agent through the tissues and disappears after recirculation. Therefore, rapid and repeated scanning of the whole volume of interest is required to make use of the specific dynamics and early distribution pattern.

The term 'nonspecific' was coined for the class of CM to which iopromide belongs at a time when radiographic imaging was either not capable of detecting the iodine concentrations in the interstitial space of tissues or not fast enough to image the very short period of contrast medium distribution before an equilibrium is reached, which equalizes fast and slow perfusion and diffusion into the tissue.

Contrast medium injection rate, concentration, and dose

With a few exceptions (e.g. display of blood-brain barrier disturbance), the specificity of non-ionic contrast agents following intravascular injection lasts only for seconds to a few minutes. Therefore in many cases rapid injection is necessary to visualize pathology (see figure 3). Since attenuation depends exclusively on iodine, the injection rate has to be related to the amount of iodine injected per second (~'iodine delivery rate'). The injection rate should be as fast as possible but it is limited by the caliber of the cannula, the outflow of the vein selected for injection and the viscosity of the contrast agent. The latter may be reduced by choosing a not too high iodine concentration and by warming up the contrast medium to 37°C. Applying hand injection, the same or higher iodine delivery rates were obtained for a 370 mg I/ml concentration than for a preparation containing 400 mg I/ml.[9] Using a different catheter, Jung et al. reached slightly higher iodine delivery rates with a 300 mg I/ml iopromide solution than with 370 mg I/ml or iopamidol 370 mg I/ml.[10] The advantage of less concentrated (e.g. 300 mg I/ml) over more concentrated low osmolar contrast media in respect of injection and iodine delivery rates at room temperature and at 37°C was confirmed.[11, 12] In vivo, a slightly slower intravenous injection of concentrated contrast media may be compensated or even overcompensated because a higher concentration may be maintained after dilution by a given rate of blood flow. In practice, this small difference is lost because concentrated

Iodinated Contrast Media: New Perspectives with Dual Source CT

contrast media do not mix well with blood and seem to pass the lung only slowly. Intravenous injection of highly concentrated contrast media may result in lower arterial iodine concentration than the same iodine dose of a less concentrated preparation delivered in the same time.

According to the literature, there is a broad range of optimal contrast medium concentrations between 300 and 370 mg I/ml providing maximal efficacy in CT if injected at the same iodine delivery rate and dose. When intravenous digital subtraction angiograph was introduced, Langer et al. compared iopromide 240, 300, 335, 370 and 400 in a randomized double blind crossover study in 78 patients.[13] Lower concentrations were injected slightly faster and at a slightly higher volume to achieve the same iodine dose and iodine delivery rate. This is possible because of the lower viscosity of less concentrated solutions. It is not surprising that very low concentrations are too diluted from

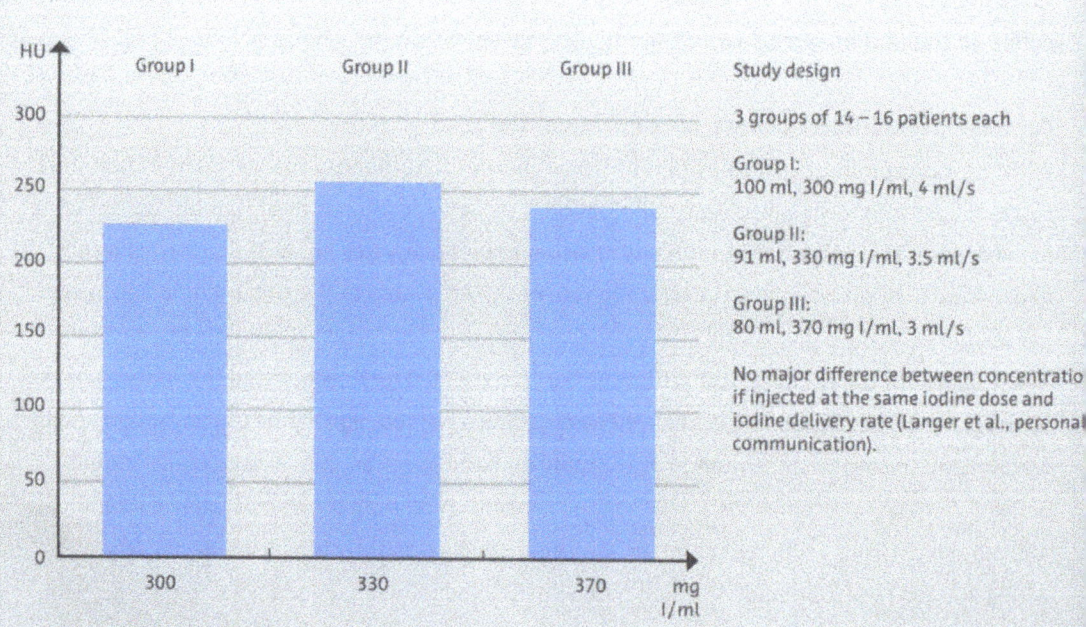

[Figure 4] Maximum contrast enhancement in the aorta following fast intravenous injection of iopromide.

the beginning and require too high injection rates whereas too high concentrations (like honey) are hard to inject, do not mix well with aqueous media and wash only slowly off the lungs. Concentrations of 300, 335 and 370 were equally effective. This has been confirmed by a study in CT (see figure 4). The results are in agreement with a similar study comparing iohexol 300 and 350 and computer simulation.[14, 15] When highly concentrated contrast media are injected at higher iodine doses than less concentrated preparations (e.g. at the same volume) or higher iodine delivery rates (i.e. same injection rate as less concentrated preparations), disadvantages of the higher viscosity may not become apparent.[16]

It is obvious that high arterial blood levels can be obtained by increasing the iodine dose.[17] This is, however, the least desirable way to increase the diagnostic yield. Increased injection rate and central position of the venous catheter further increase peak iodine concentration in arterial blood. The increase of the injection rate beyond 5 or 8 ml/s does not result in a further increase in contrast.[17, 18] Dose may be fixed for a specific diagnostic problem or adjusted to body weight or lean body weight.[19] Adjustment to body weight may not be required if arterial contrast enhancement is the primary goal because the volume of the central circulation does not increase proportionally with body weight. A variety of injection protocols has been recommended for clinical routine.[20, 21] In general, choosing a suitable iodine concentration, injection rate, a saline chasing bolus, optimal timing and the fastest possible scanning technique saves contrast medium load which may be better used to obtain additional diagnostic information.

Optimizing safety
Considering the high dose and fast intravascular injection, non-ionic x-ray contrast agents belong to the least toxic compounds known. Nevertheless, a variety of unintended (e.g. feeling of warmth) or adverse effects are known and although extremely rare, a fatal idiosyncratic reaction cannot be completely excluded.

Recognizing the risk factors of individual patients and if possible reducing the risk by appropriate pre-treatment or other safety measures is the subject of numerous research articles, reviews, book chapters and recommendations of radiological and cardiological societies.[6, 7, 22] It is not the purpose of this article to provide an overview of risks, prophylaxis and treatment of contrast media reactions.

Iodinated Contrast Media: New Perspectives with Dual Source CT

Nevertheless, one aspect is specific to CT and shall be mentioned here

In CT, contrast media are administered orally or intravenously. Whereas oral administration usually does not cause other than gastrointestinal side effects, severe reactions may occur following intravenous administration, in most cases allergoid or cardiovascular. Recently, renal tolerance of x-ray contrast media has been disputed in patients with preexisting renal insufficiency, especially if they suffer from diabetes.[23, 24, 25, 26, 27] It must, however, be noticed that almost all studies reporting contrast-induced nephropathy refer to intraarterial administration. In these patients thrombembolic complications are not rare (e.g. TIA's). Thromboembolic events may also contribute to deterioration of kidney function. Transient increases in serum creatinine in the patients who received contrast media meeting a certain definition of the investigators have been reported as contrast-induced nephropathy. This will necessarily include a proportion of changes due to the basic physiological

Author	Contrast Agent	Criteria	Administration	Result
Kennedy et al., 1988[32]	Iopromide – 370 Iopamidol – 370	Serum creatinine/ Creatinine clearance	Intravenous	No difference Tendency in favor of iopromide
Langer et al., 1989[33]	Iopromide – 370 Iopamidol – 370	Urinary enzymes	Intravenous	No difference
Carraro et al., 1998[34]	Iopromide – 300 Iodixanol – 320	Serum creatinine, urinary enzymes, protein excretion	Intraarterial	No difference
Himi et al., 1999[35]	Iopromide – 370 Iohexol – 350	Serum creatinine, ß₂-globulin, urinary enzymes	Intraarterial	No difference Tendency in favor of iopromide
Donadio et al., 2001[36]	Iopromide – 370 Ioversol – 320 Ioxaglate – 320	GFR, creatinine clearance, etc.	Intraarterial	No difference Tendency in favor of non-ionic contrast agents
Feldkamp et al., 2006[3]	Iopromide – 300 Iodixanol – 320	Serum creatinine, creatinine clearance, urinary NAG	Intraarterial	No difference

[Table 1] Renal tolerance of iopromide according to comparative clinical trials.

and pathological fluctuation of serum creatinine as well as patients whose renal function would also have deteriorated without contrast medium exposure. Few studies were performed with intravenous injection of contrast agents at dose levels typical for CT. Among these were only two controlled studies comparing creatinine fluctuations in patients following CT with and without contrast enhancement.[28, 29] In these studies, very similar serum creatinine increases (and decreases) were observed in both groups, with and without contrast medium, pointing to the limitations of uncontrolled studies in severely ill patients. Thus, the question if, in which patient population and how frequently a clinically significant impairment of renal function occurs following intravenous administration of contrast media in CT remains unanswered.[30]

A review comparing the incidence of transient increases of serum creatinine following the administration of different contrast media or prophylactic treatments in controlled studies did not suggest a preference for any of the tested non-ionic products.[31] Table 1 summarizes the results of controlled studies comparing the renal tolerance of different contrast media in various patient populations after intraarterial and intravenous administration.

Conclusion
Iodinated contrast agents are an essential component of CT. During its own development CT helped to explore the formerly unrevealed potential of contrast media as markers of pathophysiological signs of diseases. The currently dominating and most useful type of contrast medium (urographic, extracellular marker of blood vessels, perfusion, permeability and interstitial space) was discovered in the late twenties of the last century (Uroselectan), developed further to Urografin with an improved iodine content and tolerance in the fifties and then the introduction of low osmolar non-ionic contrast media in the early 80's. The class of low osmolar contrast agents is well suited for CT with optimal concentrations and low viscosity for the fastest possible iodine delivery rate and good tolerance, which allows the injection of high single and cumulative doses. Extensive experience of more than 20 years and millions of applications provide the basis for a realistic assessment of the benefits and risks associated with the use of such contras media in the broad variety of patients referred to undergo a CT examination.

Iodinated Contrast Media: New Perspectives with Dual Source CT

References

1. Rau T, Mathey D, Schofer J. High-dose tolerance of iodinated x-ray contrast media. New Developments in X-Ray and MR Angiography Symposium CIRSE, 9.9.96, Funchal, Madeira. In: Springer, Insert in Cardiovascular and Interventional Radiology 1997; 20:8-9

2. Rosovsky MA, Rusinek H, Berenstein A, et al. High-dose administration of nonionic contrast media: a retrospective review. Radiology 1996;200:119-122

3. Feldkamp T, Baumgart D, Elsner M et al. Nephrotoxicity of iso-osmolar versus low-osmolar contrast media is equal in low risk patients. Clinical Nephrology 2006;66:322-330

4. Mortelé KJ, Oliva M-R, Ondategui S, et al. Universal use of nonionic iodinated contrast medium for CT: Evaluation of safety in a large urban teaching hospital. AJR 2005;185:31-34

5. Kopp A, Mortelé KJ, Palkowitsch P, et al. Safety and tolerability of the non-ionic x-ray contrast agent , iopromide, in 74,717 patients. Radiology 2005;Suppl:Abstract No SSM11-04

6. Morcos SK, Thomsen HS. Adverse reactions to iodinated contrast media. Eur Radiol 2001;11:1267-1275

7. Morcos SK, Thomsen HS, Webb JAW, et al. Prevention of generalized reactions to contrast media: a consensus report and guidelines. Eur Radiol 2001;11:1720-1728

8. Gmelin E, Friedrich H-J. Bolusgeometrie bei unterschiedlicher zentraler und peripherer Kontrastmittelapplikation: Studie mittels Serio-CT unter Verwendung nichtionischen Kontrastmittels. Röntgen-Bl 1985;38:219-223

9. Busch HP, Stocker KP. „Iodine delivery rate" bei der Katheterangiographie unter Druckbedingungen der manuellen Injektion. Akt Radiol 1998;8:232-235

10. Jung F, Schmitt RM, Scheller B, et al. Flussraten von Röntgenkontrastmitteln verschiedener Viskosität in 4.1-Charrière-Koronarkathetern. Z Kardiol 1996;85(8):537-542

11. Hughes PM, Bisset R. Non-ionic contrast media: a comparison of iodine delivery rates during manual injection angiography. Br J Radiol 1991;64:417-419

12. Knollmann F, Schimpf K, Felix R. Jodeinbringungsgeschwindigkeit verschieden konzentrierter Röntgenkontrastmittel bei schneller intravenöser Injektion. Fortschr Röntgenstr 2004;176:880-884

13. Langer M, Felix R, Keysser R, et al. Beeinflussung der Abbildungsqualität der i.v. DSA durch die Jodkonzentration des Kontrastmittels. Digit Bilddiagn 1985;5:154-159

14. Awai K, Inoue M, Yagyu Y et al. Moderate versus high concentration of contrast material for aortic and hepatic enhancement and tumor-to-liver contrast at multi-detector row CT. Radiology 2004;233:682-688

15. Herman S. Computed tomography contrast enhancement principles and the use of high-concentration contrast media. Comput Assist Tomogr 2004;28:S7-S11

16. Fenchel S, Fleiter TR, Aschoff AJ, et al. Effect of iodine concentration of contrast media on contrast enhancement in multisclice CT of the pancreas. Br J Radiol 2004;77:821-830

17. Claussen CD, Banzer D, Pfretzschner C, et al. Bolus geometry and dynamics after intravenous contrast medium injection. Radiology 1984;153(2):365-368

18. Cademartiri F, van der Lugt A, Luccichenti G, et al. Parameters affecting bolus geometry in CT: A review. J Comput Assist Tomogr 2002;26(4):598-607

19. Ho LM, Nelson RC, DeLong DM. Determining contrast medium dose and rate on basis of lean body weight: Does this strategy improve patient-to-patient uniformity of hepatic enhancement during multi-detector row CT? Radiology 2007;243:431-437

20. Bae KT, Tran HQ, Heiken JP. Uniform vascular contrast enhancement and reduced contrast medium volume achieved by using exponentially decelerated contrast material injection method. Radiology 2004;231:732-736

21. Ichikawa T, Erturk SM, Araki T. Multiphasic contrast-enhanced multidetector-row CT of liver: contrast-enhancement theory and practical scan protocol with a combination of fixed injection duration and patients' body-weight-tailored dose of contrast material. Eur J Radiol 2006;58:165-176

22. Thomsen HS, Bush WH. Treatment of the adverse effects of contrast media. Acta Radiol1998;39:212-218

23. Aspelin P, Aubry P, Fransson S-G, et al. Nephrotoxic effects in high-risk patients undergoing angiography. N Engl J Med 2003;348:491-499

24. Liss P, Persson PB, Hansell P, et al. Renal failure in 57 925 patients undergoing coronary procedures using iso-osmolar or low-osmolar contrast media. Kidney Int 2006;70(10):1811-1817

25. Persson PB, Hansell P, Liss P. Pathophysiology of contrast medium-induced nephropathy. Kidney Int 2005;68:14-22

26. Thomsen HS, Morcos SK. In which patients should serum creatinine be measured before iodinated contrast medium administration? Eur Radiol 2005;15:749-754

27. Thomsen HS, Morcos SK. Contrast media and the kidney: European Society of Urogenital Radiology (ESUR) guidelines. Br J Radiol 2003;76:513-518

28. Heller CA, Knapp J, Halliday J, et al. Failure to demonstrate contrast nephrotoxicity. Med J Aust 1991;155:329-332

29. Rao QA, Newhouse JH. Risk of nephropathy after intravenous administration of contrast material: a critical literature analysis. Radiology 2006;239:392-397

30. Katzberg RW and Barrett BJ. Risk of iodinated contrast material-induced nephropathy with intravenous administration. Radiology 2007;243:622-628

[31] Bettmann MA. Contrast medium-induced nephropathy: critical review of existing clinical evidence. Nephrol Dial Transplant 2005; 20 (Suppl 1):i12-i17

[32] Kennedy C, Rickards D, Buckley Sharp M et al. A double-blind study comparing the efficacy, tolerance and renal effects of iopromide and iopamidol. Bri J Radiol 1988;61:288-293

[33] Langer M, Junge W, Keysser R et al. Renal and hepatic tolerance of nonionic and ionic contrast media in intravenous digital subtraction angiography. Fortschr Röntgenstr 1989;Suppl 128:95-100

[34] Carraro M, Malalan F, Antonione R et al. Effects of a dimeric vs monomeric nonionic contrast medium on renal function inpatients with mild to moderate renal insufficienc: a double-blind, randomized clinical trial. Eur Radiol 1998;8:144-147

[35] Himi K, Takemoto A, Himi M et al. Renal effects of non-ionic contrast media on adequately hydrated patients in cardioangiography – comparison of iopromide and iohexol. Eur Radiol 1999;9:S438

[36] Donadio C, Lucchesi A, Ardini M et al. Renal effects of cardiac angiography with different low-osmolar contrast media. Renal Failure 2001;23:385-396

Dual Source CT Imaging

Seidensticker
Hofmann
(Eds.)

Cardiovascular and Body Radiology
DSCT Applications

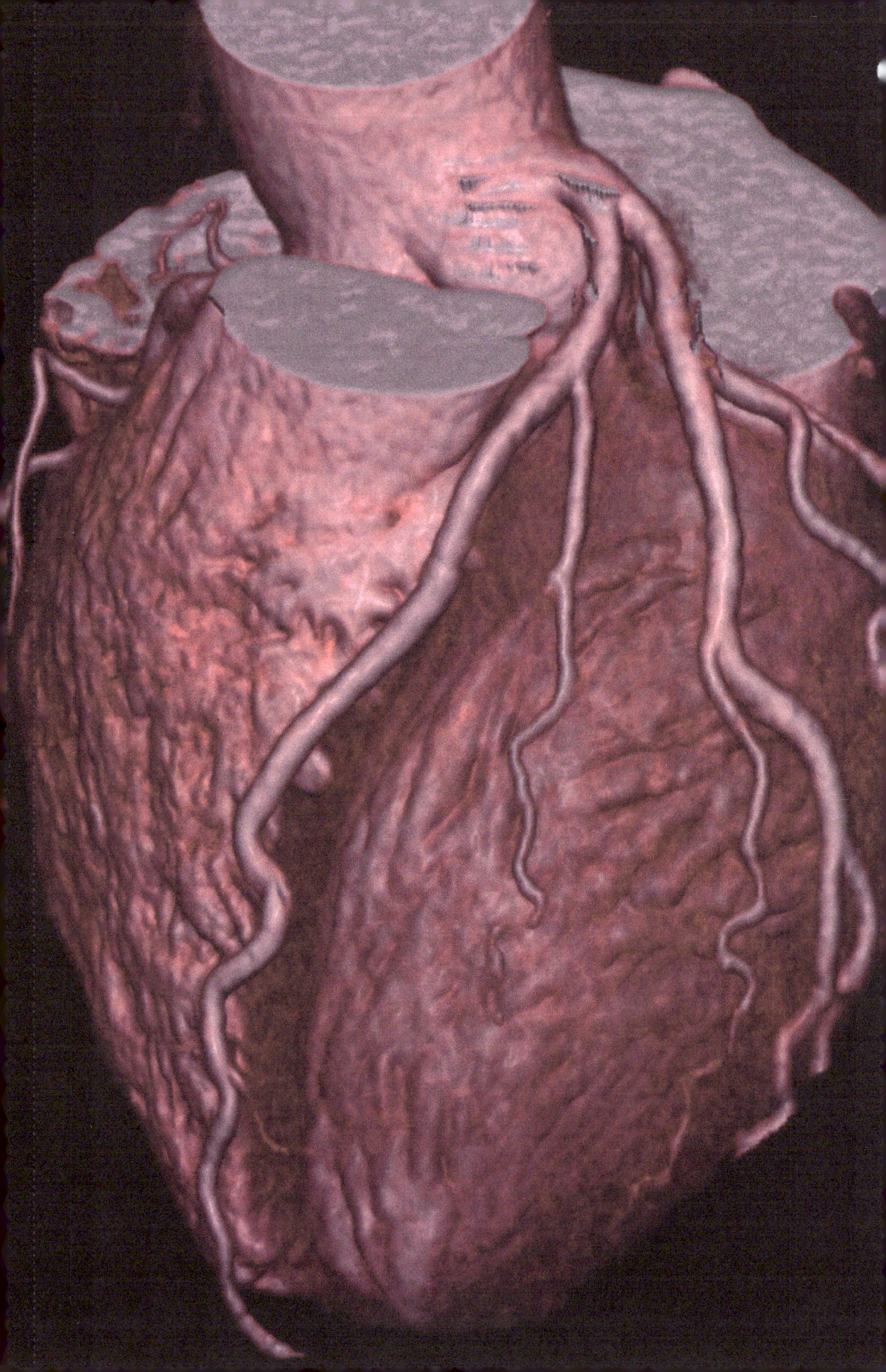

Cardiac: Coronary CT Angiography

Stephan Achenbach · Axel Kuettner · Dieter Ropers

Case 1: Ruling out Coronary Stenosis in Acute Chest Pain

Case 2: Diagnosis of a Coronary Occlusion in a Patient with Atypical Chest Pain

Visualization of the coronary arteries ("Coronary Angiography") is a central diagnostic tool in cardiology. The coronary arteries are small and move very rapidly, so that non-invasive imaging is difficult and catheter-based, invasive coronary angiography constitutes the clinical gold standard. In recent years, computed tomography technology has progressed to a stage that allows relatively reliable visualization of the coronary artery lumen after intravenous injection of a contrast agent ("coronary CT angiography", "coronary CTA"). Based on the axial cross-sections that are acquired, 2- and 3-dimensional reconstructions of the coronary arteries can be rendered and allow analysis concerning the presence of atherosclerotic lesions and coronary artery stenoses. However, temporal resolution is still a limiting factor for CT visualization of the coronary arteries. It has been convincingly demonstrated that regular and low heart rates are a prerequisite for reliable imaging of the coronary arteries by 16- to 64-slice MDCT, thus, the administration of short-acting beta-blockers prior to the MDCT scan is strongly recommended.[1] The aim is to lower heart rates to less than 65 bpm (optimally less than 60 bpm). With the new Dual Source CT scanners, which provides a heart-rate independent temporal resolution of 82 ms, it is not necessary to lower the heart rate, because diagnostic image quality can be obtained even at higher heart rates in an overwhelming majority of cases.[2,3,4] Use of sublingual nitroglycerine is also recommended for all scanners immediately before data acquisition in order to achieve coronary vasodilation, which substantially improves image quality.[1]

Numerous studies have compared the accuracy of coronary artery stenosis detection by MDCT to invasive coronary angiography. Results depend on the technology and scan protocols that were used, prevalence of disease in the patient group that was studied, and the basis for evaluation (per coronary segment, per coronary artery, or per patient). In studies performed using modern scan protocols and recent generations of 16- to 64-slice CT, the per-segment sensitivity for the detection of coronary artery stenoses in comparison with invasive coronary angiography was 83–99%, with specificities ranging from 93% to 98%.[1]

A per-patient analysis is more clinically relevant. This analysis addresses the question of whether CT coronary angiography is able to identify patients who have at least one coronary artery stenosis. In studies that have included this per-patient analysis, sensitivity ranged from 93% to 100%.

Cardiac: Coronary CT Angiography

Remarkably, the negative predictive value was found to be high across the board, ranging from 92% to 100% in both evaluation methods. Even though this may be influenced partly by a rather low prevalence of coronary artery stenoses in most of the patient groups that were studied, it does indicate the method's ability to reliably rule out the presence of coronary artery stenoses if the MDCT scan is expertly acquired and evaluated, has sufficient image quality, and fails to demonstrate coronary artery stenoses. The positive predictive value has usually been found to be somewhat lower, which indicates that MDCT, in comparison to invasive coronary angiography, tends to overestimate disease severity in some situations. Due to limitations in spatial resolution, accurate grading of the severity of a coronary lesion (percentage of stenosis) is currently not possible on a routine basis, and pronounced coronary calcifications can render images unevaluable at times. Similarly, motion or trigger artifacts as well as high image noise can degrade image quality and prevent reliable evaluation. However, preliminary experience indicates that Dual Source CTs are much more able to handle these factors than previous scanner generations. Clinically, coronary CT angiography would currently not be considered a routine replacement for the catheter-based diagnostic coronary angiogram. Clinical situations in which coronary CT angiography is especially likely to benefit are those in which coronary artery stenoses need to be ruled out but the pre-test likelihood of stenoses is not very high. If the coronary CT angiogram is then "normal" (showing no stenoses), an invasive angiogram is not necessary, which is beneficial in terms of potential complications and economic cost. Such situations may arise in patients with atypical symptoms, or in patients with equivocal stress test results (which is not uncommon). A recent scientific statement by the American Heart Association reports the potential clinical utility of coronary CT angiography in these situations.[5] Furthermore, a multi-society consensus paper on appropriateness criteria for cardiac imaging by CT and MR lists the use of CT coronary angiography as "appropriate" in patients with chest pain who have ambiguous findings in exercise testing as well as in symptomatic patients who have an intermediate likelihood of coronary artery disease but who cannot exercise or who have an uninterpretable ECG.[6] Finally, many patients with acute chest pain are also not very likely to have coronary artery disease, especially if their ECG is normal. As initial studies have shown, coronary CT angiography may be very useful in these patients to rapidly assess the presence or coronary stenoses and determine the necessity of further treatment.[6]

With their small dimensions, the coronary vessels are not easy to interpret by CT and impeccable image quality is a prerequisite to reliably detect or rule out stenoses. The use of adequate imaging technology and careful adherence to appropriate image acquisition protocols, including optimized contrast enhancement, are a necessity to obtain fully diagnostic datasets. Owing to its high temporal resolution, Dual Source CT has substantially improved image quality compared with previous scanner generations and should thus allow for reliable assessment of the coronary arteries and more widespread clinical application of coronary CT angiography.

Stephan Achenbach · Axel Kuettner · Dieter Ropers

University of Erlangen-Nuremberg

Departments of Cardiology and Radiology

Universitätsklinikum
Erlangen

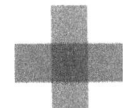

References

[1] Achenbach S, Computed Tomography Coronary Angiography. J Am Coll Cardiol 2006; 48:1919–1928

[2] Achenbach S, et al. Contrast-enhanced coronary artery visualization by dual-source computed tomography--initial experience. Eur J Radiol 2006;57:331–335

[3] Johnson TR, et al. Dual-source CT cardiac imaging: initial experience. Eur Radiol. 2006;16:1409–1415

[4] Scheffel H, et al. Accuracy of dual-source CT coronary angiography: first experience in a high pre-test probability population without heart rate control. Eur Radiol. 2006;16:2739–2747

[5] Budoff MJ, et al. Assessment of Coronary Artery Disease by Cardiac Computed Tomography: A Scientific Statement from the American Heart Association Committee on Cardiovascular Imaging and Intervention. Circulation. 2006;114:1761–1791

[6] Hendel RC, et al. ACCF/ACR/SCCT/SCMR/ASNC/NASCI/SCAI/SIR 2006 appropriateness criteria for cardiac computed tomography and cardiac magnetic resonance imaging. J Am Coll Cardiol. 2006;48:1475–149

Cardiac: Coronary CT Angiography

Basic considerations

Contrast application must be optimized in order to achieve adequate enhancement of the coronary lumen throughout the scan to avoid excessive contrast in other structures (such as the right heart cavities) and limit the amount of contrast agent given to the patients. Measures to keep the radiation dose within reasonable limits should be applied. ECG pulsing should always be activated. MinDose™ may be used to further reduce radiation dose if no information on left ventricular function is desired.

The use of 100 kV/330 mAs may be considered in patients with low body weight, for example, below 85 kg/175 lbs depending on the habitus of the patient.

In patients with high body weight, it may be useful to increase contrast flow rate and to employ the CardioObese™ mode.

Scan Parameters

Scan mode	Dual Source, ECG-gated
Heart rate control	not necessary
Scan area	mid pulmonary artery to below heart
Scan direction	cranio-caudal
Scan time	~7–12 s, depending on heart rate
Tube voltage	120 kV
Tube current	360 mAs/rotation
Dose modulation	ECG-pulsing on*
CTDI$_{vol}$	~50 mGy, depending on heart rate
Rotation time	0.33 s
Pitch	0.2–0.5, depending on heart rate
Slice collimation	0.6 mm
Acquisition	64 x 0.6 mm
Slice width	0.75 mm
Reconstruction increment	0.4 mm
Reconstruction kernel	B26f, B46f in case of excessive calcification

* Referring to ECG-pulsing table (see page 28)

Tricks

· Use nitrates if not contra-indicated.
· A reliable breathhold must be assured. A long breathhold command ("breath in-breath out-breath in-hold your breath") may be useful (requires contrast timing via test bolus).
· The best images are usually obtained in diastole for heart rates up to ~65 bpm, often in systole for higher rates.

Pitfalls

· Assure safe ECG leads – mistriggering may render scan uninterpretable.
· When patients have arrhythmias, enter a heart rate substantially lower than the actual heart rate into the scan menu – this will allow exclusion of ectopic beats while preserving the ability to reconstruct without interpolation.
· Extend scan range for patients with CABG.

Contrast Injection Protocol

	Iodine concentration 300 mg I/ml	Iodine concentration 370 mg I/ml
Injection scheme	Monophasic	Monophasic
Iodine delivery rate	1.85 g/s	1.85 g/s
CM volume	6.2 ml/s for duration of scan, ≥ 60 ml	5 ml/s for duration of scan, ≥ 50 ml
CM flow rate	6.2 ml/s	5 ml/s
Body weight adaption	no	no
Bolus timing	test bolus*	test bolus*
Bolus tracking threshold	n.a.	n.a.
ROI position	ascending aorta	ascending aorta
Scan delay	peak time plus 2 s	peak time plus 2 s
Saline flush volume	60 ml	60 ml
Saline injection rate	6.2 ml/s	5 ml/s
Needle size	18 G	18 G
Injection site	antecubital vein	antecubital vein

*Depending on the preference of the individual site, bolus tracking can be used as an alternative

Case 1 Ruling out Coronary Stenosis in Acute Chest Pain

Case history

43-year-old patient with acute chest pain, not entirely typical for myocardial infarction. ST segment elevation [fig. 1] and enzyme elevation. Echo was normal.

Question

Myocarditis versus myocardial infarction: Can coronary stenoses/occlusions be ruled out?

Diagnosis/Differential diagnosis

Chest pain and ST segment elevation are the lead symptoms of acute myocardial infarction. Here, however, the clinical presentation suggested that myocarditis might be more likely. Coronary CTA was performed in order to rapidly determine the status of the coronary arteries and thus differentiate between infarction and myocarditis.

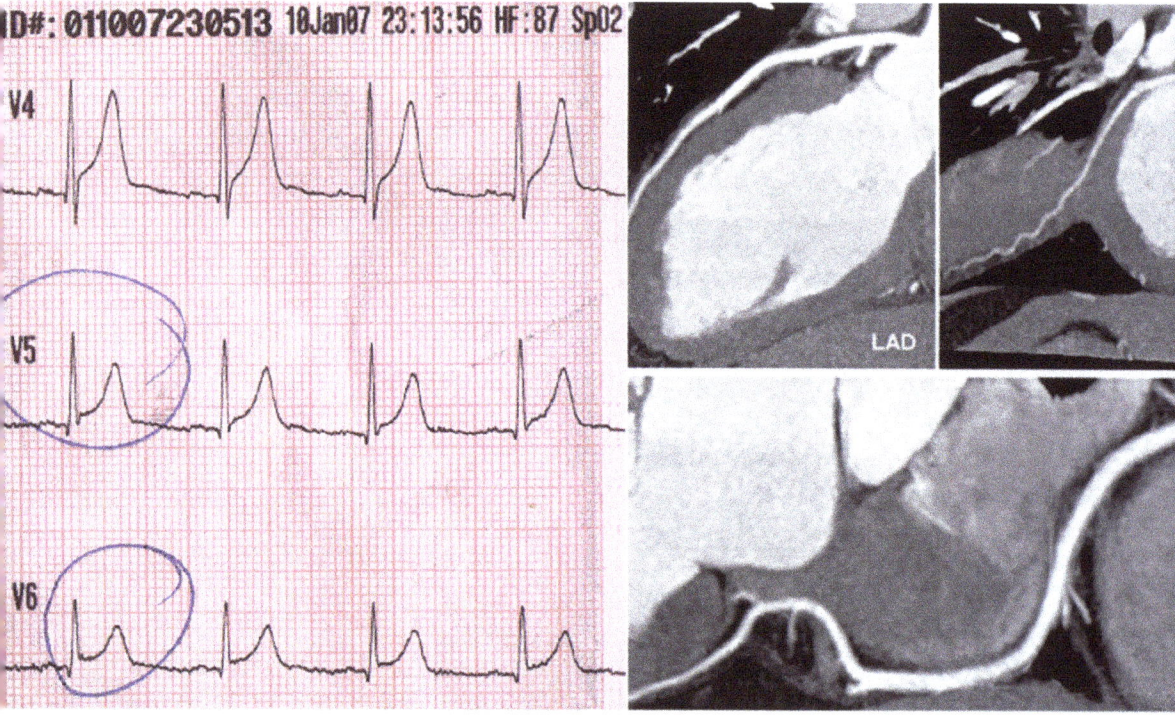

[1] ECG with ST-segment elevation.

[2] Curved multiplanar reconstructions of the coronary arteries demonstrate absence of stenoses.

Findings

In DSCT (heart rate 77 bpm), optimal image quality was achieved at 70% of the R-R interval. In the original images, multiplanar reconstructions [fig. 2] and 3-dimensional display [figs. 3 and 4], it was demonstrated that the coronary arteries were free of stenosis and atherosclerotic plaque, thus allowing the diagnosis of perimyocarditis. No invasive angiography was performed. The patient recovered uneventfully.

Take-home message

In selected situations of patients with acute chest pain, coronary DSCT angiography can be useful to rule out the presence of coronary lesions (stenoses or occlusions). In chest pain with ST segment elevation, DSCT will not usually be the test of choice. Here, however, clinical suspicion of perimyocarditis was strong and hence DSCT imaging was performed to avoid invasive angiography.

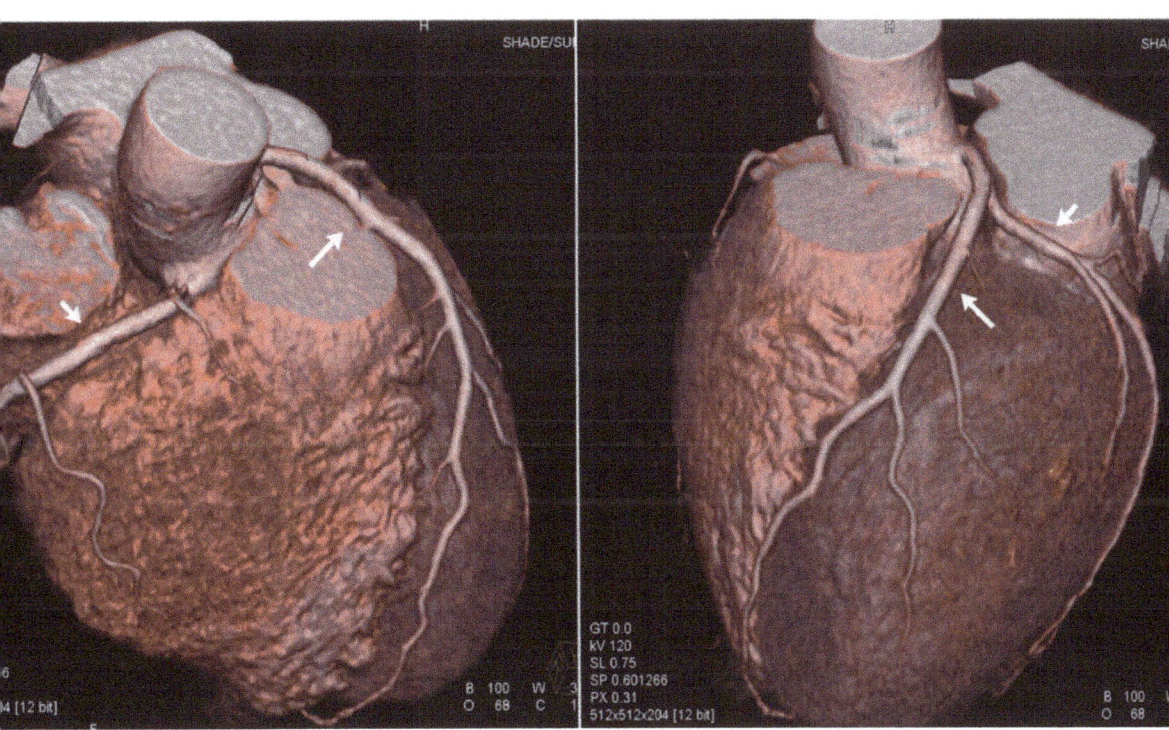

[3] Three-dimensional reconstruction of the heart and coronary arteries, here showing the left anterior descending (large arrow) and right coronary artery (small arrow).

[4] Three-dimensional reconstruction of the heart and coronary arteries, here showing the left anterior descending (large arrow) and left circumflex coronary artery (small arrow).

Case 2 Diagnosis of a Coronary Occlusion in a Patient with Atypical Chest Pain

Case history

49-year-old patient with atypical chest pain and an equivocal bicycle stress test (non-significant ST segment depression in the anterior leads).

Question

The relative young age of the patient, atypical nature of the chest pain, and equivocal stress test make coronary artery disease rather unlikely. Thus, coronary CTA was performed to rule out the presence of coronary stenoses.

Diagnosis / Differential diagnosis

In patients with atypical chest pain, coronary CTA will often demonstrate normal coronary arteries. Here, however, a relatively long, chronic total occlusion of the proximal left anterior descending coronary artery was found. The lesion contained only very little calcium.

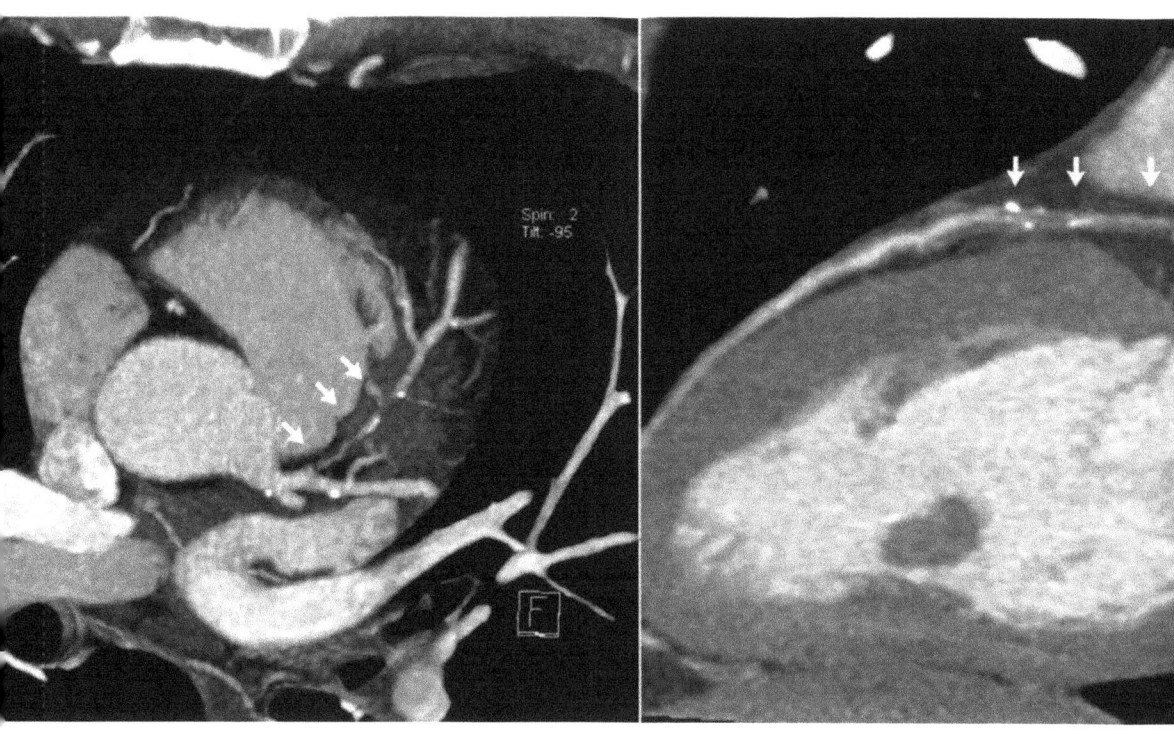

[1] Long occlusion of the left anterior descending coronary artery seen in an 8-mm thick maximum intensity projection (arrows).

[2] Curved multiplanar reconstruction of the left anterior descending coronary artery. There is relatively little calcification in the course of the occlusion (arrows).

Findings

A chronic total occlusion of the proximal left anterior descending coronary artery (LAD) was detected. DSCT demonstrated that there was relatively little calcification present in the course of this occlusion, which facilitated the decision to perform an attempt at percutaneous interventional revascularization (PCI), which was successful.

Take-home message

DSCT can be useful in patients with atypical chest pain to rule out – or rule in – the presence of obstructive coronary artery lesions.
In the context of CTO, lesion length and degree of calcification can be assessed by DSCT and may provide information on the probability of success of interventional revascularization.

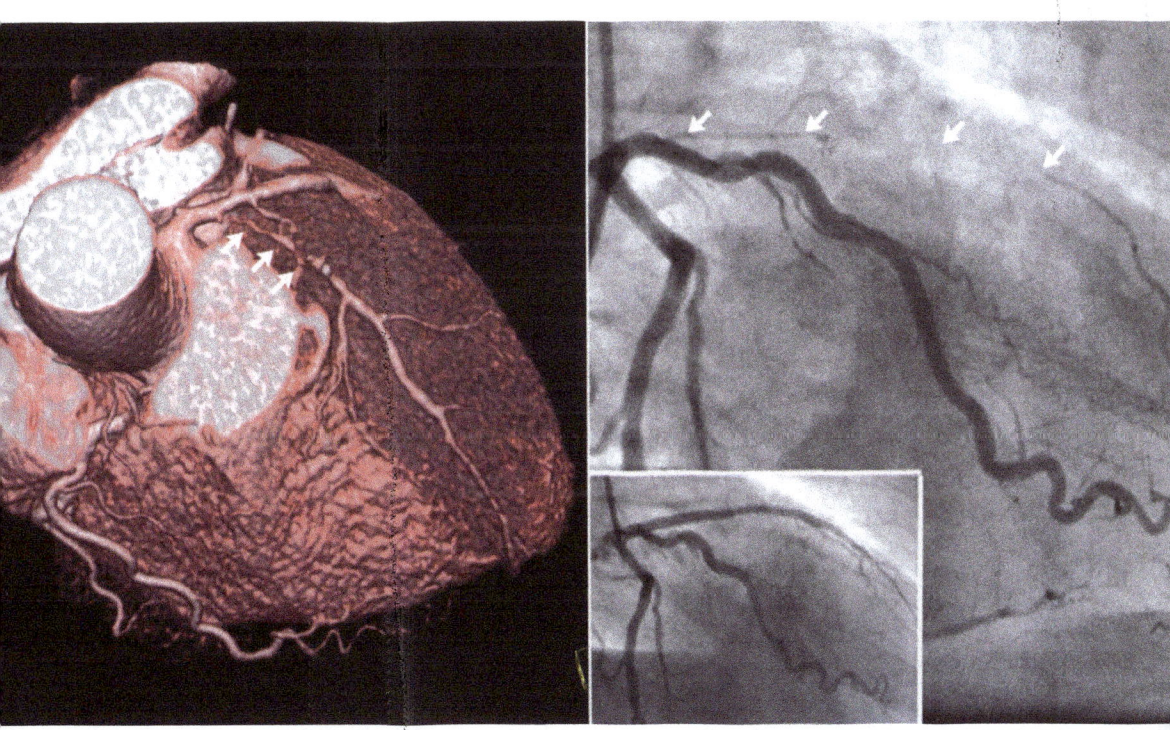

[3] Three-dimensional reconstruction of the heart and coronary arteries showing the occlusion of the LAD (arrows).

[4] Invasive coronary angiography confirms the LAD occlusion (arrows). Interventional recanalization is successful (insert).

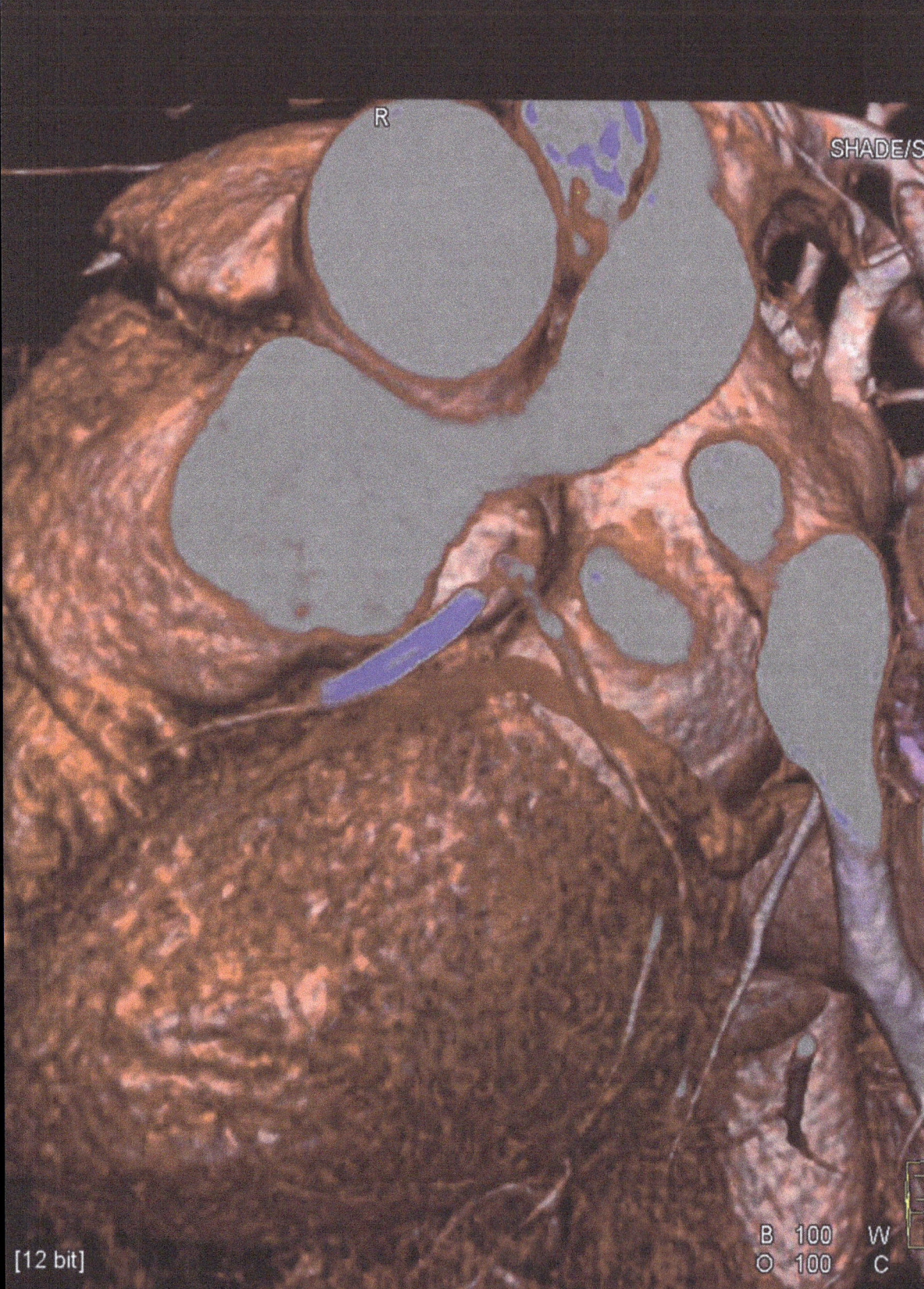

Cardiac: Coronary Stents

Stefan G. Ruehm · Cesar Arellano · Christoph Panknin

Case 1: Stent in LAD

Case 2: Stent Restenosis

Percutaneous coronary intervention (PCI) with stent placement is the leading technique for nonsurgical myocardial revascularization therapy. Despite a technical success rate of more than 95%, in-stent restenosis remains a major clinical problem. Restenosis rates of up to 46% have been described in patients receiving non-drug-eluting stents.[1] Although the incidence of early in-stent restenosis may be significantly reduced when drug-eluting stents are employed, the early detection of restenosis is important to avoid recurrent myocardial ischemia and infarction and thus to improve the long-term prognosis after revascularization therapy. Furthermore, patients who previously underwent PCI often suffer from progression of atherosclerosis at other sites and may therefore require repeated imaging studies for the assessment of arterial patency. Currently conventional catheter coronary angiography remains the reference standard for the assessment of stent patency and overall for the evaluation of coronary artery stenosis. Due to its invasiveness, conventional coronary angiography is associated with rare but potentially serious side effects such as retroperitoneal bleeding, arterial rupture, myocardial infarction or stroke. Therefore, a non-invasive alternative for imaging of the coronary artery system would be highly desirable. Coronary magnetic resonance angiography is of limited value for the assessment of stent patency due to susceptibility artifacts generated by the metallic stent material, which usually obscures the stent lumen. Electron beam computed tomography (EBCT) has been employed for the display of coronary artery stents. However, EBCT does not allow the accurate visualization of the stent lumen and is therefore of limited value for the diagnosis of stent restenosis.[2] Compared with EBCT, multi-detector computed tomography (MDCT) allows acquisition of image data with thinner slice thickness and less noise. The technique has been widely adopted for non-invasive imaging of coronary arteries. Promising results for the detection of coronary artery stenoses have been reported, particularly in patients with low heart rates and in the absence of extensive vascular calcifications.[3] However, results for the assessment of stent lumen patency have been disappointing when 4-slice MDCT scanner technology was used.[4] The introduction of 16-slice and 64-slice CT scanners with sub-millimeter resolution has resulted in improved visualization of the stent lumen at lower heart rates. However, the stent material may severely affect the image quality.[5] With Dual Source CT, the visualization of coronary stents became possible over a wide range of heart rates.[6]

Cardiac: Coronary Stents

Typically, a stent is a laser-cut stainless steel mesh formed in the configuration of a tube. It is mounted on a balloon catheter in a collapsed state. When the balloon is inflated, the stent expands and stabilizes the inner wall of the coronary artery after angioplasty. Recently drug-eluting stents have been introduced. A drug-eluting stent is coated with a pharmacologic agent to prevent restenosis. Currently available stent models are well visualized by CT and appear as bright structures on cross-sectional images. Due to blooming effects resulting in increased CT density values adjacent to the confinements of the stent, they appear significantly larger than their actual size on CT images. A combination of partial volume effects because of the limited spatial resolution in relation to the dimensions of the stent struts and beam hardening effects as well as a slightly widened slice-sensitivity profile related to spiral scanning is most likely responsible for the blooming effects. Therefore, the stent lumen is displayed with higher density. A decrease in density is generally observed from the periphery towards the center of the stent. Vessel size and stent material influence the size and pattern of stent-related artifacts. It has been shown that CT acquisitions with thinner slice collimation – available with newer scanner generations, such as the Siemens SOMATOM Sensation 64 and Definition – combined with adapted edge preserving reconstruction kernels for increased in-plane resolution, improve the visualization of the in-stent lumen.[7] A variety of post-processing techniques are available for the evaluation of coronary CT angiograms, such as multiplanar reformations (MPR), curved reformations, thin-slab maximum intensity projections (MIP) as well as various three-dimensional (3D) reconstruction techniques such as shaded surface display (SSD), volume rendering (VR) and virtual endoscopic views. In general, surface shaded or volume rendered 3D displays are not able to visualize the arterial lumen. Therefore, they are not useful for the assessment of stent patency, whereas thin-slab MIP reconstruction may be employed for the initial evaluation of coronary arteries, followed by the use of axial source images, oblique, curved and cross-sectional MPRs for the final assessment of coronary arterial and in-stent lumen patency. When a stented coronary artery segment is evaluated, the exaggerated dimensions of the stent structures due to blooming effects in combination with the associated artificially decreased luminal diameter need to be considered in order to avoid an overestimation or false positive diagnosis of in-stent restenosis. Attenuation values within the stent lumen that are significantly lower than in adjacent coronary segments generally suggest high-grade stenosis or occlusion.

In general, imaging of coronary stents requires scan protocols optimized for spatial resolution, ideally beyond the capabilities of 4- and 16-slice CT scanners. The latest 64-slice and the Dual Source CT scanner allow imaging with improved spatial resolution. These scanners feature optimized image reconstruction and post-processing techniques to further reduce stent-related image artifacts and better visualize the stent lumen. It is generally advisable to perform a sharp reconstruction (B46 kernel) in addition to a routine reconstruction (B26 kernel) to obtain more realistic intraluminal attenuation values and to increase the visible stent diameter. The introduction of new stent designs with thinner struts and less artifact prone stent materials may further reduce the current challenges of CT angiographic stent imaging.

Stefan G. Ruehm · Cesar Arellano · Christoph Panknin
David Geffen School of Medicine at UCLA
Department of Radiology

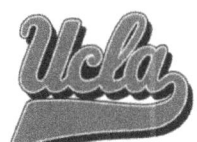

References

1. Kiemeneij F, Serruys PW, Macaya C, et al. Continued benefit of coronary stenting versus balloon angioplasty: five-year clinical follow-up of Benestent-I trial. J Am Coll Cardiol 2001; 37:1598-1603
2. Pump H, Mohlenkamp S, Sehnert CA, et al. Coronary arterial stent patency: assessment with electron-beam CT. Radiology 2000; 214:447-452
3. Achenbach S, Giesler T, Ropers D, et al. Detection of coronary artery stenoses by contrast-enhanced, retrospectively electrocardiographically-gated, multislice spiral computed tomography. Circulation 2001; 103:2535-2538
4. Ligabue G, Rossi R, Ratti C, Favali M, Modena MG, Romagnoli R. Noninvasive evaluation of coronary artery stents patency after PTCA: role of Multislice Computed Tomography. Radiol Med (Torino) 2004; 108:128-137
5. Maintz D, Seifarth H, Flohr T, et al. Improved coronary artery stent visualization and in-stent stenosis detection using 16-slice computed-to-mography and dedicated image reconstruction technique. Invest Radiol 2003; 38:790-795
6. Lell M, Panknin C, Ruehm S, et al. Evaluation of coronary stents and stenoses at different heart rates with dual source spiral CT (DSCT). Invest Radiol. 2007 Jul;42(7):536-41
7. Maintz D, Seifarth H, Raupach R, et al. 64-slice multidetector coronary CT angiography: in vitro evaluation of 68 different stents. Eur Radiol 2006; 16:818-826

Cardiac: Coronary Stents

Basic considerations

You can use an image protocol with maximal spatial and temporal resolution for optimized image quality, similar to the protocol used for standard coronary CT angiography. You can also use an injection protocol similar to the protocol used for standard coronary CT angiography. Reconstruction with a sharp kernel (B46) may help to better visualize stent lumen. Image reconstructions should include curved and multiplanar reformations.

Scan Parameters

Scan mode	Dual Source, ECG-gated
Heart rate control	not necessary
Scan area	mid pulmonary artery to below heart
Scan direction	cranio-caudal
Scan time	~7–12 s, depending on heart rate
Tube voltage	120 kV
Tube current	360 mAs/rotation
Dose modulation	ECG-pulsing on*
$CTDI_{vol}$	~50 mGy, depending on heart rate
Rotation time	0.33 s
Pitch	0.2–0.5, depending on heart rate
Slice collimation	0.6 mm
Acquisition	64 x 0.6 mm
Slice width	0.75 mm/0.6 mm
Reconstruction increment	0.4 mm
Reconstruction kernel	B46f

*Referring to ECG-pulsing table (see page 28)

Tricks

To evaluate of stented coronary artery segments, we recommend a kernel with stronger edge-enhancing characteristics (sharp B46 kernel versus soft B26 kernel). This usually increases the visible stent lumen and may help to avoid false positive readings of stent obstruction.

Pitfalls

Due to beam hardening effects, which cause increased CT values adjacent to the stent, stents appear significantly larger in CT images than their actual size. A decrease in density is generally observed from the periphery towards the center of the stent. Therefore, the size of the vessel lumen is artificially reduced in a stented coronary artery segment.

Contrast Injection Protocol

	Iodine concentration 300 mg I/ml	Iodine concentration 370 mg I/ml
Injection scheme	Monophasic	Monophasic
Iodine delivery rate	1.85 g/s	1.85 g/s
CM volume	5 ml/s for duration of scan, ≥ 60 ml	5 ml/s for duration of scan, ≥ 50 ml
CM flow rate	6.2 ml/s	5 ml/s
Body weight adaption	no	no
Bolus timing	test bolus*	test bolus*
Bolus tracking threshold	n.a.	n.a.
ROI position	left ventricle	left ventricle
Scan delay	peak time	peak time
Saline flush volume	60 ml	50 ml
Saline injection rate	6.2 ml/s	5 ml/s
Needle size	18 G	18 G
Injection site	antecubital vein	antecubital vein

*Depending on the preference of the individual site, bolus tracking can be used as an alternative

Case 1 Stent in LAD

Case history

53-year-old male with recurrent episodes of chest pain and status post stent placement in LAD.

Question

A CT angiogram was obtained to assess stent patency and overall situation of coronary arteries.

Diagnosis / Differential diagnosis

The CT angiogram shows homogeneous opacification of the lumen consistent with a widely patent stent with no evidence of restenosis. The degree of stent artifacts depends on the stent material used. False positive readings or non-diagnostic image quality of stented coronary artery segments are some of the limitations of CTA when used for the assessment of stent patency.

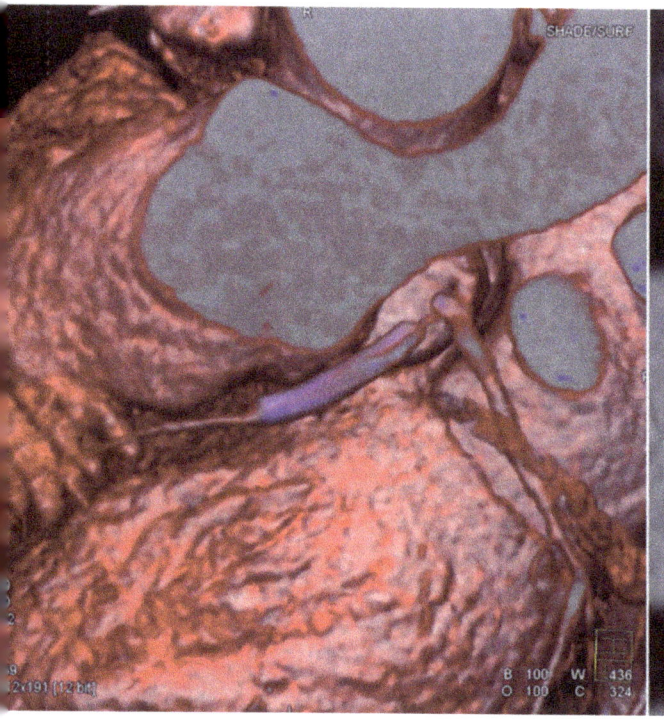

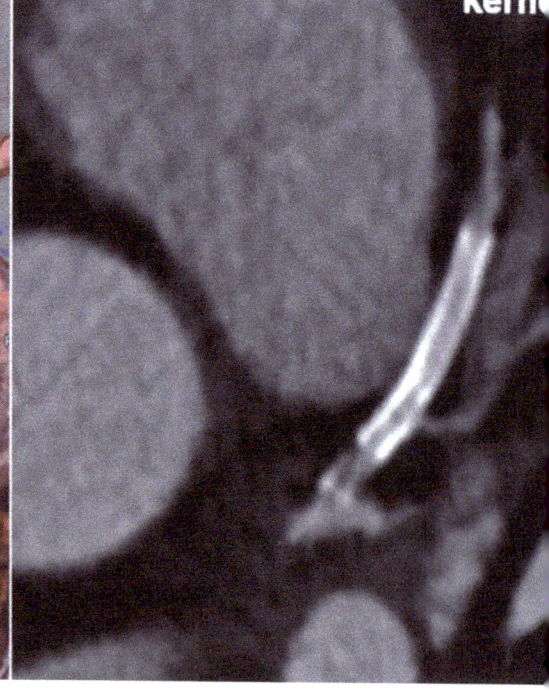

[1] Volume rendered 3D reconstruction shows stent in proximal LAD (blue color).

[2] Curved reformatted image reconstruction with soft kernel (B26) shows patent stent in proximal LAD.

Findings

Contrast enhanced CT angiogram of coronary arteries visualizes patent stent in proximal LAD. Proximal to the stent a small mixed, calcified and non-calcified plaque is visualized without significant luminal stenosis. Images were reconstructed with a soft (B26) and sharp (B46) kernel.

Take-home message

CT angiography of coronary arteries may be used to assess stent patency. Image reconstruction with sharp reconstruction filter (B46 kernel) may facilitate the assessment of stent patency. The size of the stent appears larger in CT images due to blooming effects.

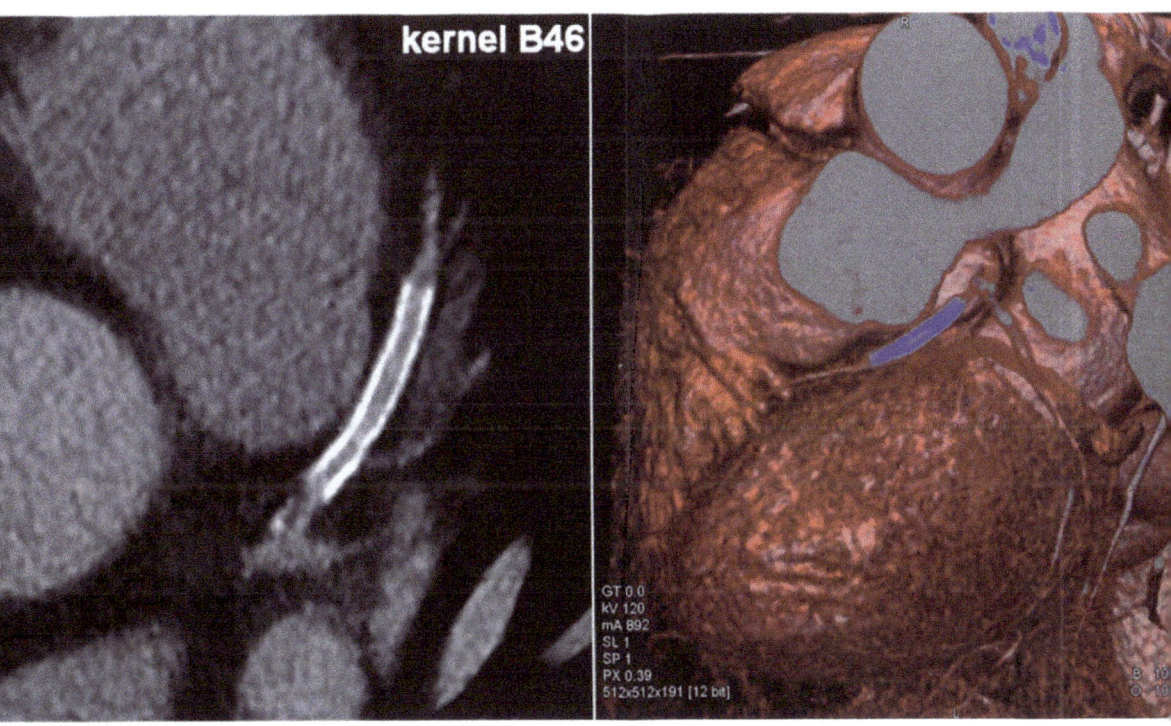

kernel B46

GT 0.0
kV 120
mA 892
SL 1
SP 1
PX 0.39
512x512x191 [12 bit]

[3] Curved reformatted image reconstruction with sharp kernel (B46) allows better delineation of stent lumen.

[4] Volume rendered 3D display of coronary CT angiogram.

Case 2 Stent Restenosis

Case history

58-year-old male with history of chest pain and percutaneous cardiac intervention presents for follow-up study.

Question

The patient is referred for the assessment of stenotic disease of coronary arteries.

Diagnosis/Differential diagnosis

A stent is noted in the proximal LAD and in the first obtuse marginal branch. The stent in the marginal branch is widely patent. The stent in the proximal LAD shows signs of restenosis. There is an area of mixed plaque immediately distal to the stent in the LAD.

Note is made of an old myocardial infarct in the inferior wall.

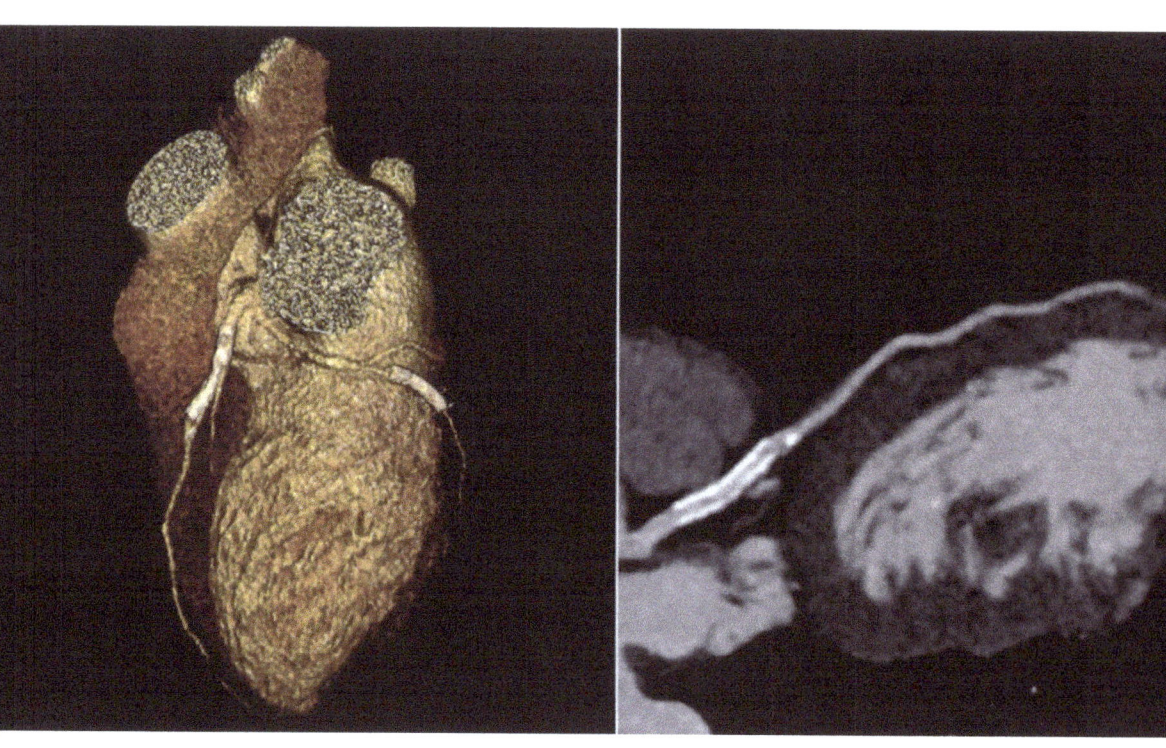

[1] Volume rendered 3D display demonstrates stent in LAD and first obtuse marginal branch.

[2] Curved reformatted image of LAD shows signs of stent restenosis. Note mixed plaque immediately distal to stent.

Findings

The lumen of the stent in the marginal branch shows rather homogeneous opacification consistent with stent patency.

The lumen of the stent in the LAD shows areas of decreased attenuation (proximal and distal aspect of stent) suggesting stent restenosis. A mixed calcified and non-calcified plaque is noted immediately distal to the stent.

Take-home message

Detection of stent restenosis still remains challenging but appears feasible with high spatial resolution acquisition protocols with DSCT. Additional findings such as myocardial perfusion defects may as well be present on standard coronary CT angiograms.

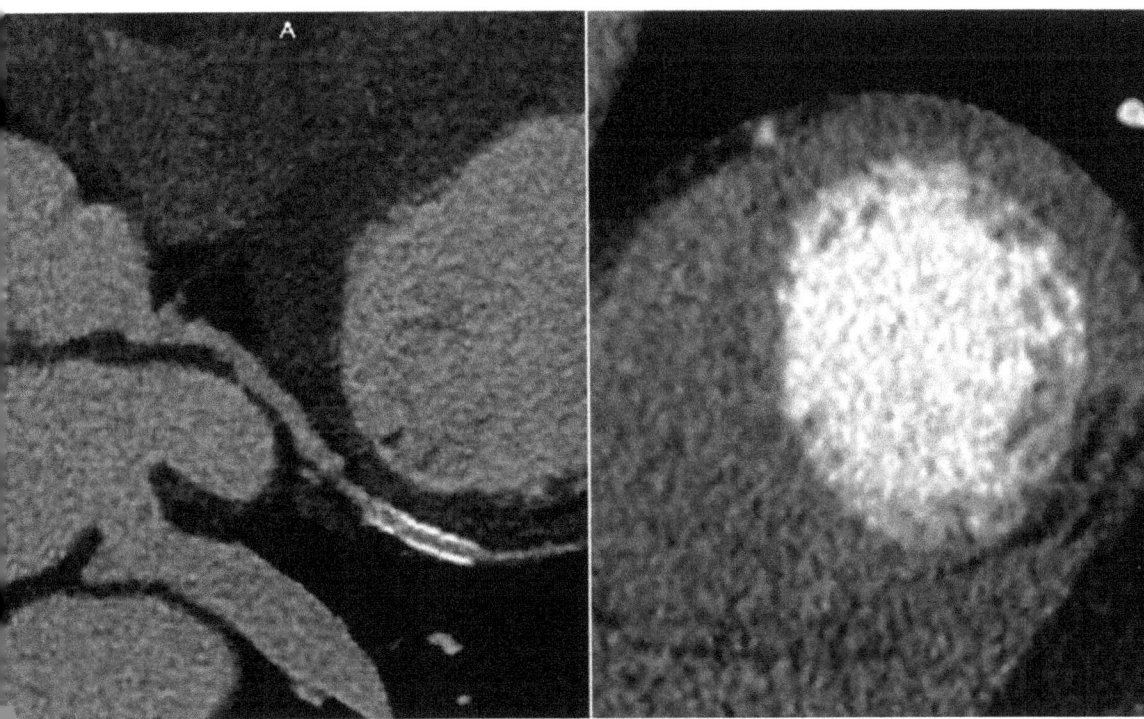

[3] Curved reformatted image of first obtuse marginal branch shows widely patent stent. Note area of decreased perfusion of inferior wall.

[4] Note area of decreased myocardial perfusion in inferior wall consistent with scar post myocardial infarction.

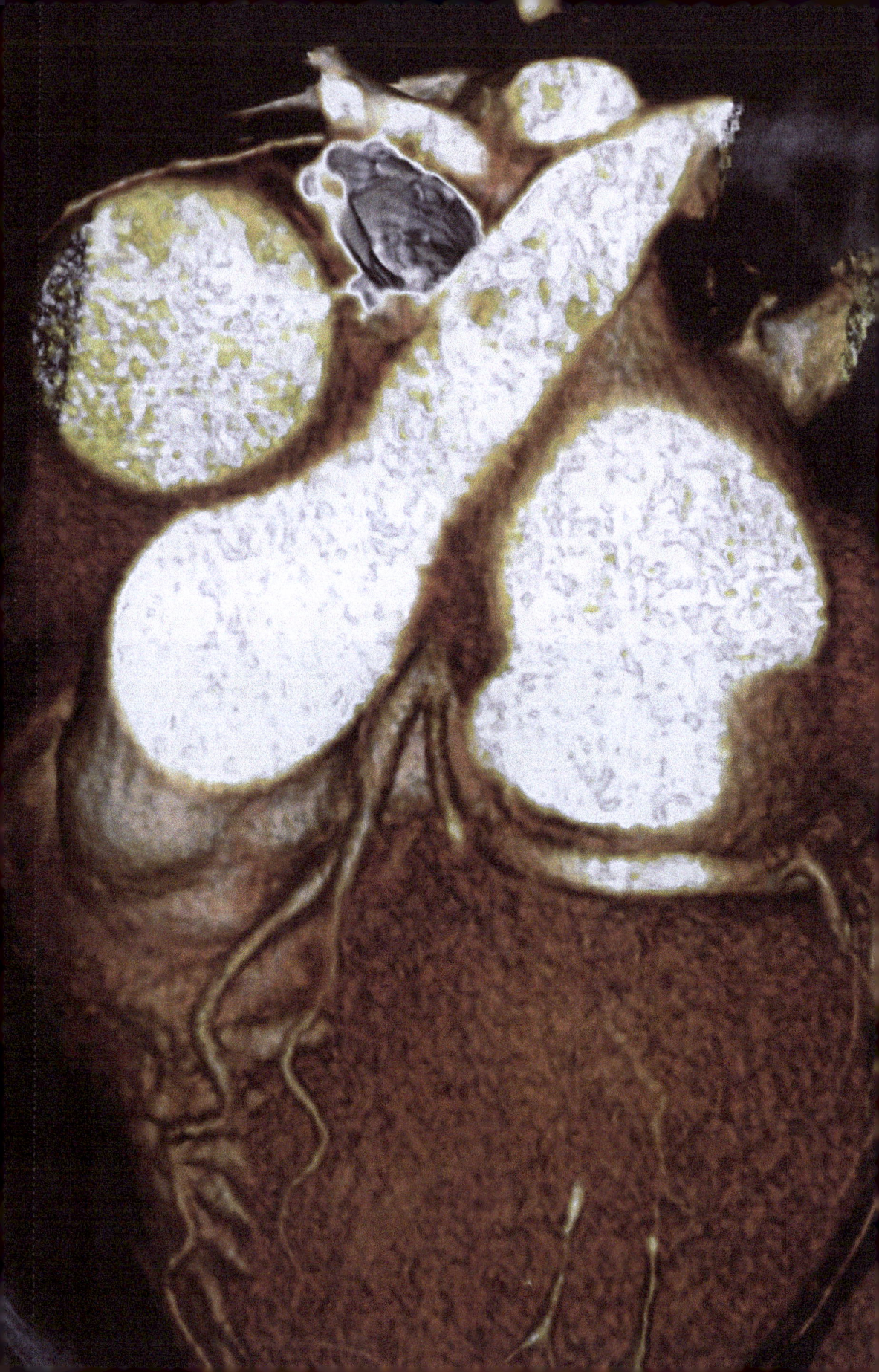

Cardiac: Coronary CTA in Obese Patients

Kavitha M. Chinnaiyan · Ralph Gentry · Gilbert L. Raff

Case 1: DSCT in a Morbidly Obese Woman Presenting with Dyspnea on Exertion

Case 2: DSCT in a Morbidly Obese Woman Presenting with Acute Atypical Chest Pain

Coronary artery disease (CAD) is the leading cause of death in the United States. Obesity is one of several known risk factors to develop CAD. In the United States, obesity is a growing epidemic, with 65% of all adults in the overweight range (BMI ≥ 25 kg/m²). This results in an increase in the prevalence of obesity by more than 75% since 1991.[1]

The obesity epidemic has become a major public health concern along with the increasing risk of cardiovascular disease. Compared with subjects of normal weight, obesity, particularly BMI > 30 is associated with increased mortality, even when the relative risks are adjusted for confounding factors such as age and smoking. With obesity being related to several coronary risk factors including hypertension, hyperlipidemia, diabetes and the metabolic syndrome, the association with CAD has been well demonstrated.[2, 3] In this patient population, diagnosing those with suspected CAD is challenging because almost all cardiac functional imaging studies of overweight and obese people are limited due to technical difficulties.[4] Using single-photon emission CT (SPECT) imaging, the majority of the morbidly obese patients can be imaged with the use of attenuation correction, dual-head cameras and high doses of the radiotracer. These techniques may not be available or applicable at all testing centers. Stress echocardiography is likewise limited because of poor acoustic windows and/or inability to achieve target heart rates with exercise. In such patients with non-diagnostic or inconclusive functional study results, diagnostic cardiac catheterization is usually performed for definitive diagnosis. Although there are no significantly increased risks of diagnostic cardiac catheterization in this population compared with patients with normal BMI, technical difficulties include achieving arterial access as well as postprocedural hemostasis and/or vascular complications.

Recent advances in multi-detector computed tomography and coronary CT angiography (CCTA) have made noninvasive diagnosis of CAD possible. In patients with normal BMI and in the presence of adequately low heart rates and low calcium scores, CCTA has demonstrated reasonably high sensitivity and specificity for detecting significant coronary stenosis.[5] However, CCTA is frequently uninterpretable or non-diagnostic in obese patients primarily due to a low signal-to-noise ratio.[6] Obesity causes increased radiation scatter within the patient's body and consequently degrades image quality due to a reduction of the signal-to-noise ratio. Using 64-slice scanners on patients

Cardiac: Coronary CTA in Obese Patients

with BMI > 30 kg/m², there is a decrease in sensitivity, specificity, positive and negative predictive value of CCTA compared with patients with BMI < 25 kg/m².

In body imaging, several methods can be utilized to improve image noise. These include use of longer gantry rotation time or thicker image slices. However, these methods severely impair the quality of CCTA due to resultant motion or partial volume artifacts. Consequently, these methods are not applicable for coronary CT imaging.

Recently, Dual Source CT scanners have demonstrated improved signal-to-noise characteristics from a special "obese mode" reconstruction. Changes in the scan protocol include effective mAs of 420, slice thickness of 0.75 mm and a higher contrast load. In addition to the increased volume of contrast bolus, it is also injected at a higher rate (6 ml/s). The higher mAs increases the penetration, resulting in higher visibility of the coronary segments. In essence, this mode permits the use of addition detector samplings (each tube 90–180 degree of the scan rotation) for image reconstruction. Although this sacrifices temporal resolution, but it can increase up to two fold the amount of information gathered during each gantry rotation. Using this mode requires adequate beta blocker doses for heart rate control, but extends effective CCTA to patients with body mass indices over 35 kg/m². Adequate heart rate control is essential because scan quality is directly determined by the heart rate during image acquisition. With heart rates of less than 60 beats per minute, the scan quality is observed to be superior and diagnostic.

Image post-processing techniques include reconstruction at various temporal resolutions (82 ms with 90 degree reconstruction to 165 ms with 180 degree reconstruction). In patients with higher heart rates, reconstruction at a temporal resolution of 82 or 105 ms results in better scan quality whereas in patients with lower heart rates (less than 60 bpm), reconstruction at 125 or 165 ms results in diagnostic scan quality. Administering the higher contrast bolus at a higher infusion rate results in higher contrast-to-noise ratios, further enhancing the quality of the scan. With use of this technique, a dramatic increase in image quality is observed in the majority of patients with BMI > 35 kg/m². However, CCTA may remain non-diagnostic in patients with BMI > 60 kg/m² due to inability to decrease image noise without a substantial increase in radiation dose. In such patients, CCTA may not be warranted and diagnostic cardiac catheterization may be needed. Further changes in protocol may make imaging this difficult population possible in the future.

CAD is highly prevalent in the obese population. The ability to accurately diagnose CAD in these patients has been challenging with traditional functional tests, primarily due to technical difficulties and attenuation artifacts. With its ability to non-invasively detect CAD, CCTA may be of use in such patients. The use of Dual Source CT scanners and the improved protocol for adequate visualization of the coronary arteries makes this possible. Diagnostic image quality can be achieved in the majority of this population with specific changes in the scan parameters. In some patients, particularly with BMI >60 kg/m², this approach is of little or no help and results in unnecessary radiation exposure.

Kavitha M. Chinnaiyan · Ralph Gentry · Gilbert L. Raff

William Beaumont Hospital

Department of Cardiology

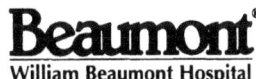

References

[1] A Nation at Risk: Obesity in the United States Statistical Sourcebook. American Heart Association

[2] Smith SC. Multiple risk factors for cardiovascular disease and diabetes mellitus. Am J Med 2007;120(3A):S3-S11

[3] Romero-Corall A, Montori VM, Somers VK et al. Association of bodyweight with total mortality and with cardiovascular events in coronary artery disease: a systematic review of cohort studies. Lancet 2006;368(9536):666-78

[4] Duvall WL, Corft LB, Corriel JS et al. SPECT myocardial perfusion imaging in morbidly obese patients: Image quality, hemodynamic response to pharmacologic stress, and diagnostic and prognostic value. J Nucl Cardiol 2006;13:202-209

[5] Raff GL, Goldstein JA. Coronary Angiography by Computed Tomography. Coronary Imaging Evolves. J Am Coll Cardiol 2007;49:1830-3

[6] Yoshimura N, Sabir A, Jubo T et al. Correlation between image noise and body weight in coronary CTA with 16-row MDCT. Acad Radiol 2006;13:324-328

Cardiac: Coronary CTA in Obese Patients

Basic considerations

Consider using CardioObese™ mode for BMI ≥ 35 kg/m². Obese patients have increased noise due to photon scattering. CardioObese™ mode improves signal-to-noise retrospectively. Temporal resolution is decreased to 165 ms/slice but the signal strength is improved. Beta-blockers are therefore administered to ensure a heart rate during acquisition of less than 65 bpm. Contrast flow rate is also increased to improve contrast-to-noise ratio.

Scan Parameters

Scan mode	Dual Source, ECG-gated
Heart rate control	<70 bpm preferable
Scan area	mid pulmonary artery to below heart
Scan direction	cranio-caudal
Scan time	~7–8 s, depending on heart rate
Tube voltage	120 kV
Tube current	420 mAs/rotation
Dose modulation	ECG-pulsing 40–70%
CTDI$_{vol}$	87.5 mGy, depending on heart rate
Rotation time	0.33 s
Pitch	0.2–0.5, depending on heart rate
Slice collimation	0.6 mm
Acquisition	64 x 0.6 mm
Slice width	0.75 mm
Reconstruction increment	0.4 mm
Reconstruction kernel	B26f, B46f in case of excessive calcification

Tricks

If the heart rate is ≤ 65 bpm, the 165 ms reconstruction is generally best. Higher iodine concentration should be used if a flow rate of 6 ml/s cannot be achieved.

Pitfalls

· Inadequate heart rate control.
· Poor sensing of ECG signal due to body mass.
· Difficulty with IV site due to subcutaneous fat.
· BMI > 50 has not been consistently tested.
· Scan should probably not be performed in this population if heart rate is > 80 bpm.

Contrast Injection Protocol

	Iodine concentration 300 mg I/ml	Iodine concentration 370 mg I/ml
Injection scheme	Monophasic	Monophasic
Iodine delivery rate	1.8 g/s	1.8 g/s
CM volume	90 ml (add 10 ml for 5 BMI points)	75 ml (add 10 ml for 5 BMI points)
CM flow rate	6 ml/s	4.9 ml/s
Body weight adaption	yes	yes
Bolus timing	bolus tracking*	bolus tracking*
Bolus tracking threshold	120 HU	120 HU
ROI position	ascending aorta	ascending aorta
Scan delay	10 s	10 s
Saline flush volume	60 ml	60 ml
Saline injection rate	6 ml/s	4.9 ml/s
Needle size	18 G	18 G
Injection site	antecubital vein	antecubital vein

*Depending on the preference of the individual site, test bolus can be used as an alternative

Case 1 DSCT in a Morbidly Obese Woman Presenting with Dyspnea on Exertion

Case history

A 64-year-old woman presents with dyspnea on exertion. She is morbidly obese (BMI of 40 kg/m²) and a former smoker.

Question

With the risk factors of smoking and obesity, coronary artery disease could be the etiology of this woman's symptoms.

Diagnosis / Differential diagnosis

· Mild calcified plaque in the proximal left anterior descending artery.
· No evidence of other coronary atherosclerotic disease.
· Cardiac size and function were normal.
· Non-cardiac structures were unremarkable.

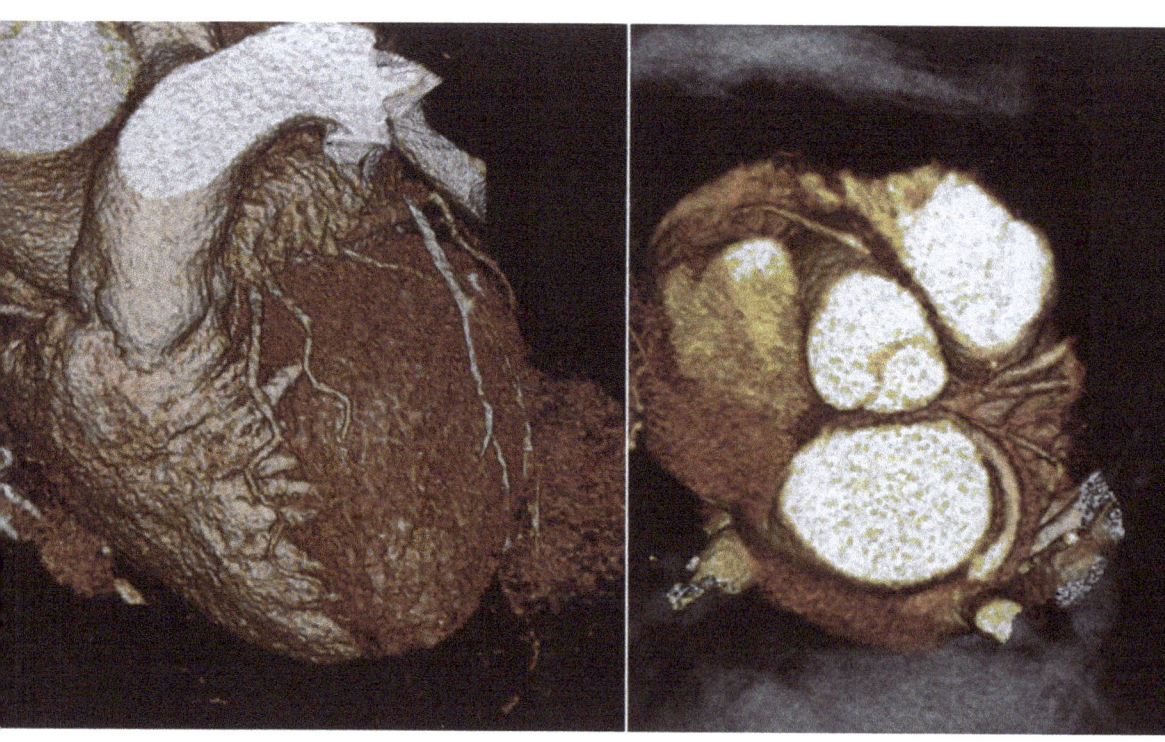

[1] Reconstruction at temporal resolution of 82 ms.

[2] Reconstruction at temporal resolution of 105 ms.

Findings

The quality of the scan was excellent. Heart rate during acquisition was 60 bpm. All coronary segments are visualized well, in all temporal resolutions. Noise measured in the proximal ascending aorta: mean 350, SD 30. Contrast-to-noise ratio was 8.8, signal-to-noise ratio was 10.5. The proximal left anterior descending artery displayed a mild calcified plaque and there was no other disease.

Take-home message

Use of the Cardio-Obese protocol results in excellent visualization of coronary arteries. For further improvement in image quality, reconstruction at various temporal resolutions (82 ms to 165 ms) is recommended.

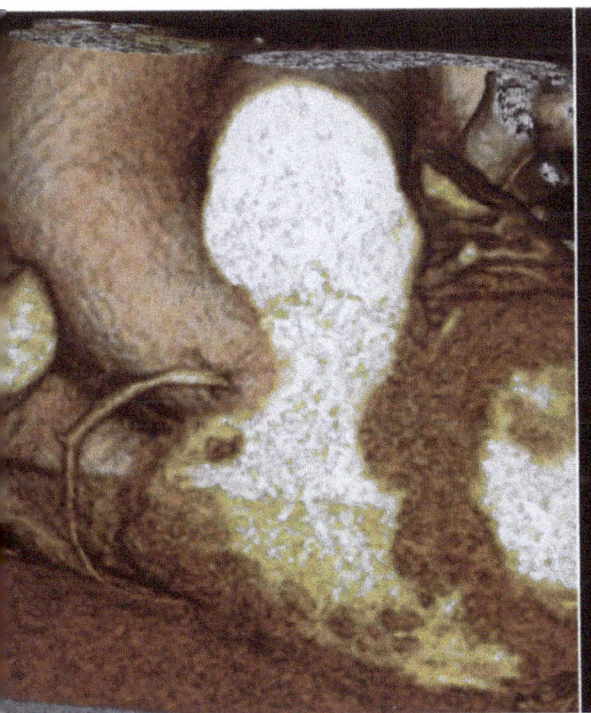

[3] Reconstruction at temporal resolution of 125 ms.

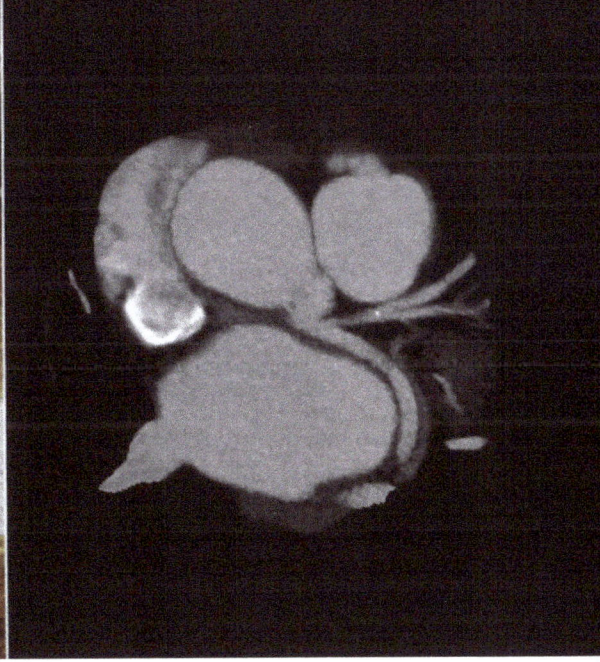

[4] Reconstruction at temporal resolution of 165 ms.

Case 2 DSCT in a Morbidly Obese Woman Presenting with Acute Atypical Chest Pain

Case history

A 51-year-old morbidly obese woman (BMI 48 kg/m²), a smoker with hypertension and hyperlipidemia presents with atypical chest discomfort and shortness of breath.

Question

This woman has a high pre-test likelihood of coronary artery disease. Would CTA help sort out the etiology?

Diagnosis/Differential diagnosis

· No evidence of coronary artery disease (calcium score = 0, no evidence of atherosclerotic disease).
· Cardiac structure and function was normal, with no CT evidence of valvular abnormalities.
· Non-cardiac structures were unremarkable.

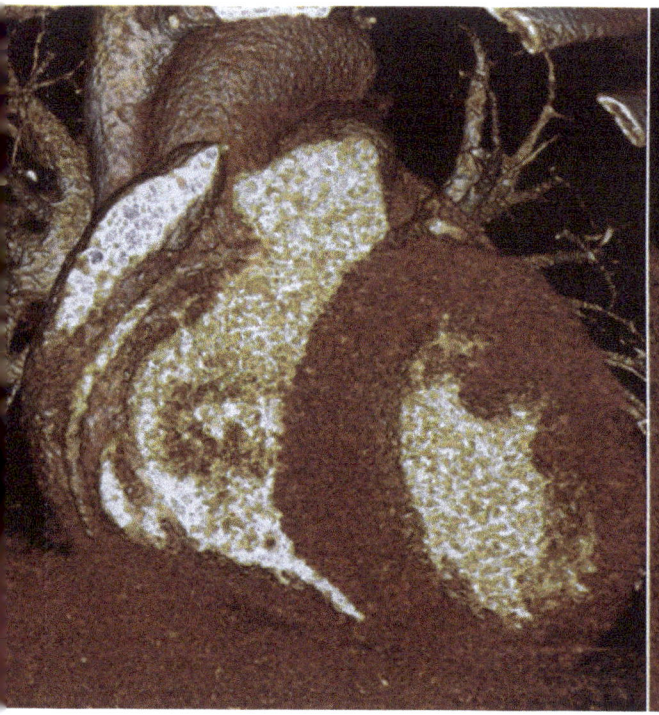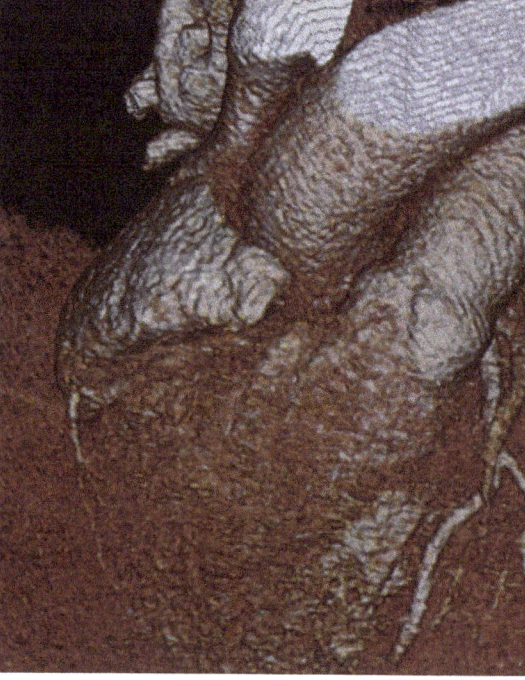

[1] Reconstruction at temporal resolution of 82 ms (Noise = 46[SD], contrast-to-noise ratio (CNR) = 5.0, signal-to-noise ratio (SNR) = 5.5).

[2] Reconstruction at temporal resolution of 105 ms.

Findings

Distal coronary segments are visualized well. Heart rate during acquisition is 56 bpm. Contrast-to-noise ratio is 5.0, signal-to-noise ratio is 5.0. Compared to temporal resolution of 82 ms, images reconstructed at a temporal resolution of 165 ms are superior in quality.

Take-home message

Reconstruction at a lower temporal resolution (165 ms) results in better image quality when heart rate during acquisition is below 60 bpm. In order to reduce noise, temporal resolution is thus sacrificed.

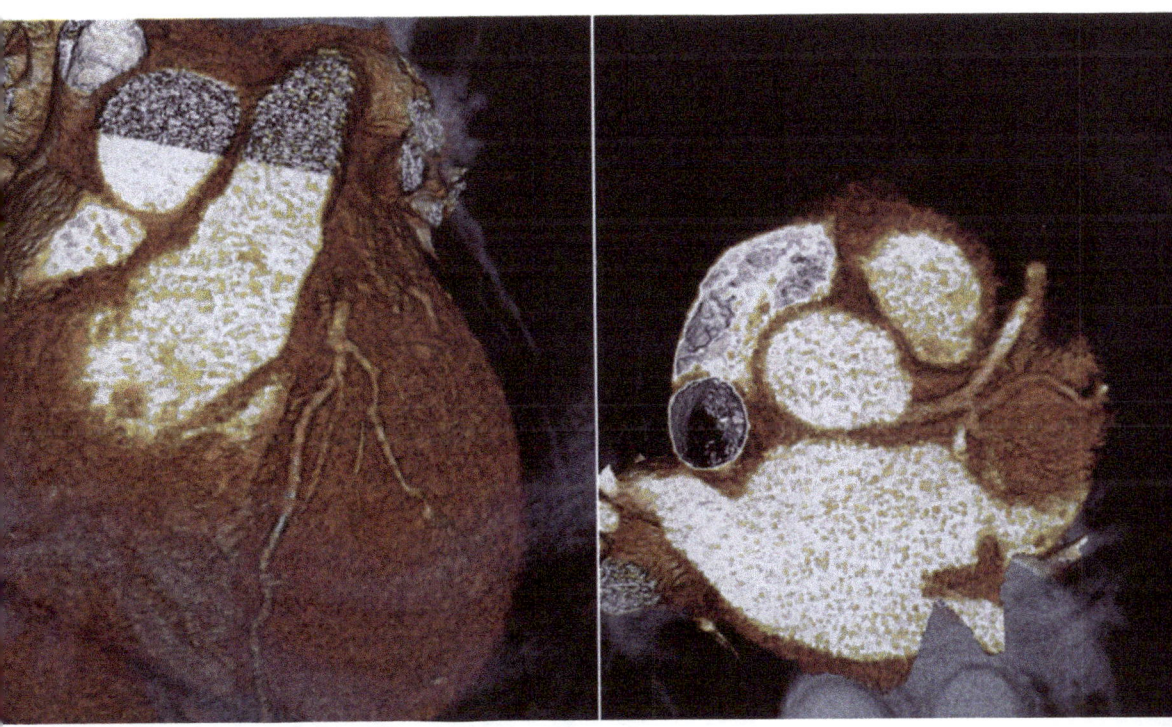

[3] Reconstruction at temporal resolution of 125 ms.

[4] Reconstruction at temporal resolution of 165 ms (Noise = 46[SD], CNR = 12, SNR = 8.3).

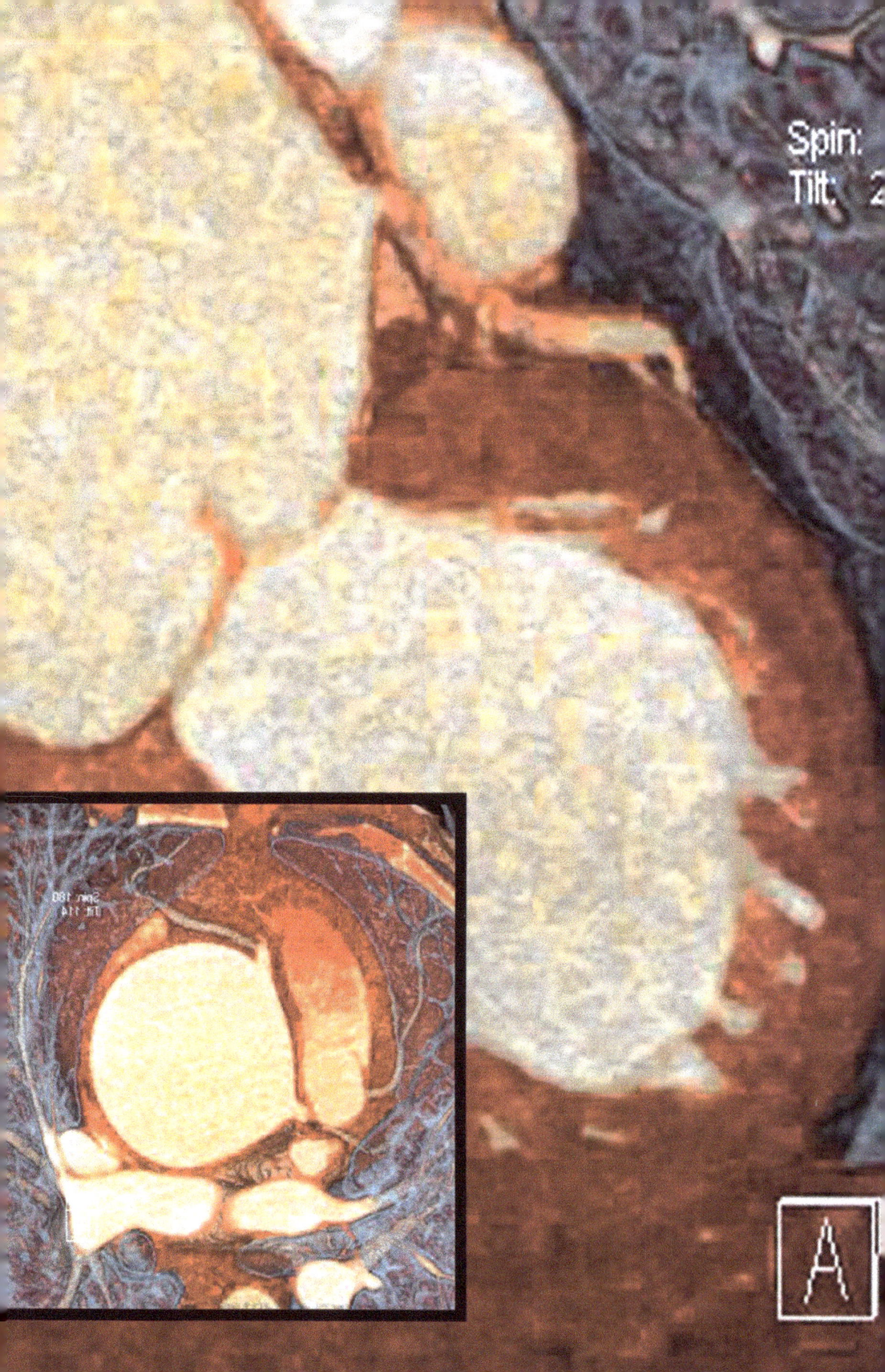

Spin:
Tilt: 2

Cardiac: Valvular Function

Hatem Alkadhi · Sebastian Leschka · Hans Scheffel · Paul Stolzmann

Case 1: Bicuspid Aortic Valve

Case 2: Mitral Regurgitation

The most important imaging modality for evaluation of cardiac valvular disease is transesophageal and transthoracic echocardiography. It allows a comprehensive workup of the patients by detecting the presence, assessing morphological abnormalities of the valves, and grading the various diseases. This information is performed by integrating information from 2D echocardiography, color flow mapping, pulsed and continuous wave Doppler as well as quantitative Doppler flow measurements into the different semiquantitative grading schemes that are available for each valvular disease. When evaluating valvular disease with echocardiography, the general rule is also to include the assessment of associated changes in chamber or aortic root dimensions in the ventricular function analysis. Echocardiography, however, has inherent limitations because it requires exact geometric alignment of the structure of interest. In addition, it often requires repetitive measurements to minimize errors, and it depends highly on patient morphologic characteristics, instrumental settings, and transducer position. Perhaps the most important limitation is that echocardiography is strongly operator dependent.

The main clinical application of cardiac CT is the evaluation of the coronary artery tree for the diagnosis or exclusion of coronary artery stenoses.[1, 2] With each cardiac CT examination, however, a huge amount of images are acquired that contain information beyond the coronary arteries alone. For example, left ventricular functional parameters can be assessed using the same dataset that was acquired for the coronary arteries with similar accuracy as the current standard of reference magnetic resonance imaging. Moreover, the accuracy of the left ventricular functional assessment with CT is higher than that of the most often used modality in clinical routine – echocardiography.

In addition, the data from each cardiac CT examination already contains morpho-anatomical and functional information regarding the cardiac valves, without the additional administration of contrast media or applying additional radiation to the patient. Thus, every cardiac CT examination should include a check for cardiac valvular disease. A number of studies have repeatedly shown that morphology of a normal and diseased mitral and aortic valve as assessed with CT correlates to a high degree with the morpho-anatomical information obtained by the clinical reference modality transthoracic and transesophageal echocardiography. Typical morphological abnormalities

Cardiac: Valvular Function

associated with valvular disease include thickening with or without calcification of the free edges of the aortic cusps or mitral leaflets, calcification of the aortic or mitral annulus, thickening of the tendinous cords and prolapse of the mitral or aortic valve. All these morphological findings of the aortic and mitral valve are delineated with a high degree of accuracy using CT coronary angiography data, and thus can indicate the possible cause and mechanism of the various valvular diseases.[3, 4]

Importantly, several studies have demonstrated that CT also provides functional information regarding valvular disease severity. Planimetric measurements of maximal opening and maximal regurgitant orifice areas of the mitral and aortic valve have shown to yield information that is similar to quantitative hemodynamic information derived from echocardiography.
- For example, planimetric measurements of the maximal opening area of the aortic valve (also called "aortic valve area") in systole correlate well with calculations obtained from echocardiography and thus allow estimation of the different degrees of aortic stenosis with CT.[3]
- Similarly, planimetric measurements of the maximal opening area of the mitral valve in diastole correlate well with measurements from echocardiography and thus allow estimation of the degree of mitral stenosis with CT.[5]
- Furthermore, planimetric measurements of the regurgitant orifice area of the mitral valve in systole significantly correlate with semiquantitative grading from ventriculography and echocardiography and thus allow estimation of the severity of mitral regurgitation with CT.[4]
- Finally, planimetric measurements of the regurgitant orifice area of the aortic valve in diastole correlate well with results from echocardiography and thus allow the grading of aortic regurgitation with CT.[6] Using a cut-off ROA size of 25 mm^2 and 75 mm^2, CT allows discrimination with a high degree of accuracy between mild, moderate and severe aortic regurgitation.

The major advantages of CT over echocardiography with regard to valvular morphology and function assessment are the lack of operator and patient morphology dependence and the lack of acoustic shadowing in association with valvular calcifications, the latter often hampering the accurate evaluation of cardiac valves with echocardiography. The major disadvantage of CT over echocardiography is the radiation exposure associated with the technique, which prevents the repeated assessment as recommended by several guidelines for patients with cardiac valvular disease.

Regarding all these valvular diseases, optimal image quality of the CT examination is the major prerequisite to ensure reliable and accurate planimetric measurements. This can only be achieved through the use of optimal CT technology together with dedicated CT data acquisition and contrast application protocols.

The primary advantage of Dual Source CT for imaging of cardiac valves derives from its high and heart rate-independent temporal resolution of 83 ms in a mono-segment reconstruction mode. At the same time, the scanner maintains the high spatial resolution of earlier 64-slice CT scanners up to 0.33 mm x 0.33 mm x 0.33 mm. This enables detailed imaging of cardiac valves even in systole or during the phases of rapid movement between mid-systole and mid-diastole.

In conclusion, CT continues to emerge as a modality that allows the comprehensive work-up of the heart by including the analysis of coronary arteries, ventricular function and cardiac valves with a high degree of accuracy within one single and short examination.

Hatem Alkadhi · Sebastian Leschka · Hans Scheffel · Paul Stolzmann
Institute of Diagnostic Radiology
University Hospital Zurich

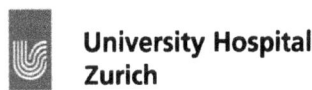

University Hospital Zurich

References

[1] Leschka S, Alkadhi H, Plass A, et al. Accuracy of MSCT coronary angiography with 64-slice technology: first experience. Eur Heart J 2005; 26: 1482-7

[2] Scheffel H, Alkadhi H, Plass A, et al. Accuracy of dual-source CT coronary angiography: First experience in a high pre-test probability population without heart rate control. Eur Radiol 2006; 16: 2739-47

[3] Alkadhi H, Wildermuth S, Plass A, et al. Aortic stenosis: comparative evaluation of 16-detector row CT and echocardiography. Radiology 2006; 240: 47-55

[4] Alkadhi H, Wildermuth S, Bettex D, et al. Mitral regurgitation: quantification with 16-detector row CT--initial experience. Radiology 2006; 238: 454-63

[5] Messika-Zeitoun D, Serfaty JM, Laissy JP, et al. Assessment of the mitral valve area in patients with mitral stenosis by multislice computed tomography. J Am Coll Cardiol 2006; 48: 411-3

[6] Feuchtner G, Dichtl W, Schachner T, et al. Diagnostic performance of MDCT for detecting aortic valve regurgitation. Am J Roentgenol 2006; 186: 1676-81

Cardiac: Valvular Function

Basic considerations

The implementation of ECG-pulsing depends on the valvular disease of interest and should always take into account considerations about the increased radiation dose when not using ECG-pulsing. ECG-pulsing must be turned off when evaluating aortic stenosis or mitral regurgitation as it requires imaging in systole. ECG-pulsing should be switched on when analyzing aortic regurgitation, mitral stenosis or morphological abnormalities in patients with infective valvular endocarditis. Consider 100 kV/330 mAs in patients with low body weight, (e.g. below 85 kg/175 lbs), depending on the patient's habitus. In patients with high body weight, it may be useful to increase contrast flow and to employ the CardioObese™ mode.

Scan Parameters

Scan mode	Dual Source, ECG-gated
Heart rate control	not necessary
Scan area	mid pulmonary artery to below heart
Scan direction	cranio-caudal
Scan time	~7–14 s, depending on heart rate
Tube voltage	120 kV
Tube current	360 mAs/rotation
Dose modulation	ECG-pulsing on*
CTDI$_{vol}$	~50 mGy, depending on heart rate
Rotation time	0.33 s
Pitch	0.2–0.5, depending on heart rate
Slice collimation	0.6 mm
Acquisition	64 x 0.6 mm
Slice width	0.75 mm
Reconstruction increment	0.4 mm
Reconstruction kernel	B26f, B46f in case of excessive calcifications

*Referring to ECG-pulsing table (see page 28)

Tricks

The scan range must be fitted to the respective indication: e.g. evaluation of the aortic valve should cover the aortic root to allow for geometric assessment of its dimensions. Patients should hold their breath in mild-inspiration. This should be trained on the scanner table immediately prior to the examination.

Pitfalls

· Images in several cardiac phases must be evaluated to define the phase with maximum opening or closing of the valve.
· Accurate multi-planar reformations exactly parallel and perpendicular to the respective valve must be performed.
· Valve opening areas and regurgitation orifice areas must be measured three times and averaged to yield accurate results.

Contrast Injection Protocol

	Iodine concentration 300 mg I/ml	Iodine concentration 370 mg I/ml
Injection scheme	Monophasic	Monophasic
Iodine delivery rate	1.85 g/s	1.85 g/s
CM volume	6.2 ml/s for duration of scan, ≥ 60 ml	5 ml/s for duration of scan, ≥ 50 ml
CM flow rate	6.2 ml/s	5 ml/s
Body weight adaption	no	no
Bolus timing	bolus tracking*	bolus tracking*
Bolus tracking threshold	140 HU	140 HU
ROI position	ascending aorta	ascending aorta
Scan delay	2 s	2 s
Saline flush volume	60 ml	60 ml
Saline injection rate	6.2 ml/s	5 ml/s
Needle size	18 G	18 G
Injection site	antecubital vein	antecubital vein

*Depending on the preference of the individual site, test bolus can be used as an alternative

Case 1 Bicuspid Aortic Valve

Case history

44-year-old male with syncope under exercise. The patient was admitted for preoperative workup of the aortic valve, aortic root and coronary arteries.

Question

What is the cause for the syncope? Coronary artery or cardiac valvular disease?

Diagnosis/Differential diagnosis

DSCT demonstrated a bicuspid aortic valve with no raphe showing unrestricted opening in systole and no coaptation defect in diastole. The aortic root including the aortic annulus, the sinus portion and the proximal ascending aorta was dilated. DSCT coronary angiography was unremarkable with no evidence of coronary plaques or stenoses.

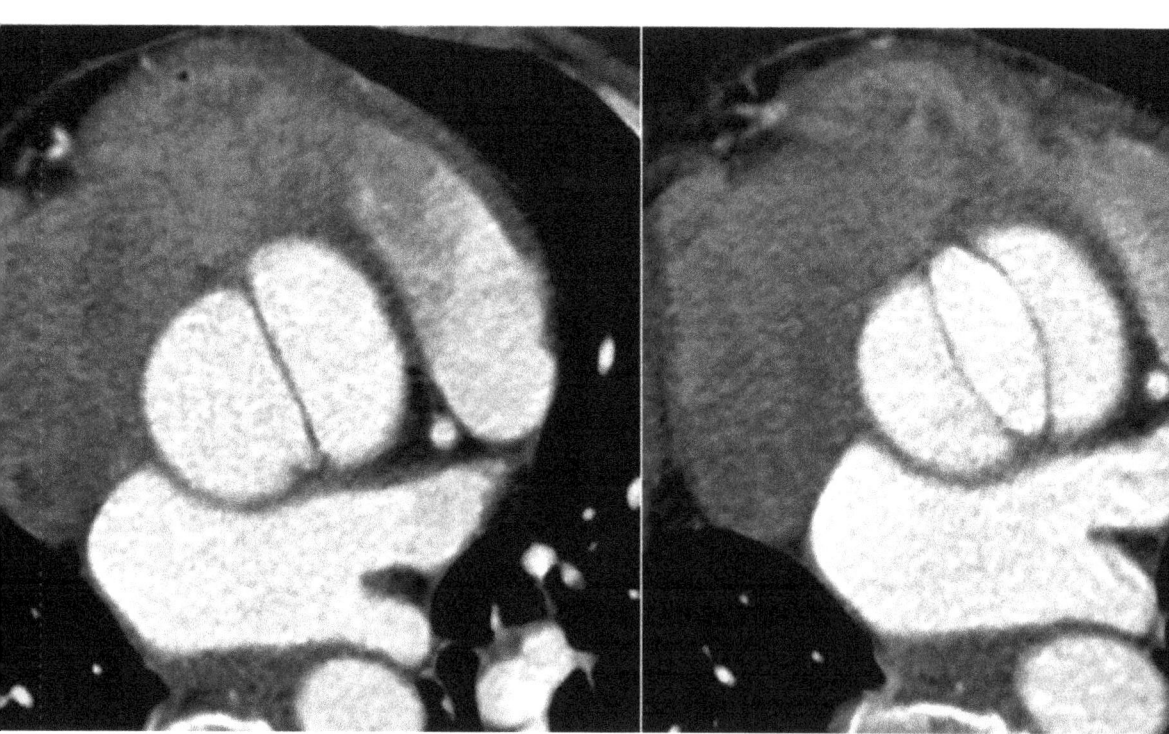

[1] Short-axis reconstruction (parallel to the aortic annulus) in mid-diastole (at 65% of the RR-interval) demonstrates closed bicuspid aortic valve with no raphe.

[2] Short-axis reconstruction (parallel to the aortic annulus) in early- to mid-systole (at 15% of the RR-interval) shows the opened bicuspid aortic valve.

Findings

Reconstructions in diastole and systole revealed a bicuspid aortic valve without a raphe and no evidence of regurgitation or stenosis. Coronary arteries were normal and showed no plaques or stenoses. The aortic root was dilated, including the aortic annulus, the sinus portion and the proximal ascending aorta. The sino-tubular junction disappeared. The left ventricular volumes and global function were normal.

Take-home message

DSCT coronary angiography allowed a comprehensive work-up of the patient with a single, short and non-invasive examination. It demonstrated aortic valve and aortic root morphology and reliably ruled-out coronary artery disease. In addition, CT allowed the accurate evaluation of the global left ventricular systolic function and end-diastolic as well as end-systolic volumes that all were in the normal range.

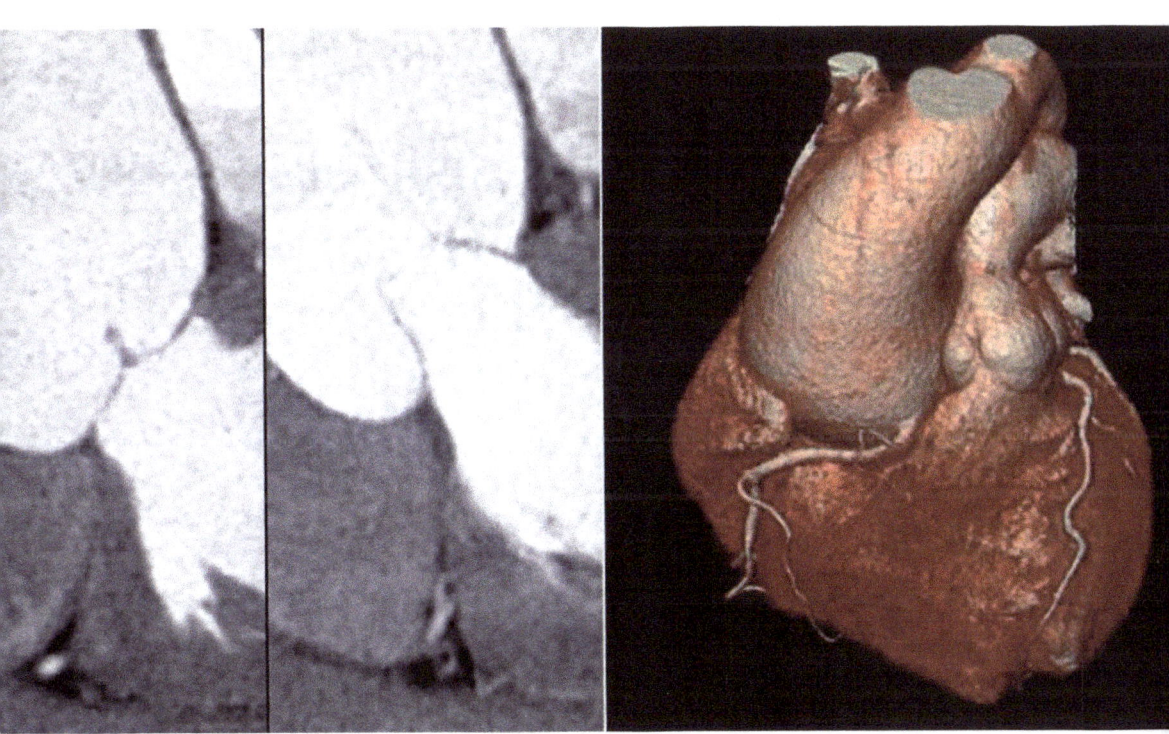

[3] Long-axis reconstruction (parallel to the left ventricle) in diastole (left) and systole (right) shows the bicuspid aortic valve with dilatation of the aortic root.

[4] Volume-rendered image demonstrates normal coronary arteries with no evidence of stenoses.

Case 2 Mitral Regurgitation

Case history
54-year-old female with atypical chest pain, intermediate cardiovascular risk profile, and inconclusive bicycle stress test

Question
Does the patient suffer from coronary artery disease, from isolated disease of the mitral or aortic valve, or from other cardiac pathology?

Diagnosis/Differential diagnosis
The diagnosis in this patient was prolapse of the anterior mitral valve leaflet leading to mitral regurgitation. The tricuspid aortic valve showed normal morphology with no restriction in opening in systole and no coaptation defect in diastole. DSCT coronary angiography demonstrated normal coronary arteries with no plaques or stenoses.

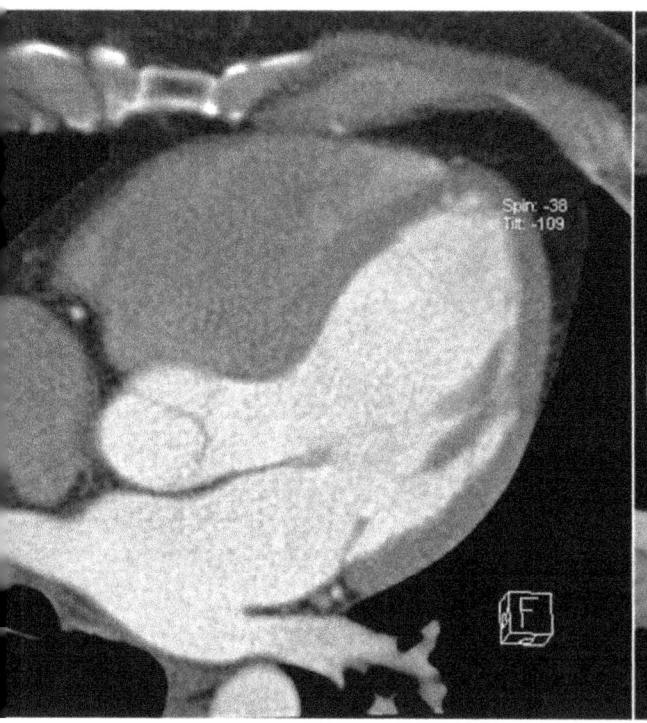

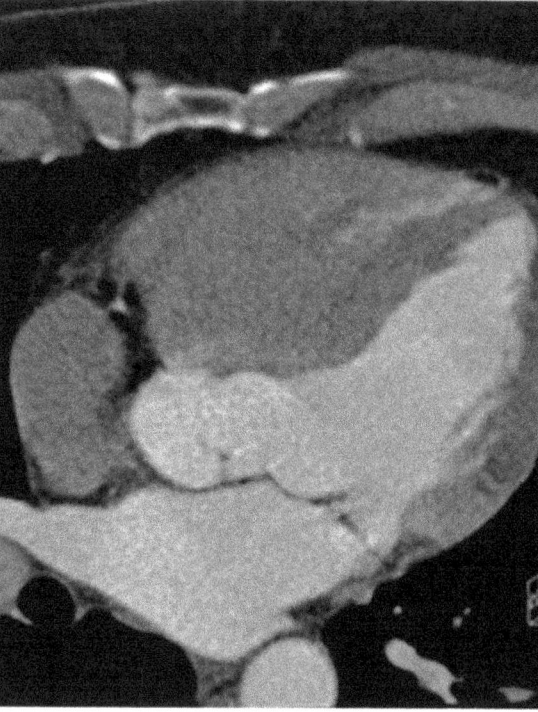

[1] Mid-diastolic reconstruction (at 65% of the RR-interval) in the long-axis of the left ventricle demonstrating a normal mitral valve with no restriction regarding opening.

[2] Early-systolic reconstruction (at 10% of the RR-interval) demonstrating prolapse of the anterior valve leaflet and regurgitant orifice indicating mitral regurgitation.

Findings

DSCT reveals prolapse of the anterior mitral valve leaflet leading to a coaptation defect of the anterior and posterior leaflet, representing the morphological correlate of mitral regurgitation. In addition, DSCT coronary angiography demonstrated normal coronary arteries with no plaques or stenoses.

Take-home message

DSCT coronary angiography allowed comprehensive work-up of the patient by demonstrating mild mitral regurgitation caused by anterior mitral valve prolapse and enabled coronary artery disease to be reliably ruled out.

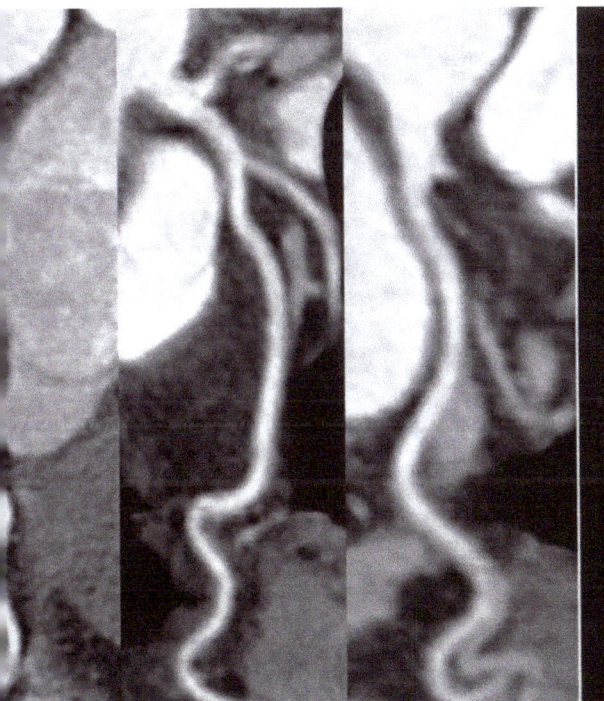 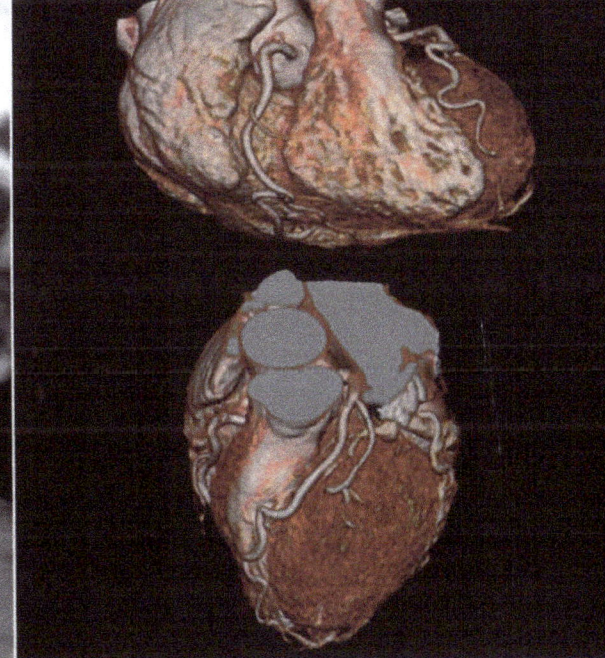

[3] Curved-planar reformations of the RCA (right), LAD (middle), and RCX (left) demonstrating normal arteries without stenoses.

[4] Volume-rendered images showing the coronary artery tree without coronary artery disease.

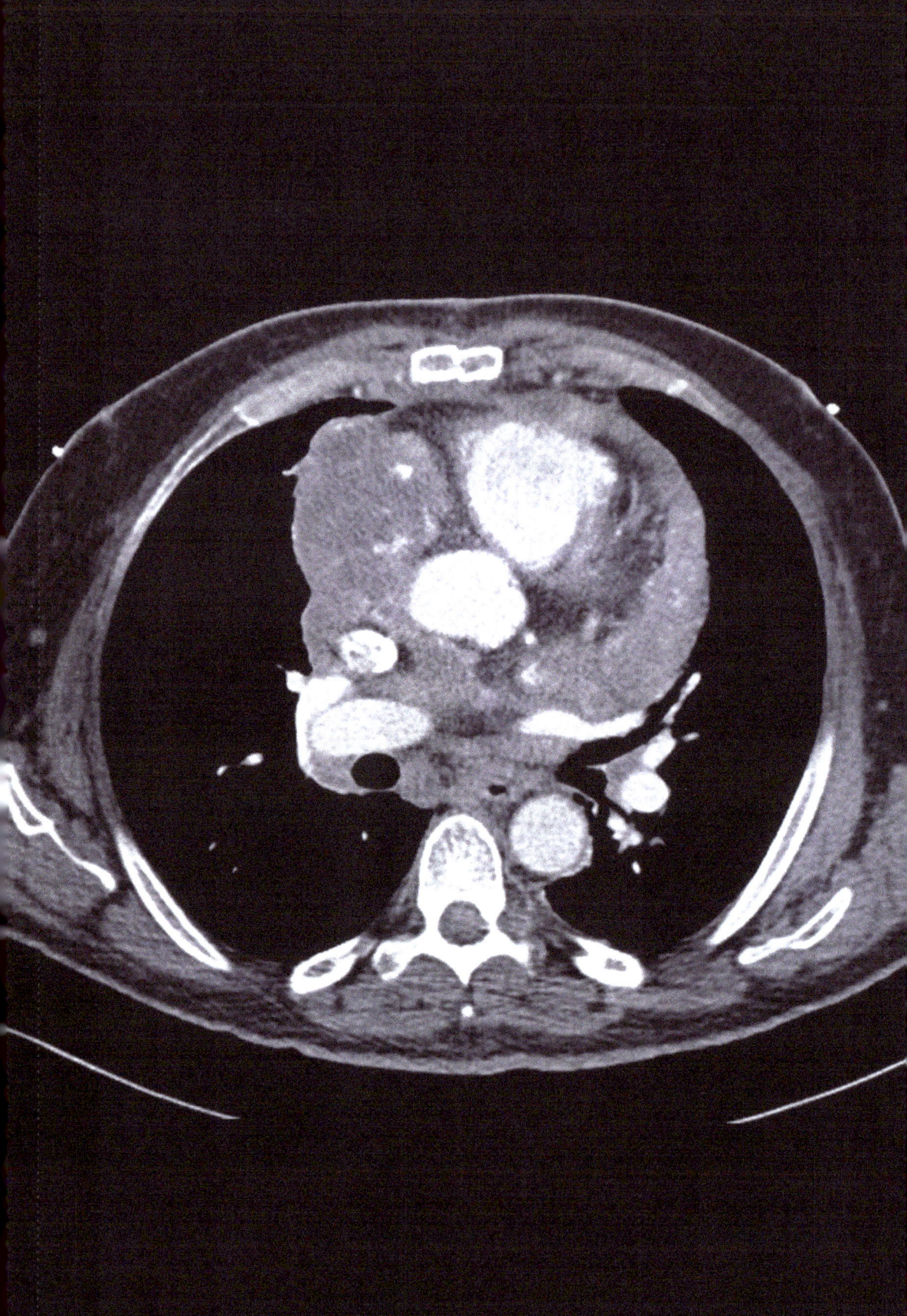

Cardiac: Morphology

Scott Harris · Cynthia McCollough · Eric Williamson

Case 1: Complex Congenital Heart Disease, s/p Repair

Case 2: Anterior MI, s/p CABG

Basics of Dual Source CT (DSCT)

As previously described, the underlying concept of Dual Source CT is the use of two x-ray tubes and two corresponding detector arrays to acquire a half gantry rotation's worth of data with only a quarter-scan gantry rotation, effectively cutting the acquisition time in half.[1] With a gantry rotation time of 0.33 seconds, the SOMATOM Definition system allows 64 channels of CT data to be acquired with a temporal resolution of 83 ms when operated in the cardiac mode. Unlike previous generations of multi-detector row CTs, the improved temporal resolution provided by DSCT is independent of patient heart rates.[1] This improved temporal resolution and the resulting ability of DSCT to provide motion-free images of the heart over a wide range of patient heart rates is the predominant advantage of DSCT over previous generations of multi-detector row CTs for the evaluation of cardiac morphology.

The improved temporal resolution of Dual Source CT versus Single-Source CT systems decreases blurring and other artifacts caused by cardiac motion. In the same way that reductions in motion-related artifacts improve the visualization of the coronary arteries for coronary CT angiography, the improved temporal resolution of DSCT allows sharper delineation of the endocardium and cardiac valves.[3]

Accurate delineation of the cardiac chambers is the foundation of cardiac morphologic analysis. Although multi-detector CT is unlikely to replace trans-thoracic and trans-esophageal echocardiography for the evaluation of cardiac morphology, the use of ECG-gated CT for the evaluation of left ventricular structure and function has become increasingly common since the development of 16-detector row CT systems. Additionally, information regarding cardiac morphology can be easily obtained from motion-free images generated as a result of ECG-gated CT performed for other indications. Such information is being increasingly utilized, especially now that the necessary post-processing workstations have become widely available, not to mention easier and less time-consuming to operate.[4] As DSCT systems become increasingly available, the evaluation of cardiac morphology and function will be utilized more and more as a part of routine ECG-gated CT of the chest and heart.

Cardiac: Morphology

Morphologic evaluation of the heart traditionally starts with evaluation of the cardiac chambers; specifically, the left ventricle. Size, orientation, and connections of the left ventricle are easily evaluable using cardiac CT and abnormalities of these parameters have important implications for cardiac diagnosis and therapy. For example, left ventricular (LV) end-systolic volume is the major determinant of survival after recovery from myocardial infarction.[2] Unfortunately, most CT studies of ventricular function are currently performed in association with coronary CT angiography, which often requires medication for heart rate control. These medications can alter cardiovascular hemodynamics and limit the clinical utility of the measurements performed at the time of the CT scan. As previously mentioned, the use of DSCT obviates the need for medical heart rate control, allowing for a more clinically relevant estimation of ventricular volumes.[5]

Evaluation of cardiac morphology also involves examination of the cardiac valves. Historically, ECG-gated CT of the heart has been somewhat limited for evaluation of the cardiac valves as compared to MRI and echocardiography. Currently, echocardiography is the primary imaging modality used for diagnosing abnormalities of the cardiac valves; however, echocardiography is mildly invasive and is limited in some patients, particularly those with extensive valvular calcifications. Cardiac MRI is also of limited utility in some patients, such as those with claustrophobia or cardiac pacemakers. Additionally, MRI is less sensitive for valve calcifications as compared to CT. For such patients, cardiac CT can serve as an effective alternative imaging modality, particularly for the aortic valve.[6]

One significant challenge for cardiac valve imaging is the rapid motion of the valve apparatus, particularly since much of this motion occurs "through" the plane of valve cross-section. As with coronary artery imaging, the improved temporal resolution afforded by DSCT should allow improved image quality of the cardiac valves as compared to Single Source CT systems. However, the routine use of tube current modulation during ECG-gated CT could impair visualization of the cardiac valves, particularly during early systole. Unfortunately, the systolic phase of the cardiac cycle is the most appropriate phase for the determination of cardiac valve area – an important imaging parameter in the evaluation of aortic stenosis. Additionally, the evaluation of mechanical cardiac valves for potential dysfunction is also dependent on imaging throughout the cardiac cycle. Still, the improved temporal resolution provided by DSCT, coupled with appropriate radiation dose reduction strategies, should make multi-phase evaluation of the cardiac valves possible without significantly increasing the radiation dose beyond what is expected for routine cardiac CT performed using earlier generations of CT scanners.

In summary, ECG-gated CT performed using DSCT appears to be a promising technique for the evaluation of cardiac morphology, either alone or in combination with CT evaluation of the heart performed for another indication.

Scott Harris · Cynthia McCollough · Eric Williamson

Mayo Clinic College of Medicine

Department of Radiology

References

[1] Flohr TG, McCollough CH, Bruder H, et al. First performance evaluation of a dual-source CT (DSCT) system. Eur Radiol 2006; 16(2):256-268

[2] White HD, Norris RM, Brown MA, Brandt PW, Whitlock RM, Wild CJ. Left ventricular end-systolic volume as the major determinant of survival after recovery from myocardial infarction. Circulation 1987; 76(1):44-51

[3] Mahnken AH, Bruder H, Suess C, et al. Dual-source computed tomography for assessing cardiac function: a phantom study. Invest Radiol 2007; 42(7):491-498

[4] Johnson TR, Nikolaou K, Wintersperger BJ, et al. Dual-source CT cardiac imaging: initial experience. Eur Radiol 2006; 16(7):1409-1415

[5] Rist C, Johnson TR, Becker A, et al. [Dual-source cardiac CT imaging with improved temporal resolution: Impact on image quality and analysis of left ventricular function]. Radiologe 2007; 47(4):287-290, 292-284

[6] Willmann JK, Weishaupt D, Lachat M, et al. Electrocardiographically gated multi-detector row CT for assessment of valvular morphology and calcification in aortic stenosis. Radiology 2002; 225(1):120-128

Cardiac: Morphology

Basic considerations

Accurate assessment of cardiac morphology is often facilitated by evaluation of the heart throughout the cardiac cycle. An ECG-pulsing window from 30–70% allows reconstruction of images in both systole and diastole. Scan coverage area is adapted depending on the indication. The entire chest should be imaged for the evaluation of congenital heart disease and cardiac masses.

Evaluation of both right- and left-sided cardiac chambers is optimized by homogeneous contrast enhancement throughout the heart. Therefore, the main contrast bolus is followed by a second bolus diluted with saline to a 30% concentration to maintain adequate cardiac enhancement while reducing artifacts from dense contrast in the SVC and brachiocephalic veins.

Scan Parameters

Scan mode	Dual Source, ECG-gated
Heart rate control	not necessary
Scan area	mid pulmonary artery to below heart
Scan direction	cranio-caudal
Scan time	~12 s, depending on heart rate
Tube voltage	120 kV
Tube current	240 mAs/rotation
Dose modulation	ECG-pulsing on*
CTDI$_{vol}$	41 mGy at 60 bpm, decreases at higher heart rates
Rotation time	0.33 s
Pitch	0.2–0.5, depending on heart rate
Slice collimation	0.6 mm
Acquisition	64 x 0.6 mm
Slice width	0.75 mm
Reconstruction increment	0.4 mm
Reconstruction kernel	B26f

* Referring to ECG-pulsing table (see page 28)

Tricks

If suspicious of pericardial disease or cardiac mass, perform non-contrast scan first to assess calcification and enhancement characteristics. For larger patients, consider increasing contrast injection rate. Cine loops in short axis and 4-chamber long axis (0–95%, every 5%) using 8 mm section width and 6 mm increment are viewed on every case.

Pitfalls

If the duration of the contrast bolus is too short, the evaluation of cardiac morphology will be compromised, particularly of the right-sided cardiac chambers. Consider performing an additional venous-phase scan for the evaluation of pericardial inflammation or cardiac mass.

Contrast Injection Protocol

	Iodine concentration 300 mg I/ml	Iodine concentration 370 mg I/ml
Injection scheme	Monophasic	Monophasic
Iodine delivery rate	1.85 g/s	1.85 g/s
CM volume	6.2 ml/s for duration of scan plus 40 ml diluted to 40%	5 ml/s for duration of scan plus 40 ml diluted to 30%
CM flow rate	6.2 ml/s	5 ml/s
Body weight adaption	yes	yes
Bolus timing	bolus tracking*	bolus tracking*
Bolus tracking threshold	150 HU	150 HU
ROI position	ascending aorta	ascending aorta
Scan delay	4 s	4 s
Saline flush volume	60 ml	60 ml
Saline injection rate	6.2 ml/s	5 ml/s
Needle size	18 G	18 G
Injection site	antecubital vein	antecubital vein

*Depending on the preference of the individual site, test bolus can be used as an alternative

Case 1 Complex Congenital Heart Disease, s/p Repair

Case history

43-year-old man presents with history of repaired complex congenital heart disease at an outside institution.

Question

What is the orientation of the cardiac chambers?
What is the position of the great vessels?

Diagnosis/Differential diagnosis

Differential diagnostic considerations would include:

· Double-outlet morphological left ventricle.
· Transposition of the great vessels.
· Ebstein's anomaly.

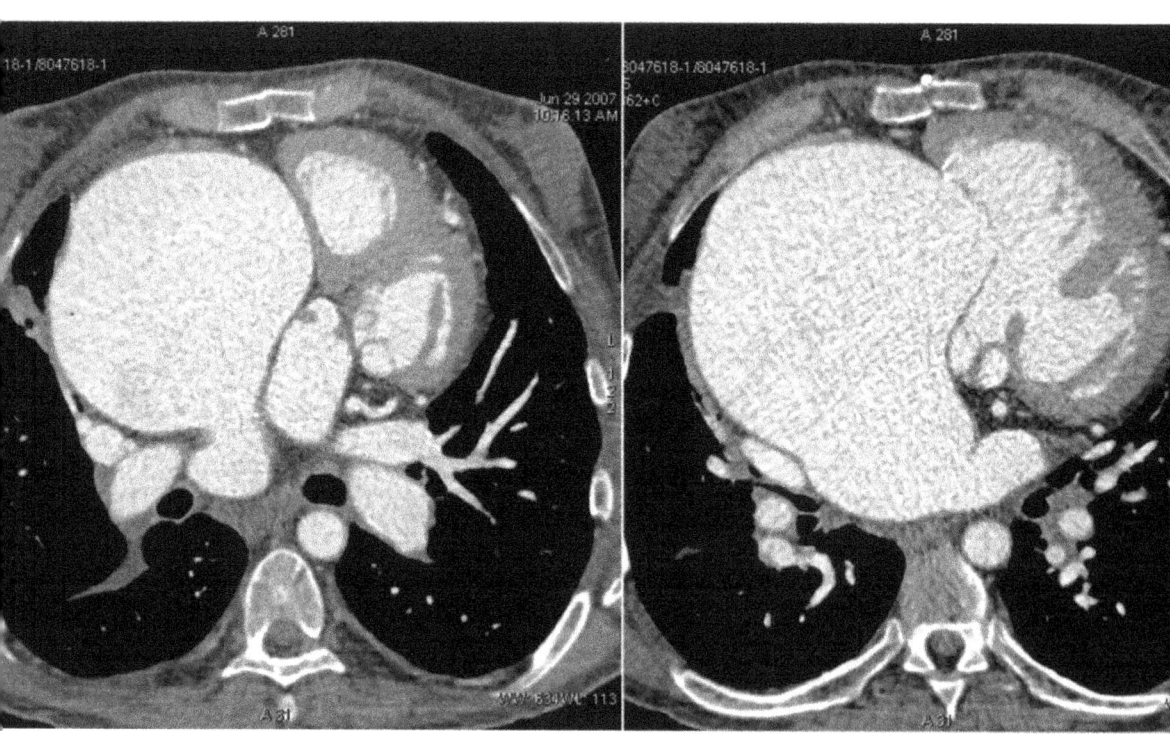

[1] Marked atrial enlargement. Transposition of the great vessels.

[2] Morphological left ventricle anteriorly positioned with posteriorly positioned rudimentary morphological right ventricle. Large VSD.

Findings

There is marked cardiomegaly with a single double outlet morphological left ventricle and transposition of the great vessels. There is a small rudimentary right ventricle and left (morphological right) atrioventricular valve. A large VSD also exists. Gross enlargement of the atria can be noticed.

Take-home message

DSCT is useful for defining cardiac morphology with its improved temporal resolution. Motion free images allow for clear delineation of the ventricular chambers and the features of the endocardium (trabeculations and moderator band) that allow characterization of each ventricle.

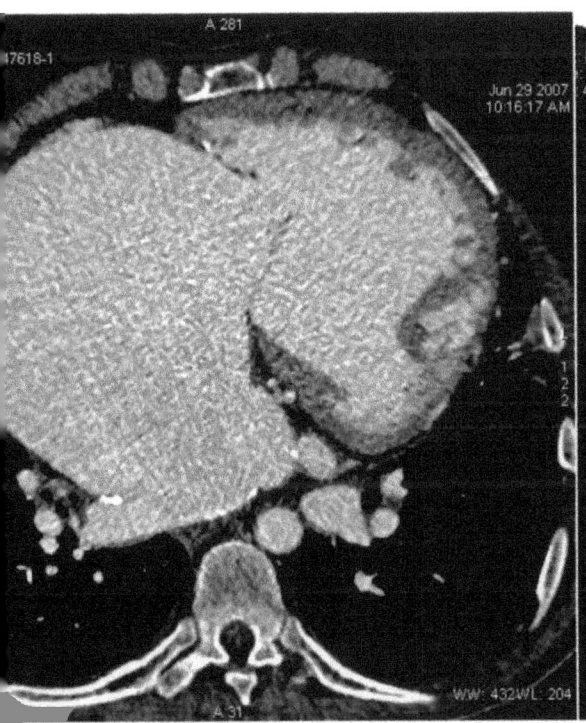

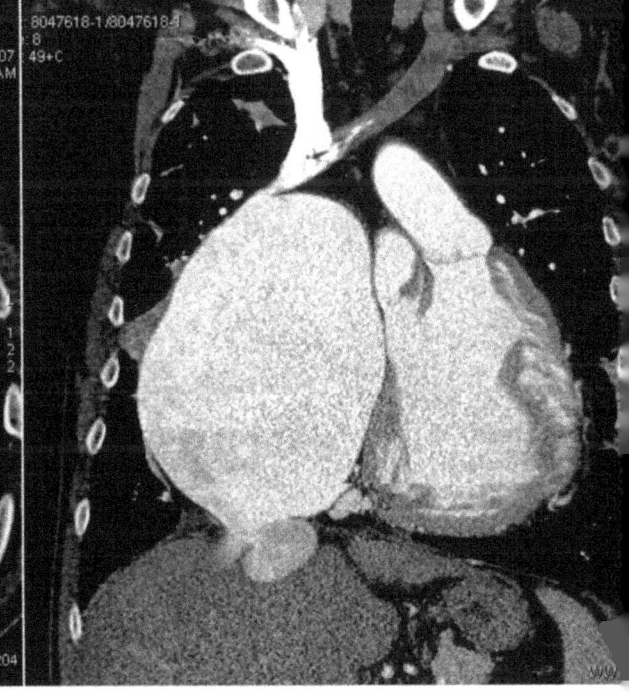

[3] Grossly enlarged single atrium and functionally single morphological left ventricle.

[4] Double outlet left ventricle with marked atrial enlargement.

Case 2 Anterior MI, s/p CABG

Case history

76-year-old woman with history of ischemic heart disease, new left bundle branch block and decreasing cardiac function.

Question

In the presence of increasing symptoms, what is the current left ventricular function?

Diagnosis/Differential diagnosis

Most likely the patient has had a recent cardiac event. Global ischemia and dysfunction is a likely possibility; however, a focal infarcted segment may result in significant cardiac dysfunction.

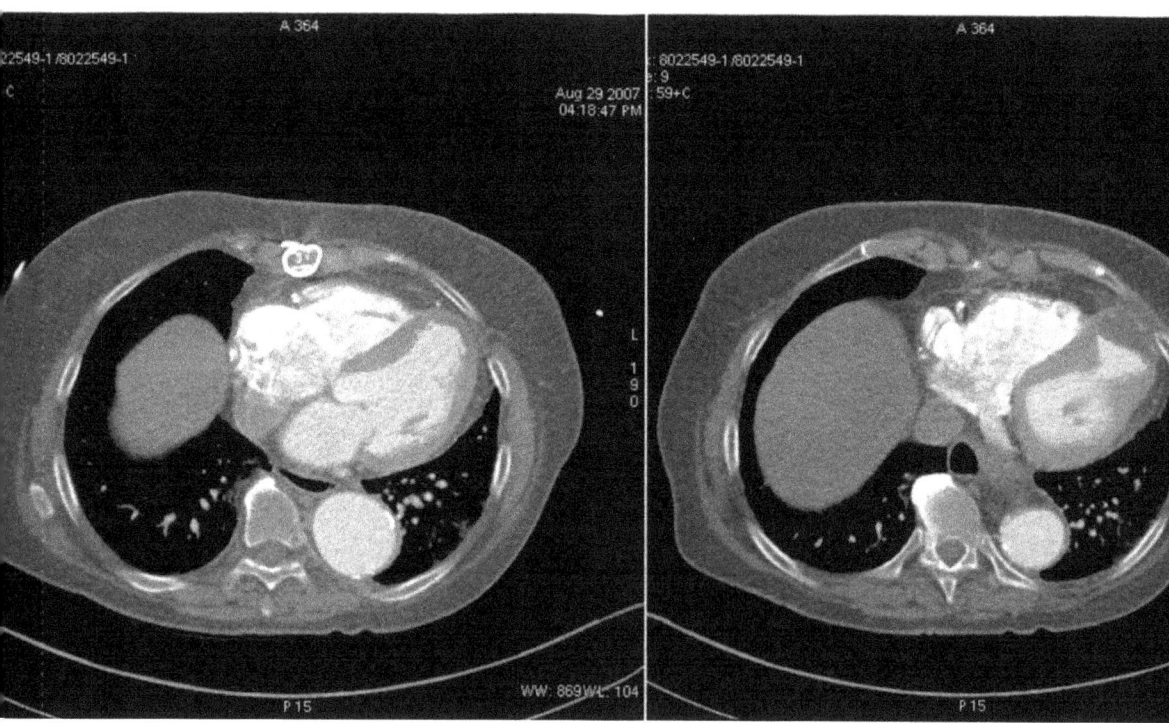

[1] Myocardial thinning with laminated apical thrombus.

[2] Akinetic apical aneurysm with myocardial thinning and laminated thrombus.

Findings

There is a dilated left ventricle with focal apical aneurysm and myocardial thinning. Overlying this akinetic segment, laminated thrombus is visualized. On this study, note was also made of occlusion of one of the patient's known bypass grafts.

Take-home message

With improved temporal resolution and ECG-gating, cine imaging of the heart can be achieved. This fast technique for functional assessment of the heart can demonstrate regional wall motion abnormalities and associated sequela (thrombus over an akinetic segment).

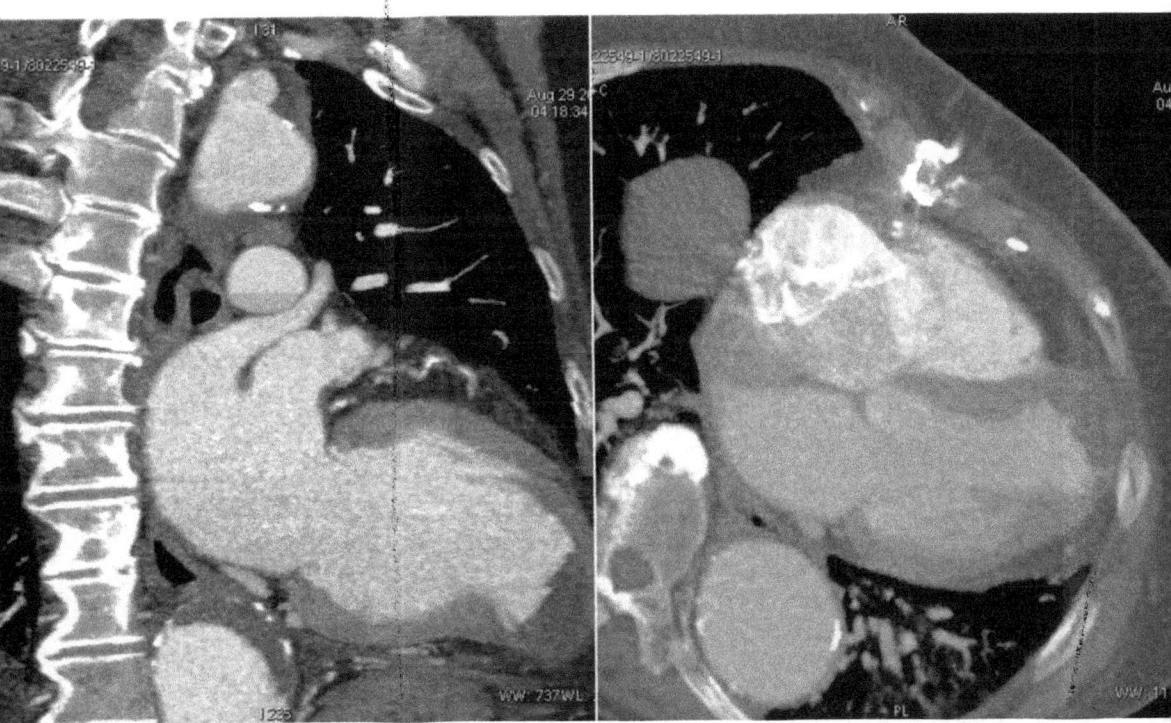

[3] Two chamber image showing apical aneurysm with prominent thrombus.

[4] Four chamber image showing apical myocardial thinning. Note the inflow mixing artifact in the right cardiac chambers, indicating imperfect bolus timing.

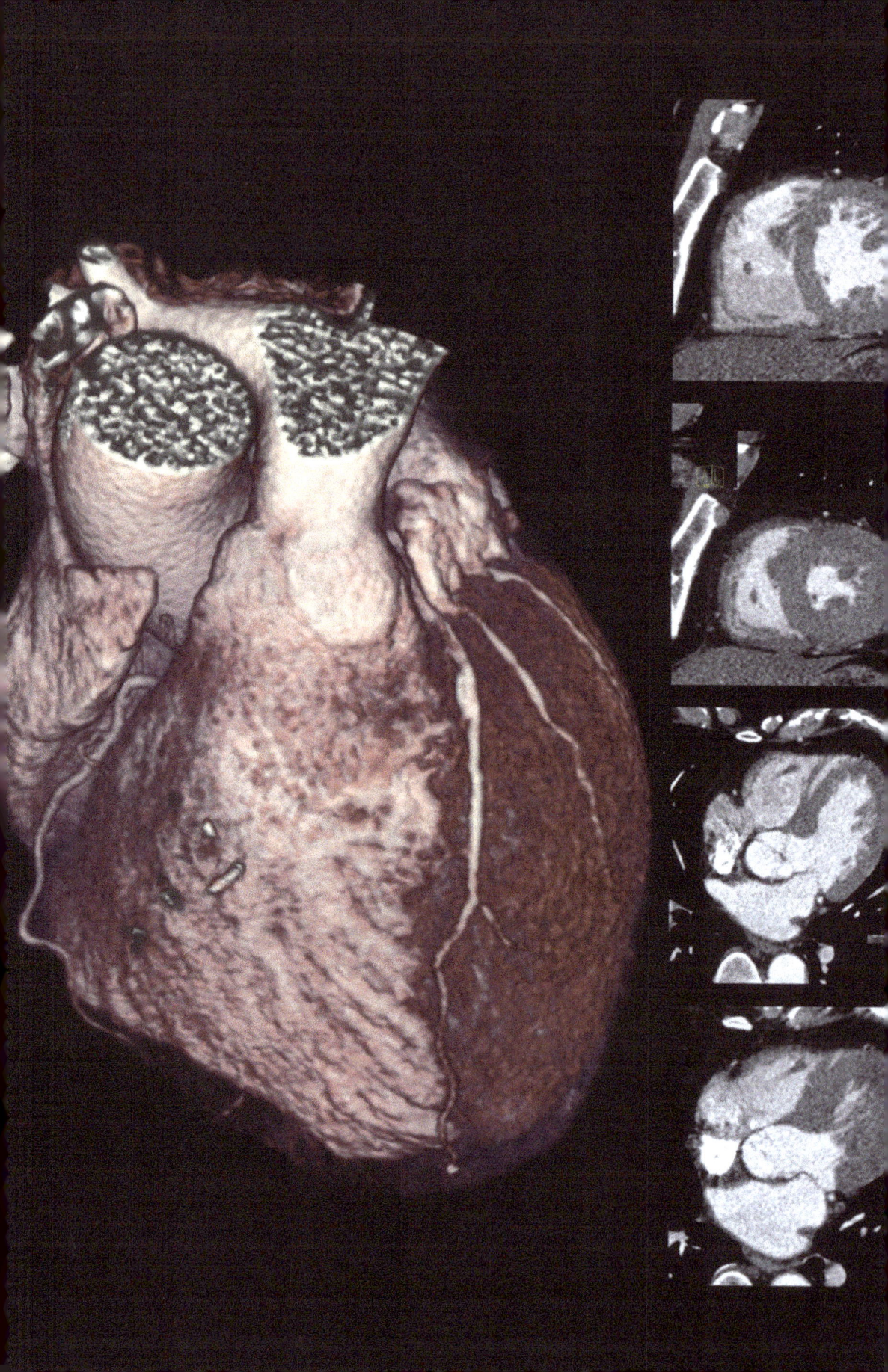

Cardiac: Left/Right Ventricular Function

Kai Uwe Juergens · Harald Seifarth · Michael Puesken · Roman Fischbach

Case 1: Dual Source CT Preceding Cardiac Resynchronization Therapy (CRT)

Case 2: Dual Source CT in Left-Ventricular Hypertrophy [A] & in ARVCM [B]

Left-ventricular volumes and myocardial mass are independent predictors of morbidity and mortality in patients with coronary heart disease, and global left-ventricular function is considered the strongest determinant of heart failure and death due to myocardial infarction. The accurate and reproducible determination of left-ventricular volumetric and functional parameters is important for clinical diagnosis and risk stratification in patients with suspected or documented coronary heart disease.[1]

In clinical practice, global and regional left-ventricular function is assessed using different invasive and noninvasive imaging modalities, such as cineventriculography and echocardiography, as well as cine magnetic resonance imaging (MRI), which is currently considered the modality of reference for assessment of cardiac function.

In 1998, ECG-gated multi-detector row computed tomography (MDCT) had been introduced as a non-invasive cardiac imaging technique primarily focusing on the detection of coronary artery stenoses and cardiac morphology. Retrospective ECG gating of a cardiac MDCT study allows for CT image reconstruction in any phase of the cardiac cycle, thus end-diastolic and end-systolic images can be generated. MDCT assessment of left-ventricular volumes is feasible applying different methodological approaches: the area-length method, the Simpson's method, as well as threshold-based direct volume measurements allowing for automated 3D-growing segmentation algorithms. Based on the acquired left-ventricular volumes, secondary function parameters such as left-ventricular ejection fraction (LV-EF), stroke volume, and cardiac output are calculated. LV-EF specifies the relative change of the end-diastolic volume to the end-systolic volume during the cardiac cycle: the normal ventricle ejects 55 to 75% of its end-diastolic volume. Thus, MDCT provides quantitative information on the left-ventricular volume changes throughout the entire cardiac cycle and, consecutively, global left-ventricular function. Global left-ventricular function parameters obtained with 4- to 16-slice CT have been measured in good agreement with results from cine MRI as well as transthoracic echocardiography.[2]

Regional left-ventricular function parameters can also be obtained from the identical CT datasets. Reconstruction algorithms developed for coronary artery visualization with 4- to 16-slice CT achieved

Cardiac: Left/Right Ventricular Function

a temporal resolution between 100 to 250 ms, which was found to be sufficient displaying diastolic and systolic phases in most patients. However, rapid volume changes during the systolic ventricular filling and ejection phases were not adequately detected, and regional left-ventricular function assessment, especially detection of diastolic dysfunction, remains limited. Currently introduced Dual Source CT (DSCT) systems providing a constant temporal resolution of 83 ms and up to 40 ms using multi-segment data reconstruction algorithms might help to overcome this limitation. Therefore, CT data post-processing for regional left-ventricular wall motion assessment should include image reconstructions of 20 phases at 5%-steps of the RR-interval from raw CT datasets to utilize the full diagnostic potential from the improved temporal resolution.

As left-ventricular function assessment is usually performed complementary to coronary CT angiography, the routine protocols used for coronary artery imaging are applied. The introduction of CT scanners with up to 64 detector rows and DSCT systems in combination with advanced power injectors for combined application of contrast-media and a saline chaser bolus enabled CT data acquisition within 6 to 12 seconds. The performance of threshold-based automated 3D-growing segmentation algorithms depends on the quality of contrast opacification. If functional parameters are to be obtained, delineation of the right atrium and ventricle and the septal myocardium is improved with a modified contrast injection scheme using either a biphasic injection or application of diluted contrast after the initial bolus injection.

Meanwhile, multiple studies on 4- to 64-slice CT systems have demonstrated that MDCT allows for reliable determination of left-ventricular volumes and global left-ventricular function parameters in good agreement with established imaging modalities. MDCT is still not considered a first-line modality for left-ventricular function assessment; however, this technique provides clinically valuable additional information in patients undergoing MDCT coronary angiography and enables a combined assessment of cardiac morphology and left-ventricular function without the need for additional radiation exposure.[3,4] Furthermore, MDCT enables left-ventricular function assessment in patients with implantable pacemakers and cardioverter defibrillators (ICD), especially in the follow-up after cardiac resynchronization therapy with MRI being contraindicated. With current improvements in MDCT post-processing and image analysis software, a further increase in clinical applicability of global left-ventricular function evaluation is expected.

Even regional left-ventricular wall motion analysis at rest is feasible from MDCT datasets in good agreement with competitive imaging modalities, as systolic and diastolic image reconstructions depict changes in left-ventricular wall thickness and multiphase reconstructions even allow analysis of left-ventricular wall motion over the cardiac cycle. Normokinetic left-ventricular segments are reliably identified with MDCT. However, sensitivity for detection and accurate classification of left-ventricular wall motion abnormalities has to be improved. Further improvement in temporal resolution as provided by 64-slice MDCT and DSCT systems seems to be mandatory to match regional LV function analysis obtained from echocardiography and MRI.[5,6]

Kai Uwe Juergens · Harald Seifarth · Michael Puesken · Roman Fischbach
University of Münster
Department of Clinical Radiology

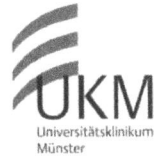

References

[1] White HD, Norris RM, Brown MA, Brandt PWT, Whitlock RML, Wild CJ. Left ventricular end-systolic volume as the major determination of survival after recovery from myocardial infarction. Circulation 1987;76:44-51

[2] Juergens KU, Fischbach R. Left ventricular function studied with MDCT. Eur Radiol 2006;16:342-357

[3] Juergens KU, Grude M, Maintz D, et al. Multi-Detector Row CT of Left Ventricular Function with Dedicated Analysis Software versus MR Imaging: Initial Experience. Radiology 2004:230:403-410

[4] Mahnken AH, Katoh M, Bruners P, et al. Acute myocardial infarction: assessment of left ventricular function with 16-detector row spiral CT versus MR imaging-study in pigs. Radiology 2005;236:112-117

[5] Fischbach R, Juergens KU, Ozgun M, Maintz D, Grude M, Seifarth H, Heindel W, Wichter T. Assessment of regional left ventricular function with multidetector-row computed tomography versus magnetic resonance imaging. Eur Radiol 2007;17:1009-1017

[6] Rist C, Johnson TR, Becker A, Leber AW, Huber A, Busch S, Becker CR, Reiser MF, Nikolaou K. Dual-source cardiac CT imaging with improved temporal resolution : Impact on image quality and analysis of left ventricular function. Radiologe 2007;47:287-294

Cardiac: Left/Right Ventricular Function

Basic considerations

The assessment of left- and right-ventricular function is usually accomplished complementary to coronary CT angiography and, therefore, is based on the routine DSCT coronary artery imaging protocols. Homogeneous and reliable opacification of the right heart is a fundamental requirement for delineation of the septum, myocardial wall thickness measurement, and myocardial mass estimation. A second bolus of 40 mL consisting of 70% of saline and 30% contrast medium injected after the main bolus yields enhancement of the right ventricular cavity and allows for a delineation of the right ventricular myocardium and septum.

Scan Parameters

Scan mode	Dual Source, ECG-gated
Heart rate control	not necessary
Scan area	mid pulmonary artery to below heart
Scan direction	cranio-caudal
Scan time	~8–14 s, depending on heart rate
Tube voltage	120 kV
Tube current	360 quality ref. mAs/rotation
Dose modulation	ECG-pulsing off, CARE Dose4D
CTDI$_{vol}$	~50 mGy, depending on heart rate
Rotation time	0.33 s
Pitch	0.2–0.5, depending on heart rate
Slice collimation	0.6 mm
Acquisition	64 x 0.6 mm
Slice width	0.75 mm
Reconstruction increment	0.4 mm
Reconstruction kernel	B30f

Tricks

Threshold-based segmentation requires sufficient opacification of the RV and LV. Therefore, correct timing of the two contrast media phases is crucial. If right ventricular function assessment is the main goal of the study, the second phase CM injection should be set to 70% CM concentration for better delineation of RV and RVOT.

Pitfalls

· If injection duration of the high concentration bolus is too long, hyperenhancement and inhomogeneous opacification of the RV will result, impairing automatic contour detection or ventricle segmentation.
· Don't use MinDose™ to ensure sufficient image quality for ventricular segmentation throughout the whole cardiac cycle.

Contrast Injection Protocol

	Iodine concentration 300 mg I/ml	Iodine concentration 370 mg I/ml
Injection scheme	Monophasic	Monophasic
Iodine delivery rate	1.85 g/s	1.85 g/s
CM volume	85 ml plus 40 ml diluted to 40%	70 ml plus 40 ml diluted to 30%
CM flow rate	6.2 ml/s	5 ml/s
Body weight adaption	no	no
Bolus timing	bolus tracking*	bolus tracking*
Bolus tracking threshold	150 HU	150 HU
ROI position	ascending aorta	ascending aorta
Scan delay	5 s	5 s
Saline flush volume	50 ml	50 ml
Saline injection rate	6.2 ml/s	5 ml/s
Needle size	18 G	18 G
Injection site	antecubital vein	antecubital vein

*Depending on the preference of the individual site, test bolus can be used as an alternative

Case 1 Dual Source CT Preceding Cardiac Resynchronization Therapy (CRT)

Case history

66-year-old man with two-vessel coronary artery disease, chronic myocardial infarction, and persistent atrial fibrillation.

Question

Assessment of cardiac morphology and left-ventricular function preceding cardiac resynchronization therapy (CRT) with ICD.

Diagnosis / Differential diagnosis

· Two-vessel coronary artery disease; chronic myocardial infarction with consecutive aneurysm of left-ventricular apex and adherent calcified thrombi.

· Severely reduced left-ventricular ejection fraction.

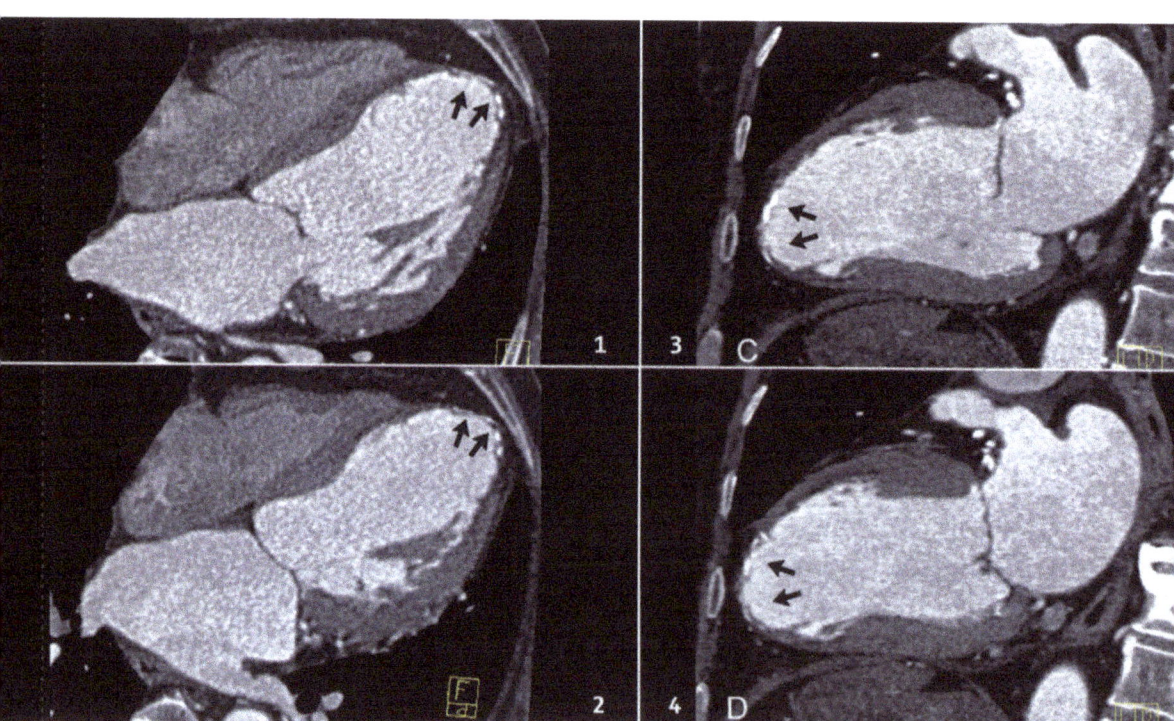

[1–6] Diastolic (1, 3, 5) and systolic (2, 4, 6) MPRs in horizontal (1, 2) and vertical (3, 4) long-axis as well as in short-axis (5, 6) orientation.

Findings

Aneurysmatic dilatation of left-ventricular apex and thinning of myocardium. Calcified thrombi within the aneurysm. Akinesis of the anterior, septal, and anteroseptal left-ventricular wall, and dyskinesis of left-ventricular apex: LV-EDV 344.9 mL, LV-ESV 268.5 mL, and LV-EF 22.2%.

Take-home message

Dual Source CT provides clinically valuable information on left-ventricular morphology and global as well as regional function in patients preceding CRT. As postinterventional cardiac MRI is contraindicated due to ICD, Dual Source CT enables follow-up evaluation of left-ventricular function to monitor any therapy effect.

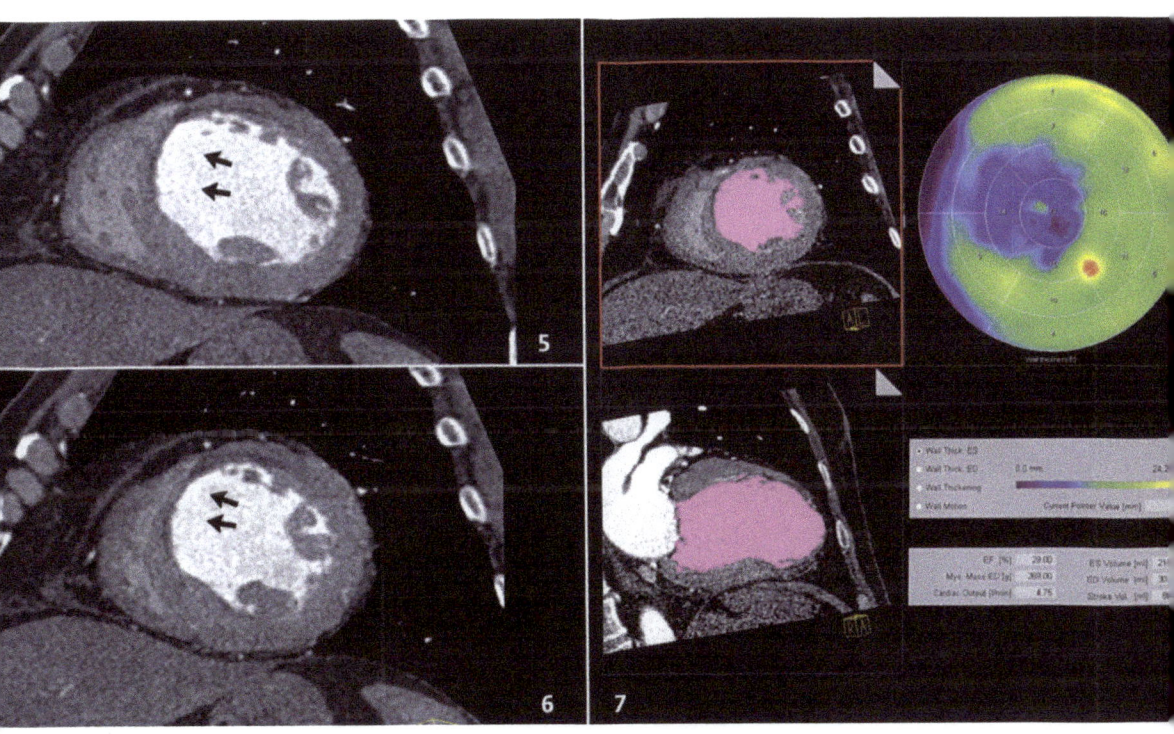

[7] Screenshot from dedicated CT evaluation software (*syngo* Circulation, Siemens AG) applying a 3D threshold segmentation algorithm: SA and vertical LA CT reformations (left column); Bull's eye plot, numerical results.

Case 2 Dual Source CT in Left-Ventricular Hypertrophy [A] & in ARVCM [B]

Case history

[A] 58-year-old men with 2-vessel CAD and several cardiovascular risk factors, e.g. long-term arterial hypertension, dyslipoproteinemia, was referred for Dual Source CT angiography.

Question

Dual Source CT angiography for re-evaluation of coronary arteries and potential detection of coronary artery stenoses.

Diagnosis / Differential diagnosis

· [A] Left-ventricular hypertrophy (LVH) most likely due to long-term arterial hypertension; 2-vessel CAD with subendocardial scar in postero-lateral and posterior left-ventricular wall due to myocardial infarction.

· [B] In the second clinical case presented morphological & functional findings of DSCT are typical for arrhythmogenic right-ventricular cardiac morphology (ARVCM).

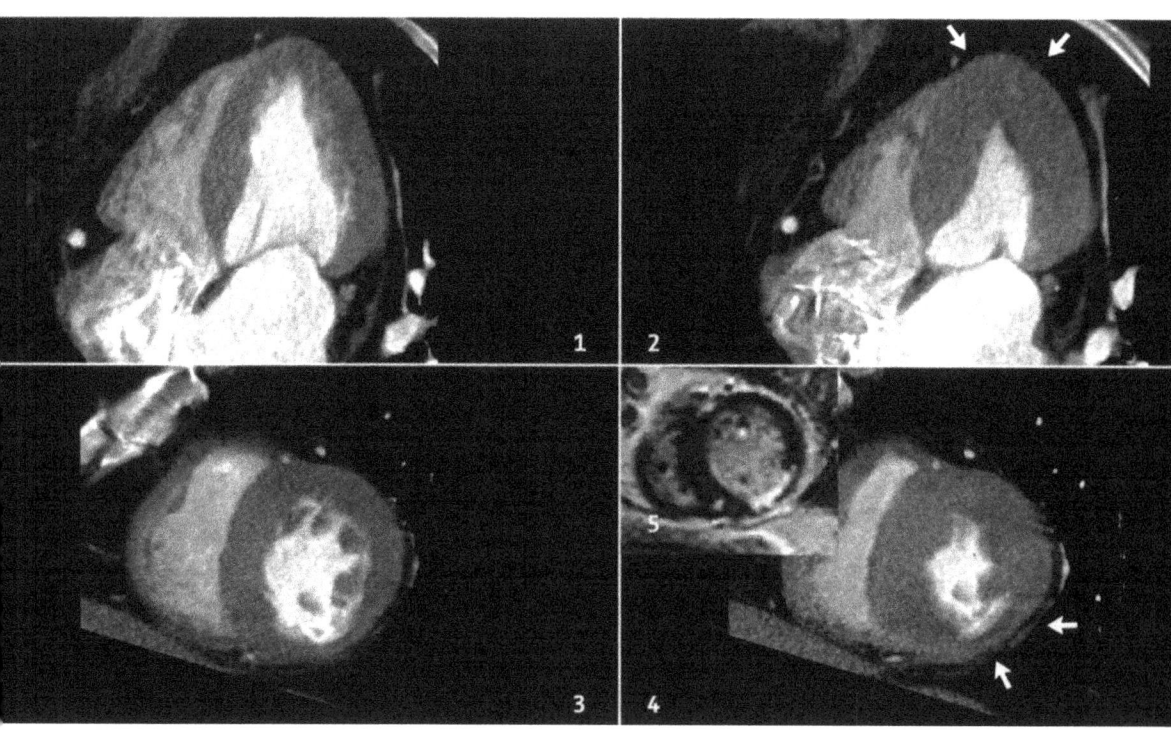

[A] [1–5] Diastolic [1, 3] + systolic [2, 4] DSCT image reformations in horizontal long-axis [1, 2] and short-axis [3, 4] orientation, short-axis image reformation from CE-MRI [5].

Findings

[A] Concentric hypertrophy of entire LV myocardium [1, 2; arrows] without obstruction of LVOT. Circumscript thinning of postero-lateral and posterior LV myocardium with hypokinesis to akinesis in systolic images [2, 4; arrows]; LV-EF was reduced (51.2%). Cardiac MRI displayed hyperenhancement in postero-lateral and posterior left-ventricular myocardial wall following iv-application of Gd-DTPA [5].

Take-home message

[A] Dual Source CT provides clinically valuable information on LV morphology and global as well as regional function in patients with LV hypertrophy and chronic myocardial infarction. [B] Typical features of ARVCM are right-ventricular (RV) dilatation, thinning of RV wall, hypertrophic RV trabeculae, and fibro-fatty replacement of RV myocardium.

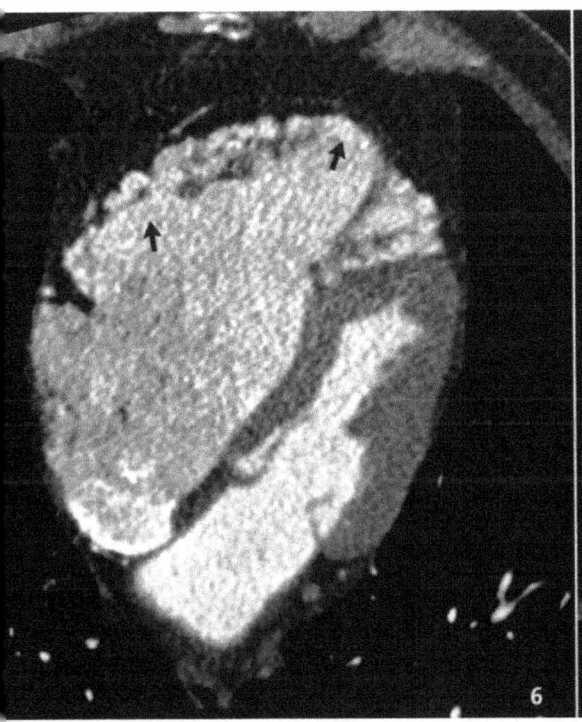
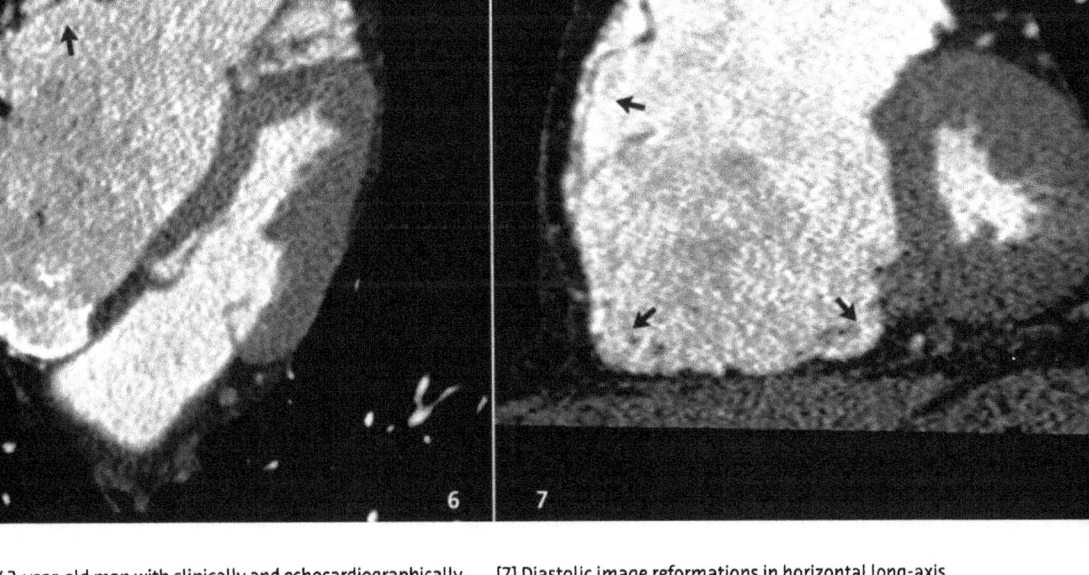

[B] [6] 42-year-old man with clinically and echocardiographically suspected ARVCM was referred for Dual Source CT angiography for non-invasive exclusion of CAD.

[7] Diastolic image reformations in horizontal long-axis ["four-chamber view"; 6] orientation and short-axis [7] orientation from Dual Source CT angiography.

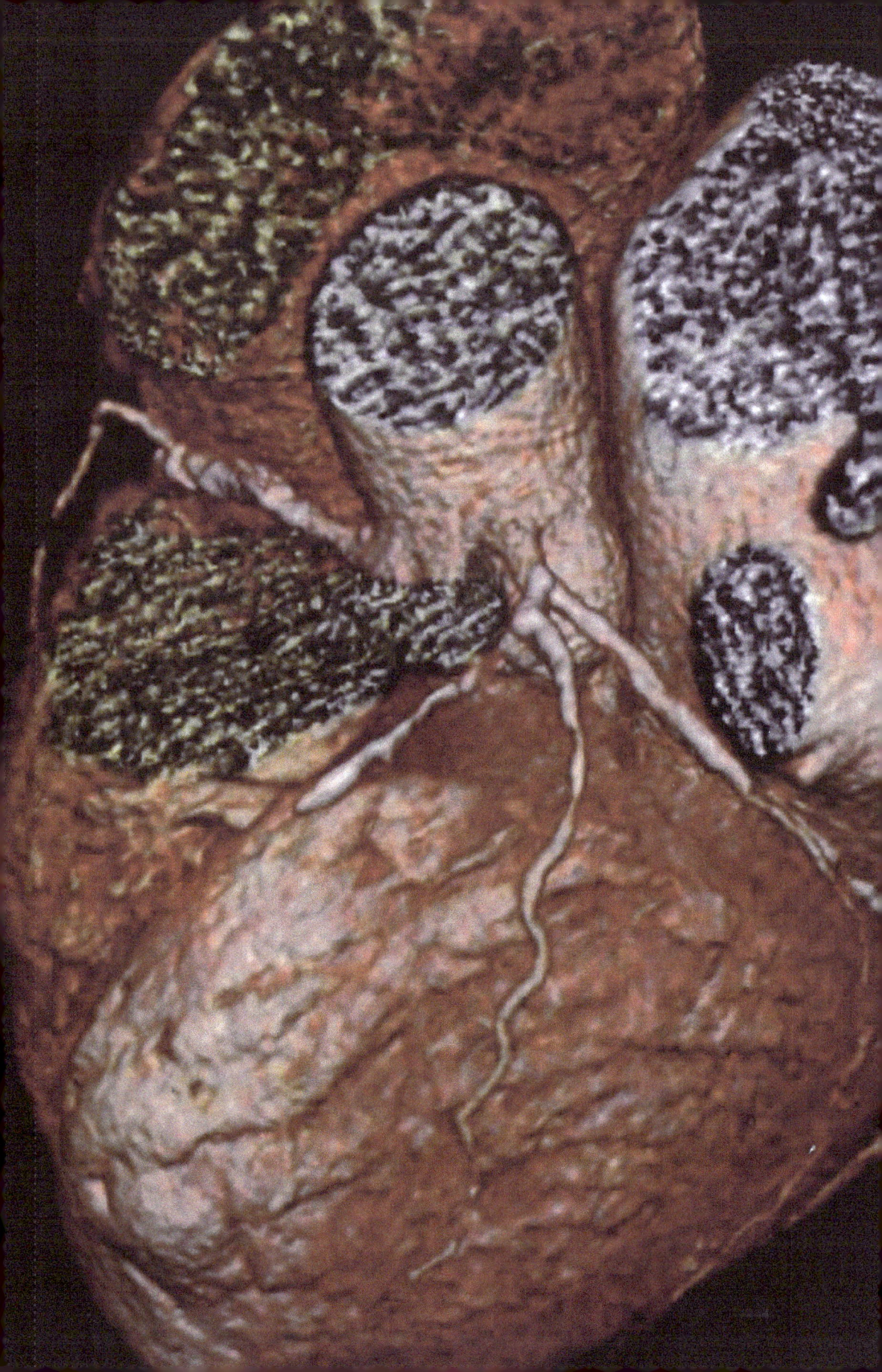

Cardiac: Atrial Fibrillation/Arrhythmia

Nico R. Mollet · Filippo Cademartiri · Gabriel P. Krestin

Case 1: Patient with Atrial Fibrillation and Atypical Chest Pain

Case 2: Patient with Atrial Fibrillation and Chronic Stable Angina Pectoris

CT coronary angiography is an emerging technique able to non-invasively detect significant coronary stenoses and non-obstructive coronary plaques. Promising results have been obtained in selected patients with low (< 70 bpm) and regular heart rates. The introduction of Dual Source CT scanners has resulted in a markedly improved temporal resolution when imaging the small and rapidly moving coronary arteries, which allows improved coronary imaging in patients with higher (> 70 bpm) heart rates. However, the improved temporal resolution of Dual Source CT scanners also allows more reliable evaluation of the coronary arteries in patients with severe heart rhythm irregularities, e.g. patients with atrial fibrillation or frequent premature beats. However, coronary imaging in arrhythmic patients remains challenging: scan protocols must be adapted on a per-patient basis and reconstruction of high quality datasets requires specific skills of the radiographer and/or radiologist. In this chapter, we will discuss tips & tricks to improve image quality in patients with severe arrhythmia, and we will present two cases of patients with atrial fibrillation and symptoms of atypical chest pain and chronic stable angina pectoris.

CT coronary angiography requires simultaneous recording of the ECG during the scan acquisition to be able to reduce coronary motion artifacts by reconstructing datasets obtained during a certain phase of the cardiac cycle when the heart moves less (generally the end-systolic and/or mid-to-end-diastolic phase of the cardiac cycle). In spiral CT coronary angiography, datasets can be flexibly reconstructed at different phases, because data is obtained throughout the entire cardiac cycle. Two image reconstruction algorithms can be applied to obtain optimal motion-free image quality. A single-segment reconstruction algorithm can be used, in which data obtained during a single heart beat is used for image reconstruction. The temporal resolution using such an algorithm in Dual Source CT is equal to a quarter of the rotation time (e.g. 83 ms). The temporal resolution can be further reduced by using a bi-segmental reconstruction algorithm that combines data obtained during two consecutive heart beats, thereby further reducing the temporal resolution to 42 ms. However, such a bi-segmental reconstruction algorithm requires a regular heart rate and therefore should not be applied in patients with severe heart rhythm irregularities. Combining the data of two consecutive heart beats without an equal R-R interval (which is the case in patients with arrhythmia) results in image blurring and may even mask the presence of clinically significant coronary stenoses.

Cardiac: Atrial Fibrillation/Arrhythmia

Different algorithms can be used to position the reconstruction windows within the cardiac cycle. A percentage approach is most commonly used, in which reconstruction windows are positioned at a certain percentage of the R-R cycle when the heart moves less (e.g. 60% of the R-R cycle). Reconstruction windows can also be positioned using an absolute reverse approach (e.g. 400 ms before the next R-wave) or an absolute forward approach (e.g. 600 ms after the last R-wave). These algorithms can be flexibly used and the operator can select the best dataset on a per-patient basis. However, a percentage approach is more sensitive to arrhythmia when compared to absolute forward or backward reconstruction algorithms.[1] The percentage approach should therefore not be used in patients with atrial fibrillation. Instead, the absolute forward approach is especially useful to reconstruct end-systolic datasets, which is often the best phase for reliable coronary imaging in patients with arrhythmia, especially if the baseline heart rate is high (above 70 bpm). End-systolic datasets generally provide optimal image quality in patients with higher heart rates.[2, 3] Moreover, the position of the end-systolic phase is typically relatively constant even if the length of the R-R interval varies among different (arrhythmic) heart beats. In contrast, the position of the diastolic phase varies significantly throughout the R-R interval, and datasets reconstructed within the diastolic phase are generally not useful in patients with arrhythmia for this reason.

Step artifacts may occur in patients with arrhythmia due to a mismatch between the selected reconstruction phase and the actual obtained data during different heart beats. The position of the reconstruction windows should therefore always be carefully checked and manually repositioned if necessary. In fact, manual repositioning of the reconstruction windows (so-called 'ECG-editing') is a key feature to obtain high quality coronary images in patients with arrhythmia. However, unrestricted use of this advanced reconstruction tool requires low pitch values. It is therefore recommended to manually select low pitch values (e.g. 0.2) irrespective of the baseline heart rate in patients with severe arrhythmia. Prospective x-ray tube modulation (so called 'ECG-pulsing') can be applied in patients with severe arrhythmia. This feature is automatically switched off in the case of a premature beat which results in a sudden change of the R-R interval and will only be switched on again if the heart rhythm is constant. On the other hand, the combination of low pitch values and less efficient reduction of the radiation exposure by ECG-pulsing results in a higher radiation dose of CT coronary angiography in patients with severe arrhythmia, such as atrial fibrillation.

Nico R. Mollet[A, B] · **Filippo Cademartiri**[A] · **Gabriel P. Krestin**[A]

Erasmus Medical Center Rotterdam

Department of Radiology[A] & Cardiology[B]

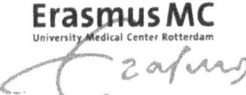

References

[1] Cademartiri F, Mollet NR, Runza G, Baks T, Midiri M, McFadden EP, Flohr TG, Ohnesorge B, de Feyter PJ, Krestin GP. Improving diagnostic accuracy of MDCT coronary angiography in patients with mild heart rhythm irregularities using ECG editing. AJR Am J Roentgenol. 2006 Mar; 186(3):634-8

[2] Sato T, Anno H, Kondo T, Harigaya H, Inoue K, Kakizawa S, Ohshima K, Sarai M, Hishida H, Katada K, Kanou M. Applicability of ECG-gated multislice helical ct to patients with atrial fibrillation. Circ J. 2005 Sep; 69(9):1068-73

[3] Herzog C, Arning-Erb M, Zangos S, Eichler K, Hammerstingl R, Dogan S, Ackermann H, Vogl TJ. Multi-detector row CT coronary angiography: influence of reconstruction technique and heart rate on image quality. Radiology. 2006 Jan;238(1):75-86

[4] Leber AW, Johnson T, Becker A, von Ziegler F, Tittus J, Nikolaou K, Reiser M, Steinbeck G, Becker CR, Knez A. Diagnostic accuracy of dual-source multi-slice CT-coronary angiography in patients with an intermediate pretest likelihood for coronary artery disease. Eur Heart J. 2007 Oct;28(19):2354-2360. Epub 2007 Jul 21

Cardiac: Atrial Fibrillation/Arrhythmia

Basic considerations

The presence of atrial fibrillation requires a fixed, low pitch (generally 0.2) irrespective of baseline heart rate, because the heart rate may vary significantly throughout the scan.

If a relatively fast pitch is selected, e.g. in patients with a high baseline heart rate during the last 10 beats prior to the start of the scan, extensive interpolation artifacts will occur if the heart rate drops more than 10 bpm during the scan. A multi-segment reconstruction algorithm should not be used in patients with arrhythmia, because the data of two consecutive heart beats at a different contraction phase will be merged, resulting in poor image quality due to blurring.

Scan Parameters

Scan mode	Dual Source, ECG-gated
Heart rate control	not necessary
Scan area	mid pulmonary artery to below heart
Scan direction	cranio-caudal
Scan time	~7–12 s, depending on heart rate
Tube voltage	120 kV
Tube current	360 mAs/rotation
Dose modulation	ECG-pulsing on, 25–70%
$CTDI_{vol}$	~50 mGy, depending on heart rate
Rotation time	0.33 s
Pitch	0.2 (fixed)
Slice collimation	0.6 mm
Acquisition	64 x 0.6 mm
Slice width	0.75 mm
Reconstruction increment	0.4 mm
Reconstruction kernel	B26f, B46f in case of excessive calcification

Tricks

· Carefully check the position of the reconstruction windows in every heart beat to avoid step artifacts.
· Edit reconstruction windows positioned in arrhythmic heart beats, if possible.
· End-systolic datasets generally provide optimal image quality, because this interval is relative constant even in arrhythmic heart beats.

Pitfalls

· A percentage reconstruction algorithm is very sensitive to arrhythmia and should therefore not be used in patients with atrial fibrillation.
· Absolute forward reconstruction (fixed delay after R-peak in ms) is especially useful to obtain end-systolic datasets, which is often the best phase in patients with arrhythmia, especially if the baseline heart rate is high.

Contrast Injection Protocol

	Iodine concentration 300 mg I/ml	Iodine concentration 370 mg I/ml
Injection scheme	Monophasic	Monophasic
Iodine delivery rate	1.85 g/s	1.85 g/s
CM volume	6.2 ml/s for duration of scan, ≥ 60 ml	5 ml/s for duration of scan, ≥ 50 ml
CM flow rate	6.2 ml/s	5 ml/s
Body weight adaption	no	no
Bolus timing	bolus tracking*	bolus tracking*
Bolus tracking threshold	100 HU	100 HU
ROI position	ascending aorta	ascending aorta
Scan delay	peak time plus 2 s	peak time plus 2 s
Saline flush volume	60 ml	60 ml
Saline injection rate	6.2 ml/s	5 ml/s
Needle size	18 G	18 G
Injection site	antecubital vein	antecubital vein

* Depending on the preference of the individual site, test bolus can be used as an alternative

Case 1 Patient with Atrial Fibrillation and Atypical Chest Pain

Case history

A 66-year-old female with atrial fibrillation and new onset of atypical chest pain was referred to CT coronary angiography.

Question

Does the patient have significant (> 50% lumen diameter reduction) coronary stenoses?

Diagnosis / Differential diagnosis

· A significant stenosis located at the proximal left anterior descending coronary (LAD) artery was observed.

· The patient was referred to conventional coronary angiography and the lesion was stented in a single-session PCI procedure.

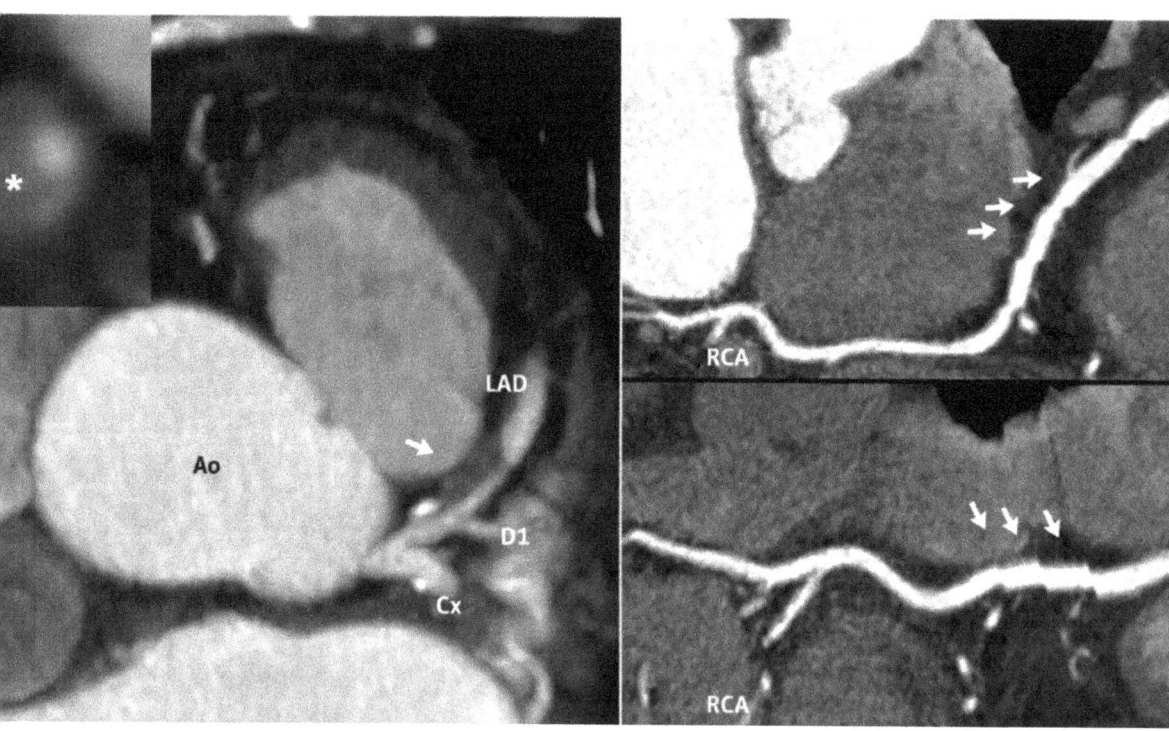

[1] CT coronary angiography shows a significant proximal LAD stenosis. Inlay: cross-sectional image of the stenosis shows a large predominantly non-calcified plaque.

[2] 2 orthogonal curved MPR's indicate the absence of significant coronary stenoses, despite the presence of residual motion (step) artifacts.

Findings

An end-systolic dataset (reconstructed +300 ms after the previous R-wave) provided optimal image quality. Except for the LAD stenosis, additional significant coronary stenoses could be reliably ruled out despite the presence of several step artifacts located at the level of the right coronary artery (RCA) and distal LAD.

Take-home message

End-systolic datasets frequently provide optimal image quality in patients with arrhythmia, especially when the heart rate is relatively high (above 70 bpm). It may not be possible to completely diminish all step artifacts, however, stenosis detection is generally not significantly affected by these artifacts.[4]

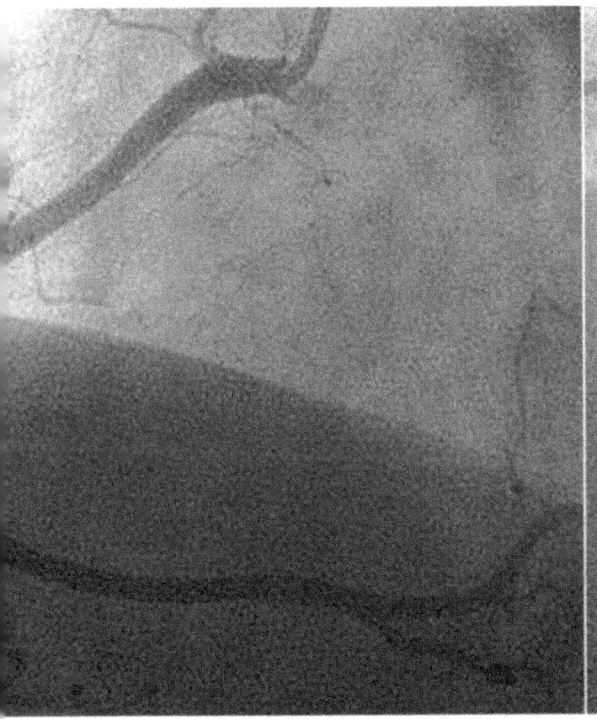 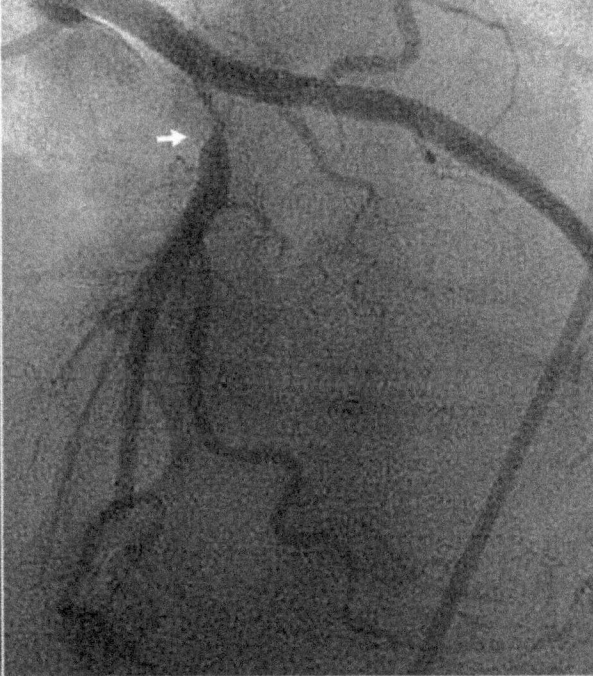

[3] The absence of significant coronary stenoses at the level of the RCA was confirmed on the conventional angiogram.

[4] The significant LAD stenosis was confirmed on the conventional angiogram and the lesion was stented in the same session.

Case 2 Patient with Atrial Fibrillation and Chronic Stable Angina Pectoris

Case history

A 73-year-old male with atrial fibrillation and symptoms of chronic stable angina pectoris was referred to CT coronary angiography to evaluate the presence of coronary stenoses.

Question

Does the patient have significant coronary artery disease which requires revascularization therapy?

Diagnosis / Differential diagnosis

· Several significant coronary stenoses were found both in the left and right coronary artery.
· Most importantly, a total occlusion at the origin of the left anterior descending coronary artery (LAD) was found.
· Percutaneous intervention was unsuccessful and the patient consequently underwent bypass surgery.

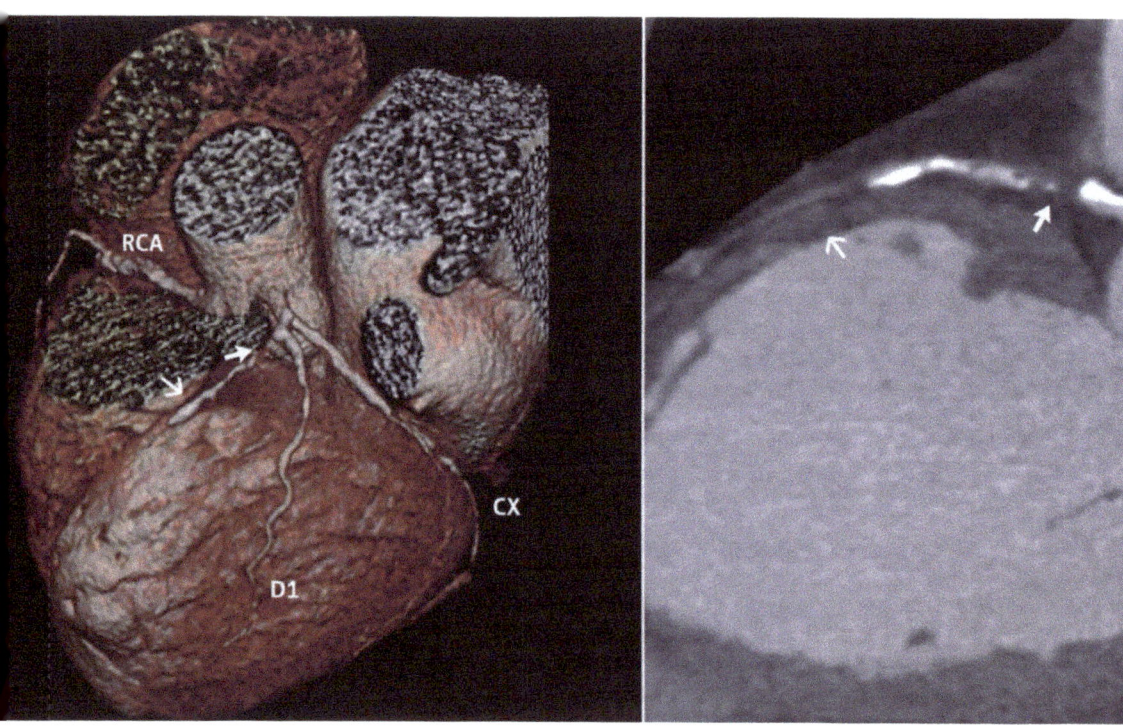

[1] Volume rendered image of the patient shows an occluded LAD at the level of the bifurcation with the first diagonal branch.

[2] A curved MPR image shows the occluded trajectory and the presence of collateral filling at the level of the distal LAD.

Findings

Chronic totally occluded coronary arteries
are found in up to 30% of patients undergoing
conventional coronary angiography. The absence
of a visible entry point and the presence of
coronary calcification are known predictors of
an unsuccessful percutaneous revascularization
procedure.

Take-home message

Step artifacts were diminished after manual
repositioning of the reconstruction windows (so-
called 'ECG-editing') at the level of the terminal
T-wave, which represents the end-systolic phase
of the cardiac cycle.

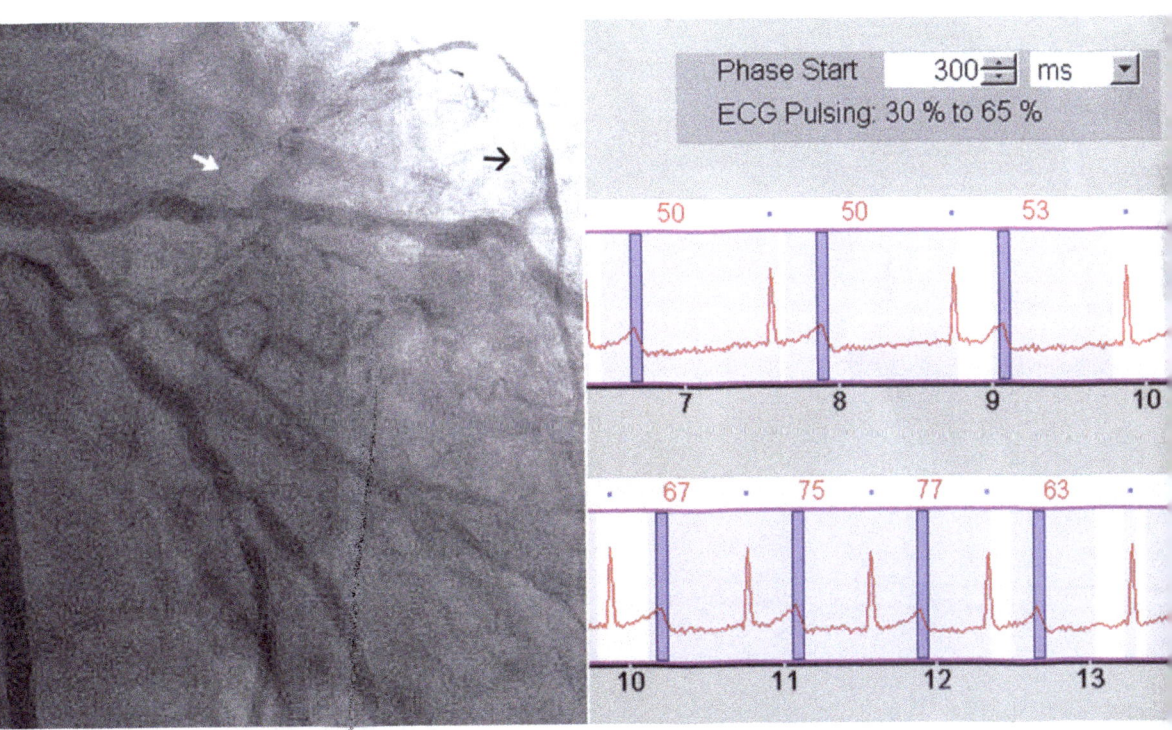

[3] The CT findings were confirmed on the conventional
angiogram (white arrow: occlusion LAD, black arrow:
collateral filling).

[4] The ECG of the patient shows atrial fibrillation. Note: the
positions of the reconstruction windows are located at the level
of the terminal T-wave (end-systolic phase).

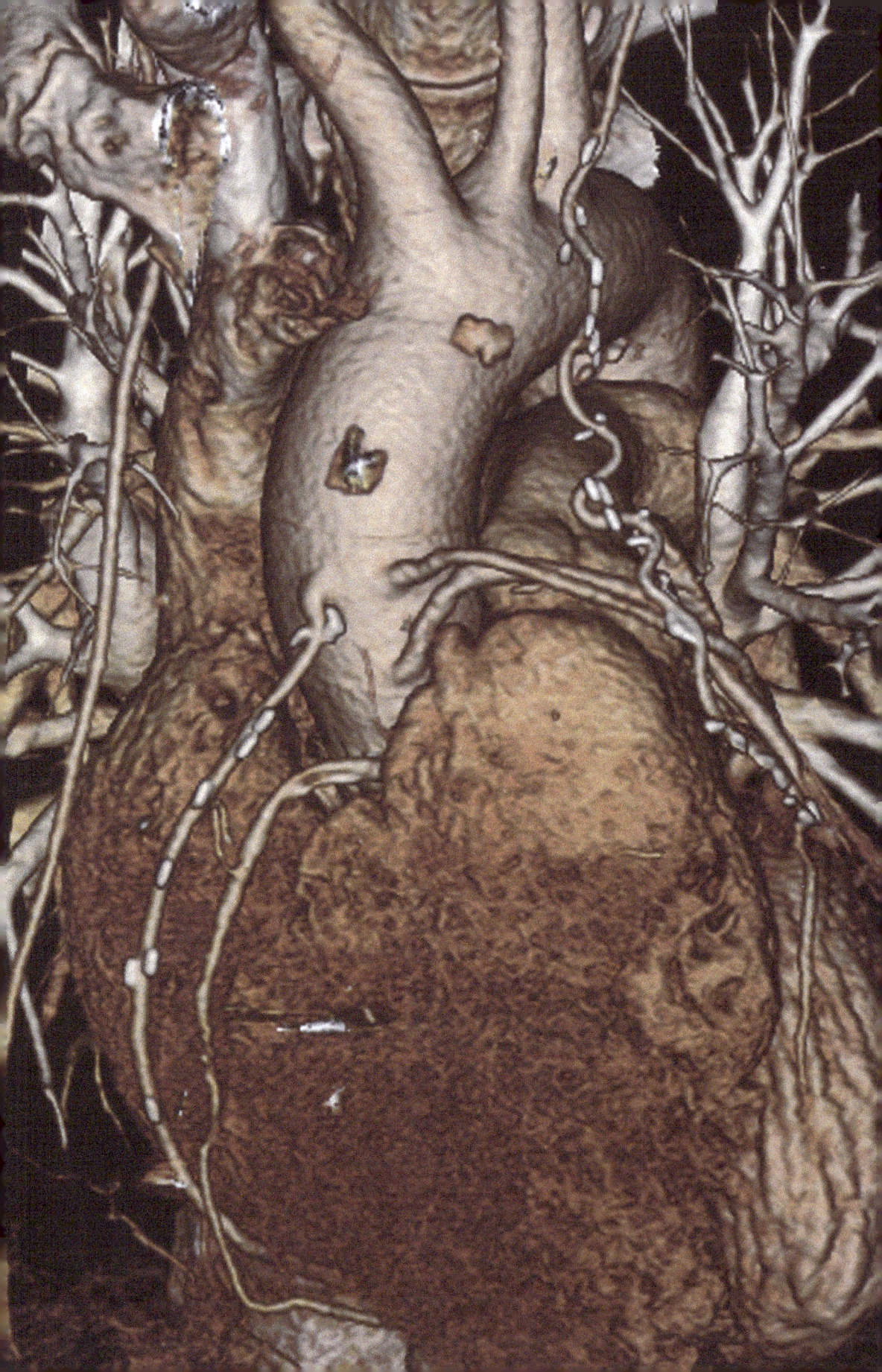

Cardiac: Bypass Grafts

Pal Suranyi · Christian Thilo · Heon Lee · U. Joseph Schoepf

Case 1: Thrombosed Venous Bypass Graft Pseudoaneurysm Following Coil Embolization

Case 2: Quadruple, Patent Coronary Artery Bypass Grafts

CT was used early on for non-invasive imaging of coronary artery bypass grafts (CABGs) in order to determine patency or occlusion because CABGs are generally larger and less mobile than native coronary arteries making them more forgiving imaging targets.[1] CABG patency could be determined with > 90% sensitivity and specificity using contrast enhanced single-slice spiral CT. Subsequent generations of CT scanners, particularly since the introduction of multi detector-row CT, have enabled even finer diagnostic assessment.[2, 3] Thus, CABG evaluation serves as a paradigm for how a diagnostic test can be shifted from an invasive procedure to non-invasive imaging.

Dual Source coronary CT angiography (cCTA) is not only faster than previous scanner generations and less invasive than cardiac catheterization, it also may, in some cases, more reliably localize unusual proximal bypass anastomoses and provide more anatomic information crucial to the success of potential redo CABG surgery. Examples for such useful information are the proximity of grafts or other vessels to the sternum, atherosclerosis of the internal mammary arteries (which would preclude their utilization as arterial bypass grafts), severe calcification of native coronary arteries (creates difficulty when suturing the distal anastomoses), pleural fluid, pericardial fluid, or sternal infection.

Occluded grafts usually present as tubular hypoattenuating structures that are denser than epicardial fat but hypoattenuating relative to myocardium. The proximal anastomoses of such occluded grafts may be found with the help of "hypass markers" (metallic rings around the proximal anastomosis) or as subtle outpouchings of the aortic wall.

Due to its excellent temporal resolution, Dual Source CT also yields valuable information regarding global and regional left and right ventricular function, which is crucial for evaluating patients before redo surgery or catheter intervention. One must remember, however, that resting regional function alone is not a reliable indicator of viability or the lack thereof, as not all of the left ventricular myocardium participates in the pump function at rest.[4]

Special considerations when imaging CABG patients can be divided into three categories: before, during and after scanning.

Cardiac: Bypass Grafts

Before scanning it is helpful to determine whether the internal mammary arteries (IMA) have been used as arterial grafts or whether this is planned during redo surgery. Since these patients already have known coronary artery disease (CAD) and generalized atherosclerosis, it is important to evaluate for ostial IMA stenosis at their origin from the subclavian arteries. Thus, in such patients it is advisable to extend the scan range to the entire chest. However, the scan range should always encompass the aortic arch.

Another important consideration is whether the patient is already on beta-blockers or nitrates, which in this patient population is highly likely. Furthermore, a priori knowledge about the patient's blood pressure and LV ejection fraction may also be useful, especially if additional beta blockers are to be used to control heart rate and rhythm. Due to the high temporal resolution of DSCT, however, it is possible to generate excellent quality diagnostic images even in patients with heart rates above 100 beats per minute. Thus, in our practice, we have abandoned the use of rate-controlling agents entirely with DSCT. The administration of nitrates can be beneficial, since they may increase vessel diameters (by 12 to 21%) and improve visualization, but this should be done carefully to avoid reflex tachycardia or hypotension.

Knowledge about previous stenting may be useful in choosing the appropriate reconstruction kernel (B46f) following the acquisition.

During imaging one should avoid pre-contrast scanning, as Calcium-scoring is regarded as a screening/risk-stratification tool and is not indicated in patients with known CAD.

For the scenarios described above, it is advisable to extend the scan range to the origins of the IMAs. Particularly if the entire chest is scanned, it is imperative to keep radiation as low as possible, while using ECG-pulsing (tube modulation) at all times. While use of ECG-pulsing with 64-slice CT had been reserved for patients with slow and steady heart rates, the improved temporal resolution of DSCT now enables routine application of this beneficial tool to all patients. Reduced tube currents during systole are sufficient for functional assessment, while the full tube current is only used during a portion (typically diastole) of the cardiac cycle. In patients with faster heart rates (HR > 65), a wider pulsing window is used (35–75% of the R-R interval). This enables reconstruction of high-quality systolic images, which are especially useful for assessing the right coronary artery. For lower heart rates, a narrower window may be used (55–75%). Some experts recommend scanning at 70–70%

only. In reality this results in nearly full current at ±5% of the cardiac cycle (from about 65 – 75%), which yields diagnostic results in most patients with slow and steady heart rates.

Although still under scientific investigation, one may consider acquiring low-dose, low-kV delayed images (for assessment of viability) 5 – 10 minutes following contrast media injection, especially if the patient has shown well defined areas of hypoattenuation during the cCTA acquisition.[5] Therefore, a precursory reconstruction and review of the cCTA images for potential hypoattenuation in the myocardium is advisable while the patient is still on the scanner table.

During image review it is important to disable automated segmentation of the heart. Segmentation algorithms might not recognize grafts and sculpt them away from the 3D volume rendered view. Nevertheless, 3D rendering is very useful to understand the overall anatomy before reviewing the transverse source images, multiplanar reformatted (MPR) views or curved MPRs. This is especially true for some of the more creative bypass configurations or grafts with serial anastomoses to several vessels ("jump grafts").

Pal Suranyi · Christian Thilo · Heon Lee · U. Joseph Schoepf
Medical University of South Carolina
Department of Radiology and Division of Cardiology

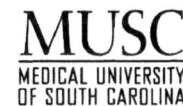

References

[1] K. Anders, U. Baum, M. Schmid et al.: Coronary artery bypass graft (CABG) patency: Assessment with high-resolution submillimeter 16-slice multidetector-row computed tomography (MDCT) versus coronary angiography. Eur. Journal of Radiology, 2006 Volume 57, Issue 3, Pages 336-344

[2] C. Herzog, P. L. Zwerner, J. R. Doll, C.D. Nielsen, S.A. Nguyen, G. Savino, T. J. Vogl, P. Costello, and U.J. Schoepf: Significant Coronary Artery Stenosis: Comparison on Per-Patient and Per-Vessel or Per-Segment Basis at 64-Section CT Angiography. Radiology 2007;244:112-120

[3] R. Jabara, N. Chronos, L. Klein et al.: Comparison of multidetector 64-slice computed tomographic angiography to coronary angiography to assess the patency of coronary artery bypass grafts. JACC 2007 Jun 1;99(11):1529-34. Epub 2007 Apr 13

[4] E. Balcells, E. R. Powers, W. Lepper et al.: Detection of myocardial viability by contrast echocardiography in acute infarction predicts recovery of resting function and contractile reserve. JACC Volume 41, Issue 5, March 2003, Pages 827-833

[5] Gabriele A. Krombach, Thoralf Niendorf, Rolf W. Günther and Andreas H. Mahnken: Characterization of myocardial viability using MR and CT. Eur Radiol, 2007 Jun;17(6):1433-44. Epub 2007 Jan 6

Cardiac: Bypass Grafts

Basic considerations

No calcium-scoring needed because there is established coronary disease. Scan entire chest from above the clavicles through the diaphragm to include the entire IMA if bypass situation is unknown or there is a known IMA graft. Start at the aortic arch if only venous grafts are present. ECG-pulsing should be used to reduce radiation exposure. Use MinDose™ if functional information is not of concern. If myocardial hypoattenuation is seen upon coronary CTA, consider acquiring a thick section (1.2 mm collimation) low kV (80 or 100 kV) scan for delayed enhancement and viability assessment.

Scan Parameters

Scan mode	Dual Source, ECG-gated
Heart rate control	not necessary
Scan area	clavicle (or arch) to diaphragm
Scan direction	cranio-caudal
Scan time	~12–15 s, depending on heart rate
Tube voltage	120 kV
Tube current	360 mAs/rotation
Dose modulation	ECG-pulsing on*
CTDI$_{vol}$	~50 mGy, depending on heart rate
Rotation time	0.33 s
Pitch	0.2–0.5, depending on heart rate
Slice collimation	0.6 mm
Acquisition	64 x 0.6 mm
Slice width	0.75 mm/1.5 mm for function
Reconstruction increment	0.4 mm/1 mm for function
Reconstruction kernel	B26f, B46f for stent, in case of excessive calcifications

* Referring to ECG-pulsing table (see page 28)

Tricks

· Increase mAs in obese patients.
· Use smoother kernels (B20f) and thicker sections for obese patients. Use sharper kernel (B46f) for reconstruction in patients with stents and/or heavy calcifications.
· Start with 3D (VRT) view to understand overall graft anatomy, then review MPRs and curved MPRs.

Pitfalls

· Automatic segmentation of heart may remove some of the bypass grafts.
· Shell-like circumferential calcifications may look like stents.
· Inappropriate windowing may make it difficult to differentiate vessel lumen filled with high attenuation contrast media from calcifications.
· Preferably, use right arm for IV, to avoid proximal left IMA being obscured by streaks.

Contrast Injection Protocol

	Iodine concentration 300 mg I/ml	Iodine concentration 370 mg I/ml
Injection scheme	Monophasic	Monophasic
Iodine delivery rate	1.85 g/s	1.85 g/s
CM volume	6.2 ml/s for duration of scan, ≥ 60 ml	5 ml/s for duration of scan, ≥ 50 ml
CM flow rate	6.2 ml/s	5 ml/s
Body weight adaption	no	no
Bolus timing	test bolus*	test bolus*
Bolus tracking threshold	n.a.	n.a.
ROI position	ascending aorta	ascending aorta
Scan delay	test bolus peak time	test bolus peak time
Saline flush volume	60 ml of CM/Saline (30/70%)	60 ml of CM/Saline (30/70%)
Saline injection rate	6.2 ml/s	5 ml/s
Needle size	18 G	18 G
Injection site	right antecubital vein	right antecubital vein

* Depending on the preference of the individual site, bolus tracking can be used as an alternative

Case 1 Thrombosed Venous Bypass Graft Pseudoaneurysm Following Coil Embolization

Case history

This 67-year-old patient post CABG was admitted due to recurrent chest pain following microcoil embolization of his saphenous venous graft pseudoaneurysm performed at another institution.

Question

What is the cause of the persistent chest pain? Are any of the bypass grafts occluded/stenotic, or is the source of the pain extra-cardiac?

Diagnosis/Differential diagnosis

· Acute graft thrombosis, myocardial infarction, myocardial ischemia due to graft stenosis, aortic dissection, pulmonary embolism, pericarditis, lung tumor.

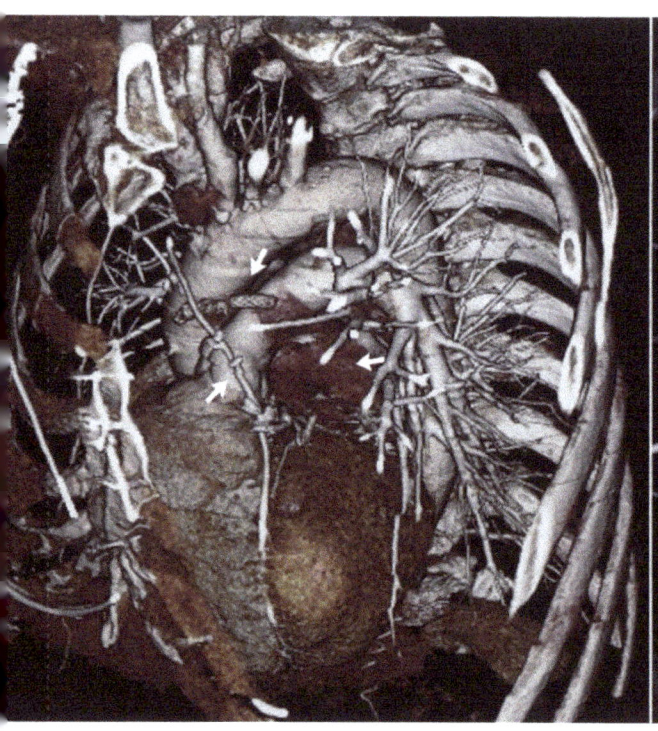

[1] 3D overview of the heart. The stented, occluded bypass graft that developed a pseudoaneurysm can be seen behind a LIMA which appears to be patent and feeding the LAD.

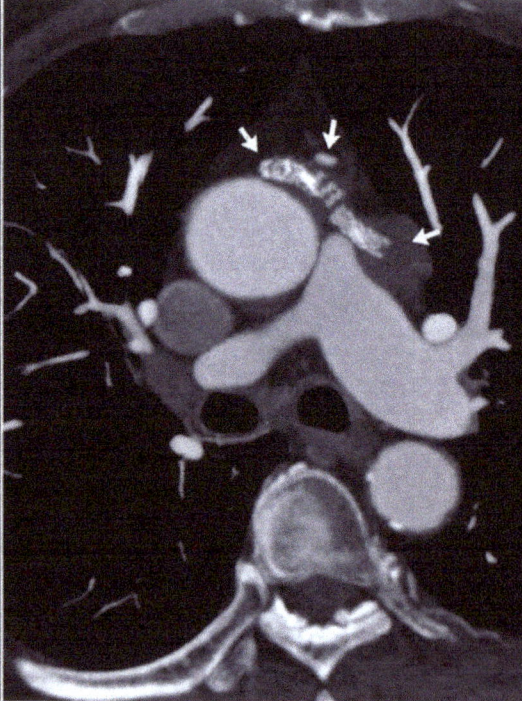

[2] Axial 5 mm MIP of the proximal portion of the stented (two stents), occluded graft continuing into a thrombosed pseudoaneurysm. LIMA is also shown anterior to the stents.

Findings

Thrombotic occlusion of previously stented
venous graft (to the left circumflex artery) with
large pseudoaneurysm without evidence of
contrast enhancement and with numerous
microcoils in place.

Patent LIMA to the severely diseased mid LAD
with good distal runoff.

Take-home message

In patients with persistent chest pain of unknown
origin following CABG surgery, coronary CTA is
an excellent tool for differential diagnosis. Acute
graft occlusion can be quickly and efficiently
diagnosed with Dual Source CT, while additional
valuable information is also gained about the
chest wall, lungs, other thoracic vessels and the
native coronary arteries.

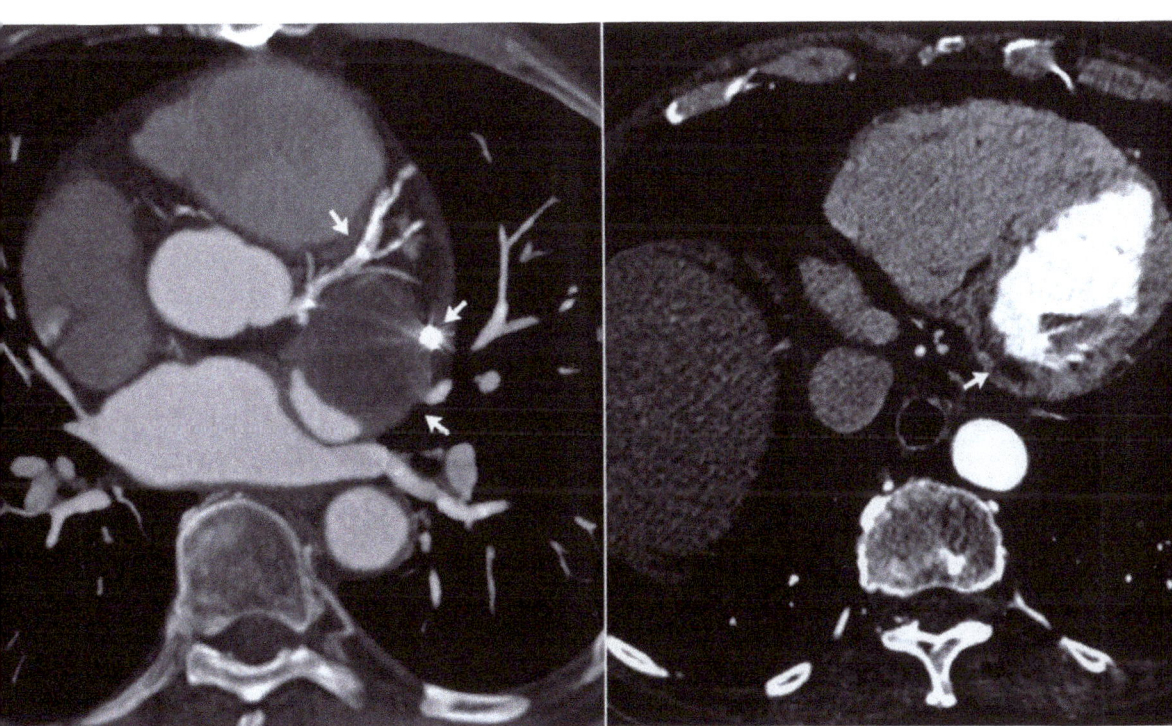

[3] Axial MIP at the level of the severely diseased LAD. The coil
used for embolizing the pseudoaneurysm can be seen in the
center of this large, thrombosed mass.

[4] Distal MPR (0.75 mm) of the heart reveals severe
hypoattenuation of the myocardium posteriorly, corresponding
to infarct in the region once supplied by the occluded graft.

Case 2 Quadruple, Patent Coronary Artery Bypass Grafts

Case history

Five years following quadruple CABG surgery, this 64-year-old patient started experiencing atypical chest pain.

Question

Are any of the bypass grafts or anastomoses stenotic or occluded? Is there an extra-cardiac cause behind the patient's symptoms?

Diagnosis / Differential diagnosis

· Acute graft thrombosis, myocardial infarction, myocardial ischemia due to graft stenosis, aortic dissection, pulmonary embolism, pericarditis, lung tumor.

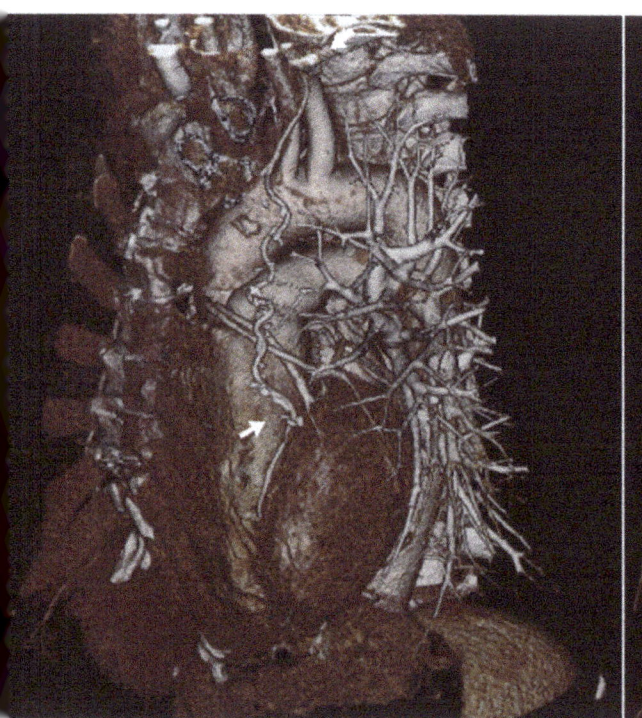

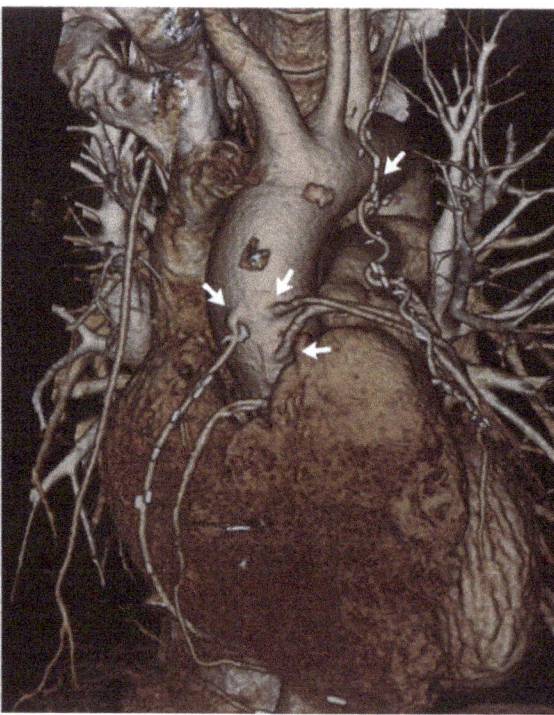

[1] 3D overview of vascular anatomy. The origin of the LIMA from the subclavian artery can be assessed, as well as the proximity of this graft to the sternum.

[2] After carefully "removing" the chest wall, the configuration of this complicated anatomy can be easily reviewed. All four bypass grafts appear patent.

Findings

Although all four grafts appeared patent, there was a mild stenosis at the proximal anastomosis of one of the venous grafts (to the first obtuse marginal branch (OM1) of the LCx) with atretic distal runoff. In the posterolateral region, supplied by this vessel, myocardial hypoattenuation was found, suggesting ischemia (see figure 3).

Take-home message

Dual Source Cardiac CT can detect graft stenosis or tight anastomoses and consequent myocardial ischemia efficiently. The data can be used to plan intervention (stent size, approachability) or redo surgery if it is deemed necessary by the clinician.

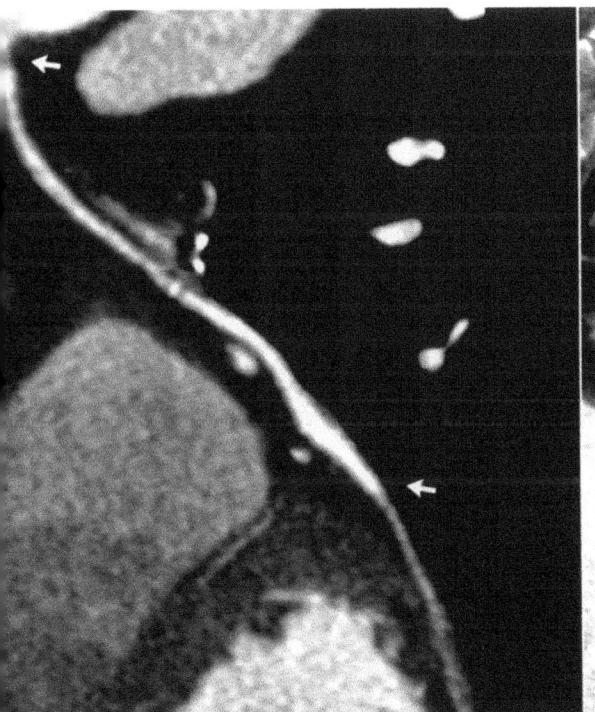

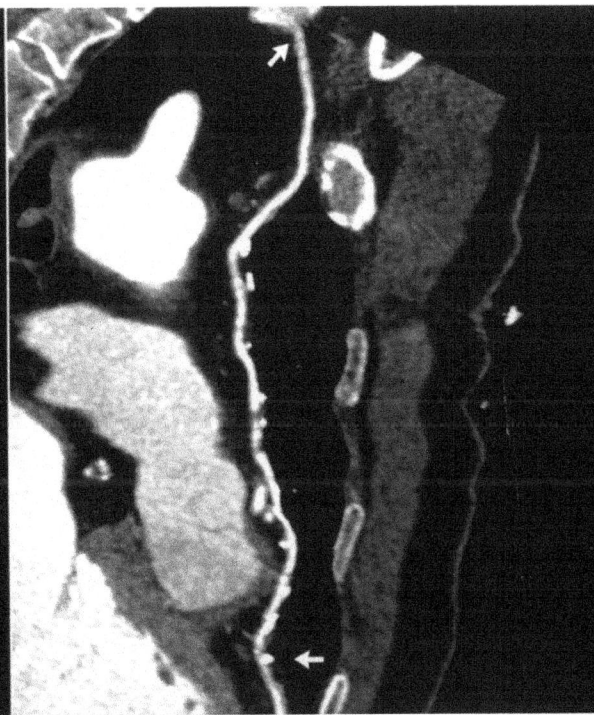

[3] Curved MPR of the vein graft to the OM1, showing a slight ostial stenosis and an atretic runoff. The myocardium supplied by this vessel appears hypoattenuating.

[4] Curved MPR of the LIMA, originating from the subclavian artery, and anastomosing with the LAD with satisfactory runoff. Note the surgical clips along the LIMA.

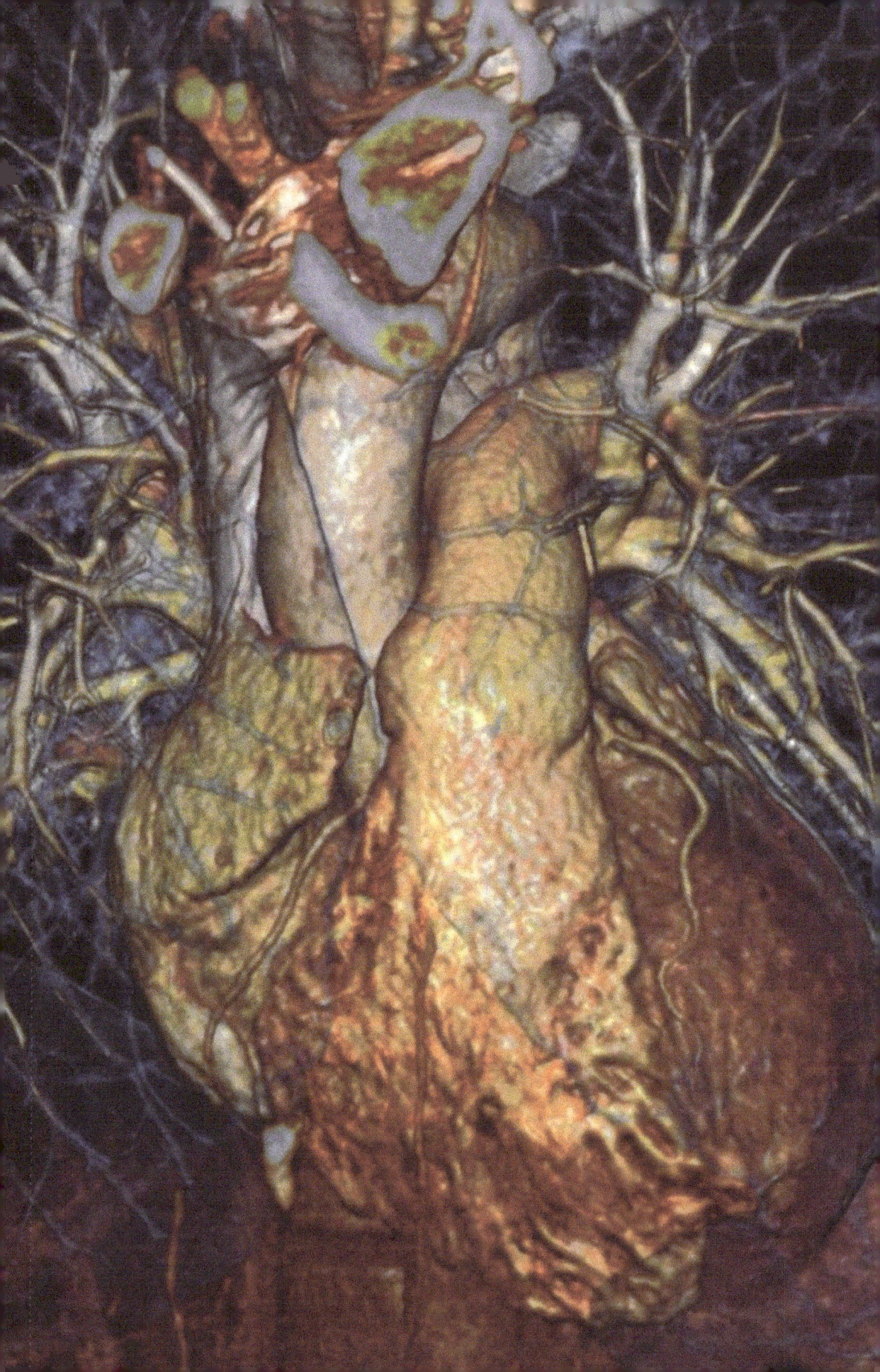

Vascular: Extended Chest Pain Protocol

Thorsten R. C. Johnson · Konstantin Nikolaou · Christoph R. Becker

Case 1: Ruling Out of Cardiovascular Causes in Acute Unclear Chest Pain

Case 2: 50-Year-Old Male with Unclear Chest Pain

The most important differential diagnoses of acute chest pain include myocardial infarction, aortic dissection or aneurysm and pulmonary embolism. The first diagnostic measures recommended by the American College of Emergency Physicians guidelines as well as the American College of Radiology Appropriateness Criteria on Acute Chest Pain are electrocardiograms (ECG) and serum cardiac markers. Further examinations, such as chest x-ray, ventilation/perfusion scan, resting myocardial perfusion scan, echocardiography, CT, aortic imaging or pulmonary angiography depend on the patient's history. However, patients' initial symptoms often do not display the characteristic signs, and the various examinations needed to make a diagnosis can be very time consuming and expensive. Therefore, examinations should focus initially on ruling out acute life-threatening conditions, including acute ischemic heart disease, aortic dissection and pulmonary embolism.

ECG-gated, CT angiography (CTA) protocols enable simultaneous assessment of pulmonary arteries, coronary arteries and the aorta within one single breathhold period. As a result, pulmonary embolism, coronary artery disease and aortic aneurysm or dissection can be ruled out in one combined examination. Many studies now show that it is feasible to evaluate these vascular territories simultaneously in one single breathhold scan and thereby identify the cause of chest pain with good sensitivity. Moreover, recent studies indicate that coronary CT angiography can be helpful for fast and cost-effective triage of chest pain patients. The images of coronary arteries acquired with ECG gating should have a similar diagnostic accuracy as a specific coronary CT angiography. However, conventional, single source CT scanners are limited in this approach, especially in acutely ill patients, due to the often reduced image quality of the coronary arteries in patients with high heart rates. Currently, the general practice is to administer beta-blockers to lower the heart rate for 16- and 64-slice CT scans. This approach is time consuming, limited by contraindications and the heart rate cannot be sufficiently reduced in many acutely ill patients.

Initial studies of Dual Source CT (DSCT) cardiac imaging have shown that it can provide robust image quality and very good diagnostic accuracy for coronary CT angiography even in high heart rates. In addition, DSCT makes more comprehensive cardiac assessment possible, including wall motion and valve function.[5]

Vascular: Extended Chest Pain Protocol

CT angiography is the modality of choice for assessing pulmonary embolism and aortic disease in acute care. The fast volume coverage that recent CT technology affords has triggered efforts to combine the evaluation of these pathologies. Adding an examination of the coronary arteries would make the DSCT protocol a universal tool for diagnosing chest pain. Many earlier studies showed the feasibility of this approach based on 64-slice CT technology with temporal resolution in the area of 165–200 ms. However, they also indicated that coronary CTA is still limited by higher heart rates, which are found frequently in this patient population.[1,2] More recent studies demonstrate that DSCT can obtain reliable diagnostic images of the coronary arteries even in high heart rates.[3,6] Based on these results, Dual Source CT was expected to greatly improve the diagnostic accuracy of the combined chest pain CT protocol, and our experience confirms that this assumption was correct. Recently, we evaluated 47 patients in a chest pain study using this combined protocol and found that robust image quality can be obtained even in acutely ill patients with high heart rates.[4] The diagnoses we observed were spread quite evenly over the different vascular territories: Eight patients were found to have pulmonary embolism and chronic secondary pulmonary hypertension. The majority of the patients were diagnosed with coronary pathologies: seventeen patients had coronary atherosclerosis, eleven patients presented significant stenoses, one case showed acute complete occlusion and three patients had recent myocardial infarction. One patient had a long segment of myocardial bridging and a systolic reconstruction was able to show a relevant compression. Three patients had valvular disorders. The aortic pathologies we observed included type A dissection and a long intramural hematoma. Of course, diagnoses were not limited to vascular causes of chest pain but also included pulmonary metastases, pneumonia, pneumothorax, pericardial or pleural effusions and esophageal cancer. Not one case of relevant coronary artery disease went overlooked in these patients, which affirms the diagnostic accuracy of DSCT. This modality can be used to reliably exclude coronary artery disease and will be helpful for fast patient triage. We must, however, acknowledge that stenoses are quite frequently rated as 'potentially relevant' in CTA so that invasive angiography remains necessary for definite diagnosis and intervention. In our study, one coronary artery stenosis was over-estimated at CTA and did not require intervention. The strength of CT is not necessarily to accurately grade stenoses, but to reliably rule out significant disease. The combined chest pain protocol does require a higher dose of radiation compared with sole coronary or aortic CTA. However, the alternative diagnostic approaches for evaluating chest pain (pulmonary CTA, aortic CTA and invasive coronary angiography) would result in a higher total patient dose.

In conclusion, the specific Dual Source CT protocol for chest pain assessment has proven to be a very helpful tool, offering a fast diagnostic workup and patient triage. Due to its heart rate insensitivity, DSCT further increases the diagnostic accuracy of coronary artery assessment.

Thorsten R. C. Johnson · Konstantin Nikolaou · Christoph R. Becker

University of Munich-Grosshadern

Department of Clinical Radiology

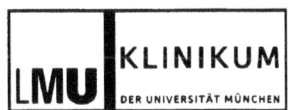

References

[1] Johnson TRC, Nikolaou K, Wintersperger BJ, Knez A, Boekstegers P, Reiser MF, Becker CR (2007) ECG gated 64 Slice CT Angiography for the Differential Diagnosis of Acute Chest Pain. AJR Am J Roentgenol 188:76-82

[2] Johnson TRC, Nikolaou K, Wintersperger BJ, Fink C, Rist C, Leber AW, Knez A, Reiser MF, Becker CR (2007) Optimization of Contrast Material Administration for Electrocardiogram-gated Computed Tomographic Angiography of the Chest. J Comput Assist Tomogr 31(2):265-71

[3] Johnson TR, Nikolaou K, Wintersperger BJ, Leber AW, von Ziegler F, Rist C, Buhmann S, Knez A, Reiser MF, Becker CR (2006) Dual-source CT cardiac imaging: initial experience. Eur Radiol 16:1409-1415

[4] Johnson TR, Nikolaou K, Fink C, Becker A, Knez A, Rist C, Reiser MF, Becker CR (2007) Dual-source CT in chest pain diagnosis. Radiologe 47(4):301-309

[5] White CS, Kuo D, Kelemen M, Jain V, Musk A, Zaidi E, Read K, Sliker C, Prasad R (2005) Chest pain evaluation in the emergency department: can MDCT provide a comprehensive evaluation? AJR Am J Roentgenol 185:533-540

[6] Schertler T, Scheffel H, Frauenfelder T, et al. (2007) Dual-source computed tomography in patients with acute chest pain: feasibility and image quality. Eur Radiol;17(12):3179-88

Vascular: Extended Chest Pain Protocol

Basic considerations

The aim of this contrast injection protocol is to achieve a simultaneous opacification of the whole vasculature of the chest to depict pulmonary arteries, coronary arteries and the aorta in one spiral scan. Therefore, a rather large bolus has to be injected at a comparably low rate. Bolus tracking in the ascending aorta ensures a sufficient opacification of pulmonary and coronary arteries. For the CT scan, ECG gating makes it possible to freeze the motion of the coronary arteries, the aortic root and the para-cardiac pulmonary vessels. Aggressive tube current modulation with MinDose™ helps to limit radiation exposure. Caudo-cranial scan direction helps to obtain good images of the heart at stable inspiration.

Scan Parameters

Scan mode	Dual Source, ECG-gated
Heart rate control	not necessary
Scan area	diaphragm to lung apex
Scan direction	caudo-cranial
Scan time	~10–18 s, depending on heart rate
Tube voltage	120 kV
Tube current	360 mAs/rotation
Dose modulation	ECG-pulsing on* with MinDose™
CTDI$_{vol}$	~40 mGy, depending on heart rate
Rotation time	0.33 s
Pitch	0.2–0.5, depending on heart rate
Slice collimation	0.6 mm
Acquisition	64 x 0.6 mm
Slice width	3 mm/0.75 mm for coronary arteries
Reconstruction increment	2.5 mm/0.4 mm for coronary arteries
Reconstruction kernel	B30f/B26f for coronary arteries

*Referring to ECG-pulsing table (see page 28)

Tricks

Plan the range precisely from the diaphragm to the lung apex to limit radiation exposure. Keep ECG cable connector out of scan range. Do not instruct patients to take a deep breath in, but just to hold their breath after mild inspiration. Reconstruct thin slices with a limited FoV of the heart to provide sufficient detail and stack of 3 mm images for assessment of the chest.

Pitfalls

Placing the ECG cable connector in the scan range causes ECG artifacts and failure to correctly gate the reconstruction. Fast and deep inspiration can interrupt the contrast bolus due to inflow of non-enhanced blood from the inferior vena cava, often causing insufficient pulmonary opacification.

Contrast Injection Protocol

	Iodine concentration 300 mg I/ml	Iodine concentration 370 mg I/ml
Injection scheme	Monophasic	Monophasic
Iodine delivery rate	1.7 g/s	1.7 g/s
CM volume	160 ml	130 ml
CM flow rate	5.7 ml/s	4.5 ml/s
Body weight adaption	yes	yes
Bolus timing	bolus tracking*	bolus tracking*
Bolus tracking threshold	200 HU	200 HU
ROI position	ascending aorta	ascending aorta
Scan delay	4 s	4 s
Saline flush volume	100 ml	100 ml
Saline injection rate	5.7 ml/s	4.5 ml/s
Needle size	18 G	18 G
Injection site	antecubital vein	antecubital vein

*Depending on the preference of the individual site, test bolus can be used as an alternative

Case 1 Ruling Out of Cardiovascular Causes in Acute Unclear Chest Pain

Case history

A 65-year-old female presents with unclear chest pain and dyspnea. The symptoms are non-specific. Initial troponin test and ECG are normal.

Question

Is there an acute cardiovascular condition requiring immediate intervention? Is there evidence of the cause of chest pain?

Diagnosis / Differential diagnosis

The most important and potentially life-threatening causes of chest pain can be assessed in this single-breathhold scan. These include pulmonary embolism, coronary artery stenosis, aortic dissection, pulmonary edema, pneumonia or pneumothorax.

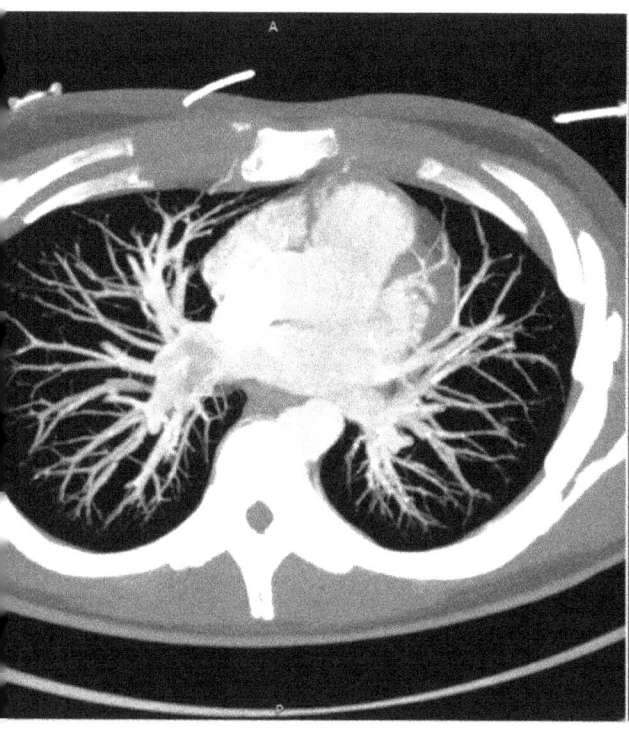

[1] The pulmonary arteries are well opacified and show no evidence of emboli.

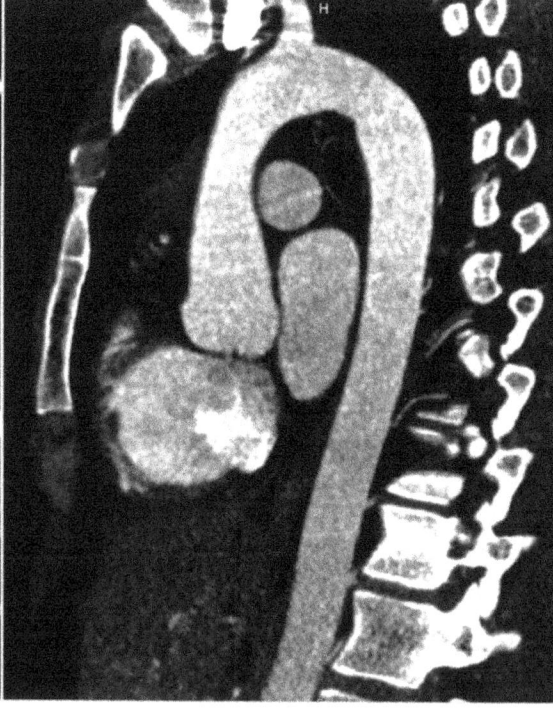

[2] The aorta is not enlarged. There is no dissection membrane.

Findings

Pulmonary embolism can be ruled out reliably in CT angiography. The image quality of the coronary arteries is sufficient to extract the whole coronary artery tree automatically and assess them with curved multiplanar reconstructions. Aortic dissection or aneursym can also be ruled out. The condition of the patient improves and she is discharged one day later without any specific intervention.

Take-home message

CT angiography can be used to rule out cardiovascular causes of chest pain and can thus provide a comprehensive and fast patient triage. This protocol can replace separate exams of the different vascular districts and thus help to reduce radiation exposure and the amount of required contrast material. The heart rate insensitivity of DSCT is very beneficial in these patients who frequently have high heart rates.

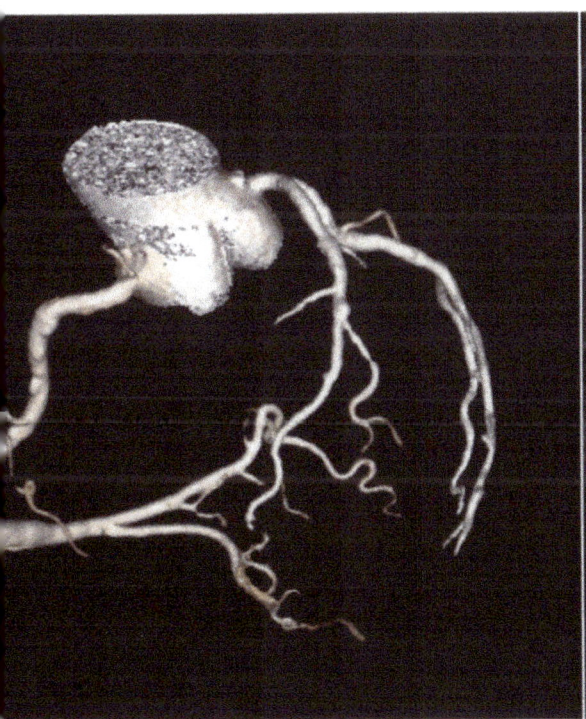

[3] The coronary arteries can be segmented automatically. There is no evidence of a stenosis or an occlusion.

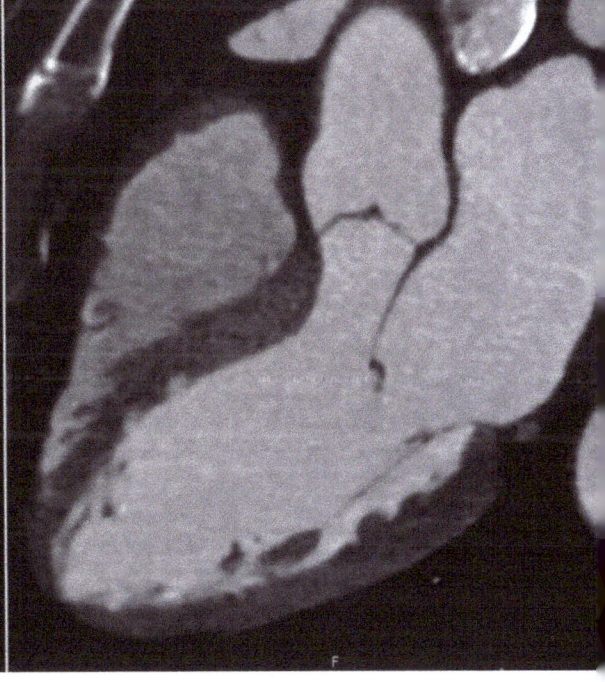

[4] The dynamic reconstruction shows a normal valve morphology and motion as well as no wall motion abnormalities.

Case 2 50-Year-Old Male with Unclear Chest Pain

Case history

A 50-year-old male with known coronary artery disease presents with acute chest pain two weeks after stenting of the left anterior descending coronary artery.

Question

Is the stent occluded? Is there a restenosis or another coronary artery stenosis? Is there another cause of chest pain?

Diagnosis / Differential diagnosis

The differential diagnoses in this patient with known coronary artery disease include stent thrombosis, in-stent restenosis due to intimal hyperplasia, other coronary artery stenosis or myocardial infarction and aortic or pulmonary causes.

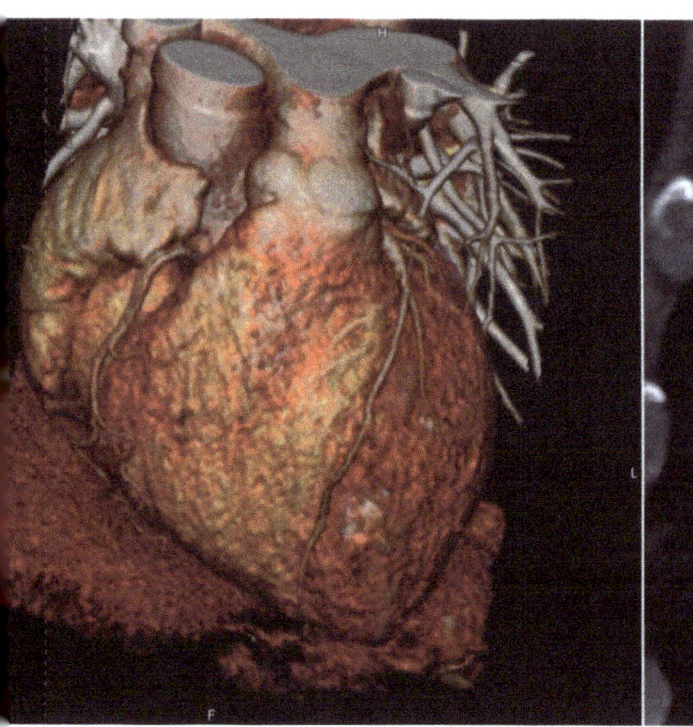

[1] Even at the high heart rate of 92 bpm, the heart is depicted without motion artifacts.

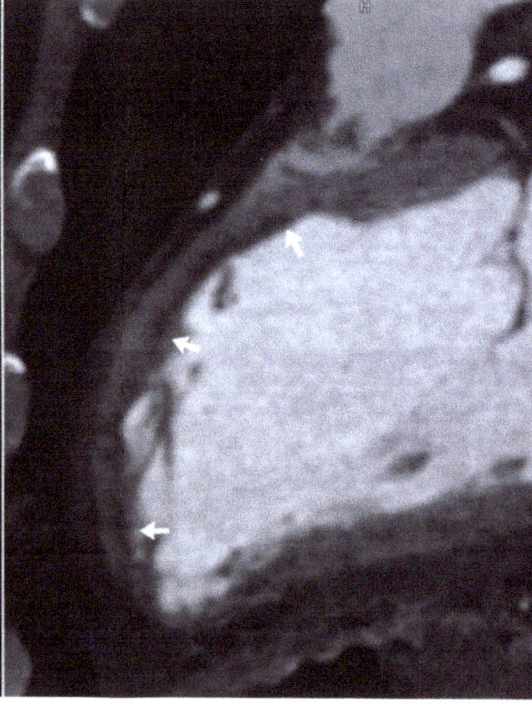

[2] The hypodense subendocardial area in the anterior wall of the left ventricle (arrows) corresponds to a scar from myocardial infarction.

Findings

CT angiography confirms stent patency. However, a non-transmural scar from infarction is evident in the anterior wall of the left ventricle, presumably due to the previously stented stenosis. Additionally, there is a moderate stenosis further distal in the LAD.

Take-home message

This comprehensive protocol not only provides high-detail morphology of the vasculature but also of the myocardium. Combined with dynamic information from multiphase reconstructions, many parameters of cardiac diseases can be assessed.

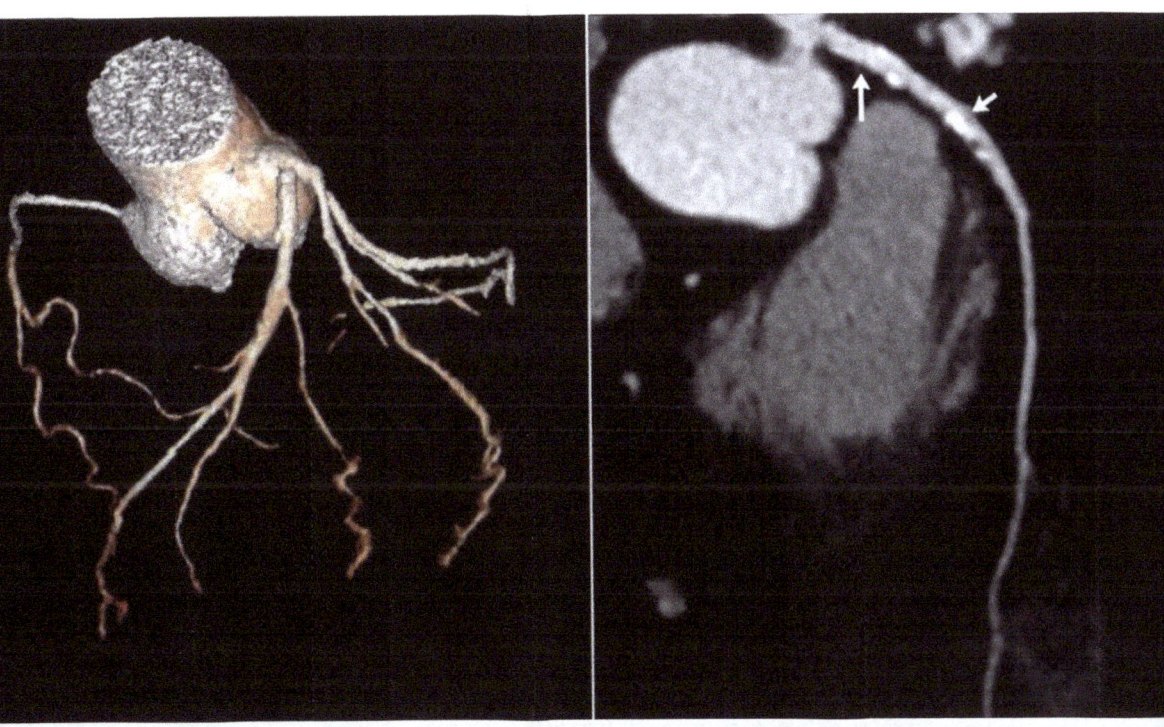

[3] The whole coronary artery tree can be extracted automatically using the *syngo* Circulation software (Siemens AG). There is no occlusion.

[4] A very radiolucent and fully patent stent is visible in the proximal LAD (arrows). Additionally there is a moderate, partly calcified stenosis further distal.

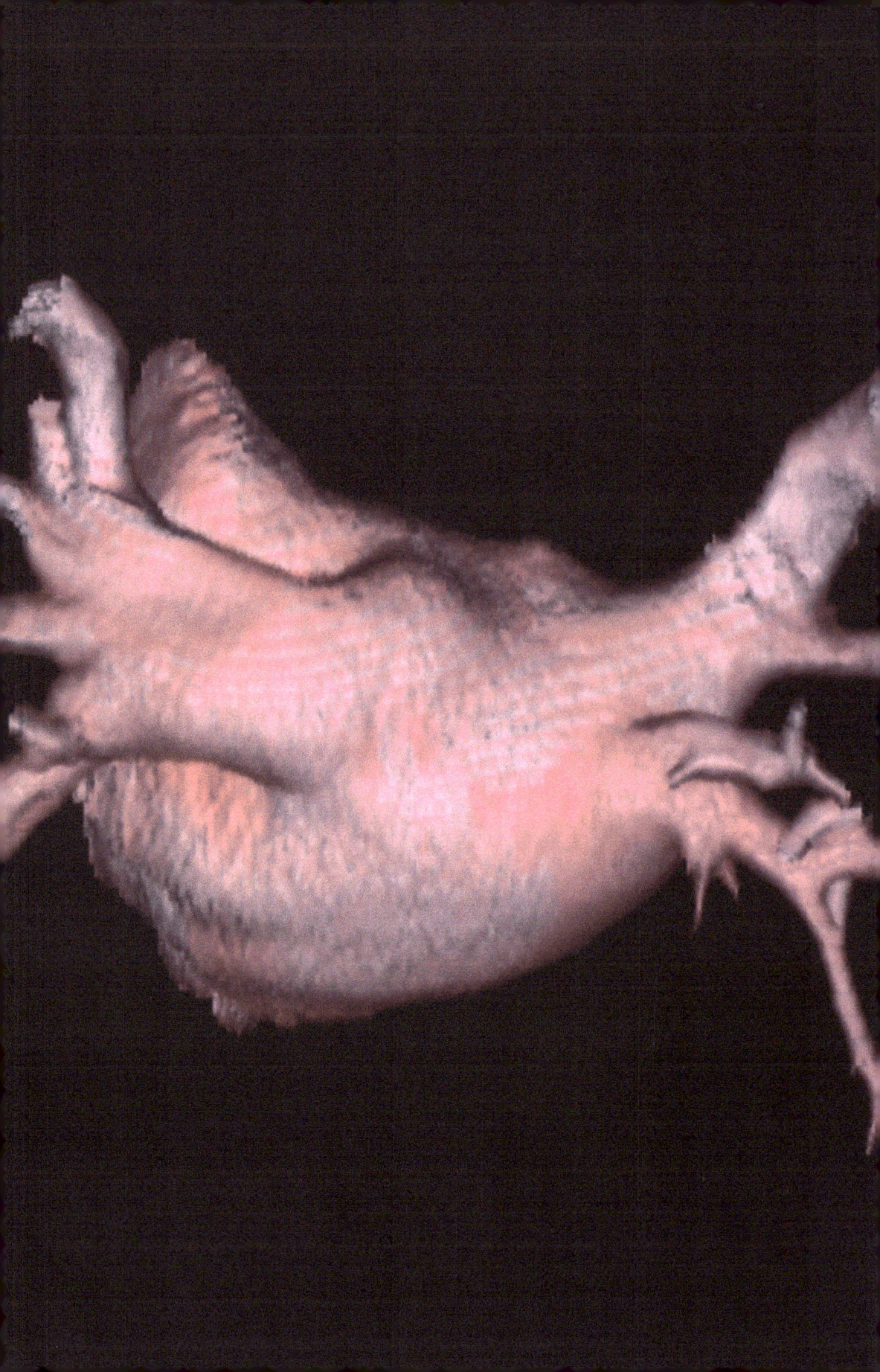

Vascular: Pulmonary Veins

Harald Brodoefel · Martin Heuschmid · Andreas F. Kopp

Case 1: Minor Pulmonary Vein Stenosis Post RFCA

Case 2: Significant Pulmonary Vein Stenosis

This chapter describes a Dual Source CT (DSCT) protocol for accurate visualization of the left atrium and pulmonary veins preceding and following radio-frequency catheter ablation for chronic atrial fibrillation (AF).

AF is the most common type of cardiac arrhythmia and an important contributor to cardiovascular morbidity and mortality.[1] The condition is classified into the acute and the chronic form, while the latter is subdivided into paroxysmal, persistent and permanent.[2]

While pharmacological AF management and cardioversion remain controversial, non-pharmacological interventions, notably radio-frequency catheter ablation (RFCA), have revolutionized the treatment of chronic AF.[3] The procedure is based on the perception that the pathophysiological mechanism of AF is frequently based on sources of ectopic atrial electric activity within the pulmonary veins.

In fact, ablation of these foci may be a curative approach. However, the procedure is subject to numerous limitations. This is especially true with the traditional technique which relies on electrophysiological identification and ablation of individual foci. Since multiple arrhythmogenic origins may be distributed over several veins, recurrence rates were found to be as high as 65%. A second strategy creates circumferential lesions at the venous ostia. It aims at complete electrical isolation of all pulmonary veins from the atrium and is associated with better outcome.

The rationale for using CT prior and post RFCA is threefold: First, the effectiveness of the technique is based on accurate mapping and complete disconnection of electrical foci from the atrial myocardium.[4] Hence, detailed knowledge of the pulmonary venous anatomy is required during ablation procedure. This includes information on number, location and angulation of the distal veins as well as the size of their ostia. Although venous or atrial anatomy was defined fluoroscopically in the past, CT has proven to be more accurate and time-saving.

Secondly, it has been shown that the pulmonary venous drainage pattern is not uniform and that variant anatomy is met in 31% to 38% of patients. While most patients will present with only two

Vascular: Pulmonary Veins

ostia for upper and lower lobe veins, Marom et al. identified three ostia as being the most frequent variant of the right pulmonary veins. On the left side, a common trunk and a single ostium for upper and lower lobe veins has been proven to be the most likely variation.[5]

With conventional pre-ablation assessment, many of the variant veins are not detected and may be the source of AF recurrence. CT has lately been appreciated as an excellent tool in the identification of variant venous anatomy and may, therefore, greatly enhance success rates of the procedure. At the same time, pre-interventional CT examination has proven its role in the exclusion of atrial thrombi, which are considered to be an absolute contraindication to the technique.

Finally, post-interventional CT is usually requested to rule out complications of RFCA. Thereby, potentially devastating complications such as pulmonary vein dissection or perforation, hemopericardium and stroke are very rare. By contrast, post-interventional stenosis of the distal pulmonary veins represents a distinct complication of RFCA and is reported to occur in 8.8–24% of the cases.[6] Hemodynamically significant stenosis may be linked to pulmonary veno-occlusive disease, including the development of pulmonary atrial hypertension. Since permanent stenosis of the ostia is the result of collagenous scar, CT should preferably be performed between 2 or 3 months following procedure.

Any CT protocol designed to visualize the distal pulmonary veins aims to deliver high contrast to the atrium and display the venous anatomy as motionless as possible. Indeed, with its unprecedented temporal resolution of a heart-rate-independent 83 ms, retrospectively gated DSCT has the potential to provide superior visualization of the ostia and distal veins. However, in a routine examination the use of such a high temporal resolution might not be necessary. While 4- or 16-slice CT still requires ECG-gating for elimination of motion artifacts, most investigators consider the temporal resolution of 64-slice systems to be high enough to provide accurate depiction of the atrium in a non-gated mode. In view of the difference between radiation dose of non-gated and gated DSCT, we therefore propose to primarily examine pulmonary veins in a non-gated single source mode. In this case, the scanner is virtually operated just like a 64-slice system and its temporal resolution is 165 ms. Exceptions to this first line approach may be severe tachycardia (above 100 bpm) in the absence of ventricular arrhythmia. Gating should then be performed according to the protocols outlined in the relevant chapters of this book. Notably, with use of retrospective gating, tube-current modulation is essential to limit radiation dose. The optimal phase for reconstruction will almost always be late diastole, in most cases between 60% or 70% of the cardiac cycle. In general, for maximum control of heart rate and conduction, we suggest administering beta blockers to any patient without contraindication.

To achieve optimal contrast in pulmonary veins and atrium, both bolus tracking and test bolus techniques will usually provide comparable results. Nevertheless, in case of arrhythmia, the test bolus is susceptible to changes in cardiac output. Therefore, bolus tracking should be preferred in this application.

For precise visualization of atrial anatomy, we suggest reconstructing between 0.75 to 2 mm MPRs in three orthogonal planes. Epicardial volume rendering as well as oblique coronal thin MIPs focused on the long axes of each pulmonary vein are valuable in the visualization of complex venous anatomy and the exact assessment of ostia. The latter should be measured in two perpendicular planes. In our institution, the Marom classification of venous drainage pattern has been adopted for reports and has greatly facilitated communication with the referring electrophysiologists.[5]

Harald Brodoefel · Martin Heuschmid · Andreas F. Kopp
Eberhard-Karls-University Tübingen
Department of Diagnostic and Interventional Radiology

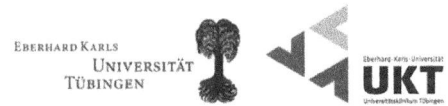

References

[1] McNamara RL, Tamariz LJ, Segal JB, Bass EB. Management of atrial fibrillation: review of the evidence for the role of pharmacologic therapy, electrical cardioversion, and echocardiography. Ann Intern Med. 2003;139:1018−1033

[2] Ryder KM, Benjamin EJ. Epidemiology and significance of atrial fibrillation. Am J Cardiol. 1999;84:131R−138R

[3] Marrouche NF, Dresing T, Cole C, et al. Circular mapping and ablation of the pulmonary vein for treatment of atrial fibrillation: impact of different catheter technologies. J Am Coll Cardiol. 2002;40:464−474

[4] Lacomis JM, Wigginton W, Fuhrman C, Schwartzman D, Armfield DR, Pealer KM. Multi-detector row CT of the left atrium and pulmonary veins before radio-frequency catheter ablation for atrial fibrillation. Radiographics. 2003;23 Spec No:35−48; discussion S48−50

[5] Marom EM, Herndon JE, Kim YH, McAdams HP. Variations in pulmonary venous drainage to the left atrium: implications for radiofrequency ablation. Radiology. 2004;230:824−829

[6] Jongbloed MR, Bax JJ, Lamb HJ, et al. Multislice computed tomography versus intracardiac echocardiography to evaluate the pulmonary veins before radiofrequency catheter ablation of atrial fibrillation: a head-to-head comparison. J Am Coll Cardiol. 2005;45:343−350

Vascular: Pulmonary Veins

Basic considerations

When compared to other cardiac applications, examination of pulmonary veins follows a fairly straightforward, easy and highly robust protocol. The reasons for this robustness are twofold: First, since the target vessels are large and controlled, washout from the right ventricle is not an issue and considerations regarding contrast kinetics are of minor importance. Second, heart beat induced atrium motion is only small in comparison to coronary arteries. Hence, motion artifacts are a less significant issue and the examination may primarily be performed in a non-gated single source mode. Use of 100 kV/180 mAs may be considered in patients with low body weight (BMI < 25).

Scan Parameters

Scan mode	Single Source, non-gated
Heart rate control	not necessary
Scan area	tracheal bifurcation to diaphragm
Scan direction	cranio-caudal
Scan time	~5 s
Tube voltage	120 kV
Tube current	140 quality ref. mAs
Dose modulation	CARE Dose4D
CTDI$_{vol}$	~10 mGy
Rotation time	0.33 s
Pitch	1
Slice collimation	0.6 mm
Acquisition	64 x 0.6 mm
Slice width	1–2 mm for heart / 3 mm for lung
Reconstruction increment	0.7–1.5 mm for heart / 2.5 mm for lung
Reconstruction kernel	B30f

Tricks

· Gated exams should be reserved for patients with severe tachycardia and sinus-rhythm or regular conduction.
· With highly irregular conduction, non-gated scan should be preferred 'irrespective of patients' heart rate.

Pitfalls

In principle, both bolus tracking or test bolus may be used for timing of the contrast injection. However, in case of irregular heart beat, cardiac output may change rapidly and test bolus procedure may provide insufficient results. Therefore, we suggest using bolus tracking in these patients.

Contrast Injection Protocol

	Iodine concentration 300 mg I/ml	Iodine concentration 370 mg I/ml
Injection scheme	Monophasic	Monophasic
Iodine delivery rate	1.48 g/s	1.48 g/s
CM volume	85 ml	70 ml
CM flow rate	4.9 ml/s	4 ml/s
Body weight adaption	no	no
Bolus timing	bolus tracking*	bolus tracking*
Bolus tracking threshold	130 HU	130 HU
ROI position	left atrium	left atrium
Scan delay	2 s	2 s
Saline flush volume	60 ml	60 ml
Saline injection rate	4.9 ml/s	4 ml/s
Needle size	18 G	18 G
Injection site	antecubital vein	antecubital vein

*Depending on the preference of the individual site, test bolus can be used as an alternative

Case 1 Minor Pulmonary Vein Stenosis Post RFCA

Case history

Six weeks after circumferential ablation of all PVs a 48-year-old male is referred to CT for follow-up. On CT examination, the patient was not in AF and heart rate was 68 bpm.

Question

Presence of post-interventional pulmonary vein stenosis. Exclusion of rare complications such as atrial thrombi or pulmonary vein dissection.

Diagnosis/Differential diagnosis

· Common pulmonary venous drainage pattern with exclusion of variant veins.
· Post-interventional non-significant stenosis of the upper right pulmonary vein.
· Normal presentation of all other ostia and exclusion of atrial thrombi.

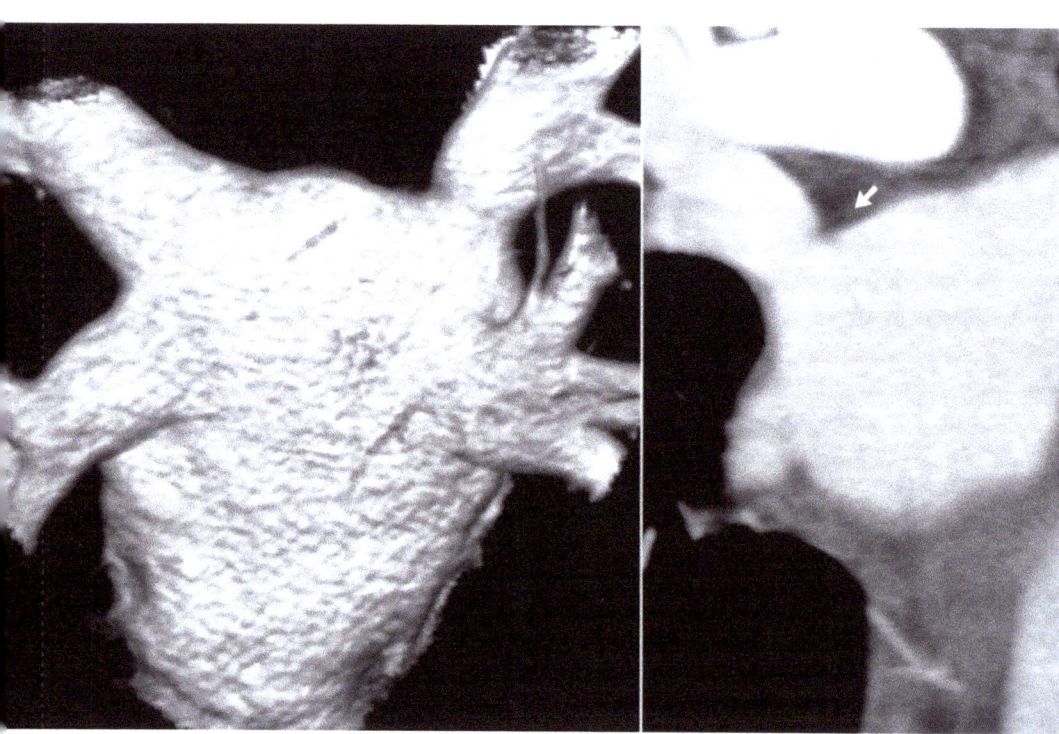

[1] Epicardial VR of the left atrium.

[2] Coronal MIP is showing a mild, non-relevant post-interventional lumen narrowing of the right upper pulmonary vein (arrow). The lower left pulmonary vein is visualized without pathology.

Findings

The epicardial volume rendering shows a normal pulmonary venous drainage pattern without variant ostia. Thin MIPs which are focused on the long axes of pulmonary veins reveal a non-significant post-interventional stenosis of the upper right pulmonary vein (arrow). Normal venous ostia are shown for the lower right and the upper left pulmonary vein.

Take-home message

Even in a non-gated single source mode, Dual Source CT provides excellent image quality and, thereby, allows for accurate depiction of left atrial anatomy or proximal pulmonary veins.

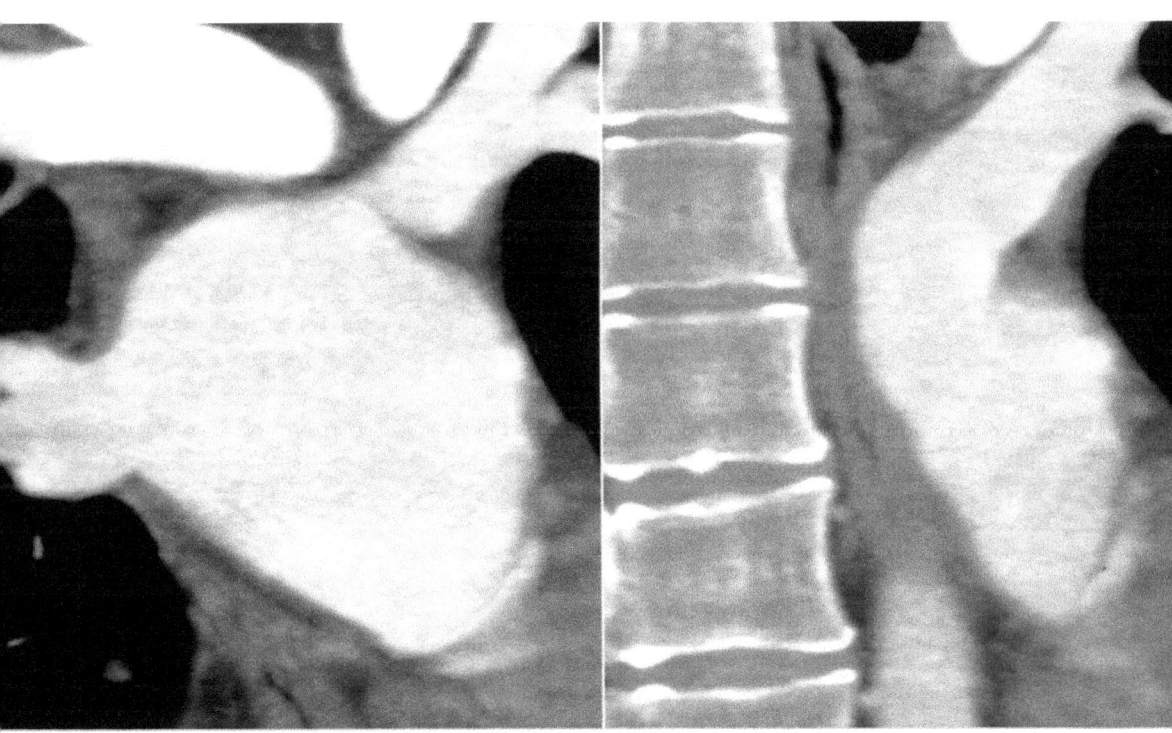

[3] Angulated MIP displaying the lower right pulmonary vein.

[4] Angulated MIP showing the normal upper left vein.

Case 2 Significant Pulmonary Vein Stenosis

Case history

Following successful RFCA a 51-year-old female was presented to CT for exclusion of pulmonary vein stenosis. The patient was clinically asymptomatic.

Question

Presence of post-interventional pulmonary vein stenosis or exclusion of further complications.

Diagnosis / Differential diagnosis

· Post-procedural 70% high grade stenosis of the proximal upper left pulmonary vein.
· No evidence of further post-procedural complications, including arterial thrombi.
· Separate ostium for the right middle lobe vein.

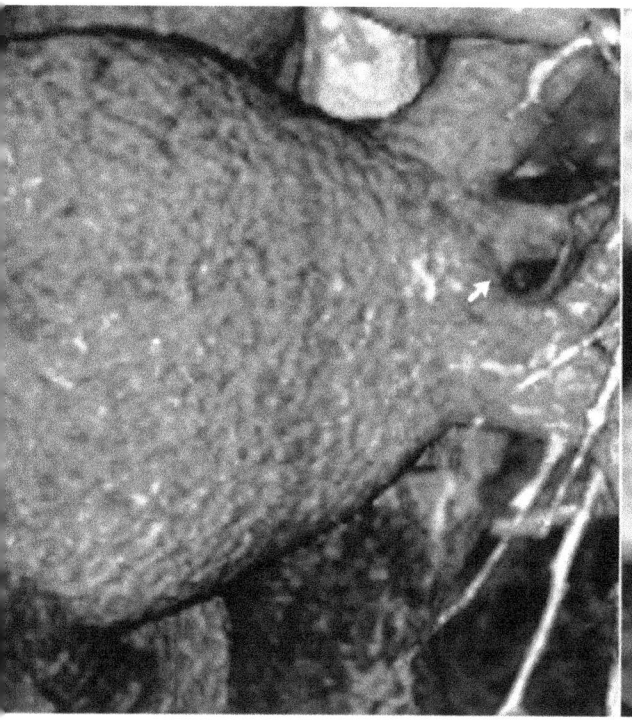

[1] Epicardial VR of the left atrium. The arrow hints at a variant vein on the right side, notably an additional ostium for the middle lobe vein (see arrow).

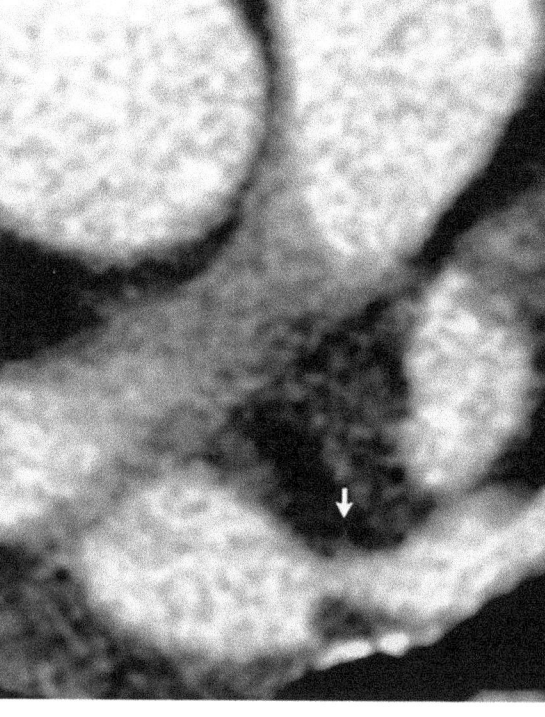

[2] Axial MPR showing a high-grade stenosis of the upper left pulmonary vein (arrow).

Findings

The epicardial volume renderings reveal separate ostia for upper, middle (arrow) and lower lobe veins on the right side. Axial and parasagittal MPRs reveal a high grade stenosis of the upper left pulmonary vein.

Take-home message

CT proves to be a reliable tool for detection of post-interventional complications such as stenosis of pulmonary veins.

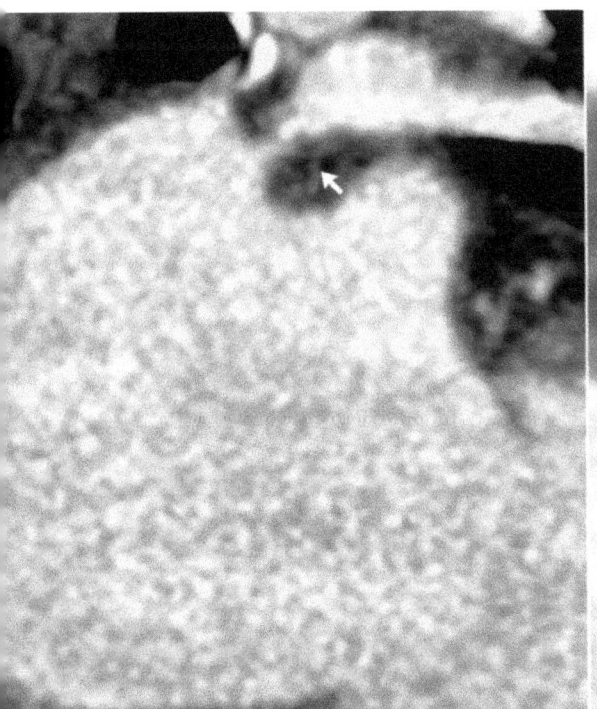
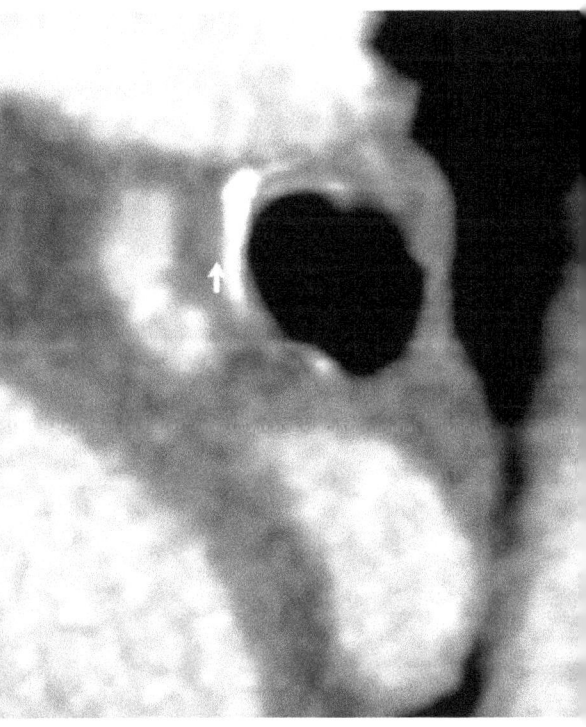

[3] MPR angulated on the main axis of the upper left pulmonary vein (arrow).

[4] Parasagittal MPR, orthogonal to the main axis of the vessel (see arrow).

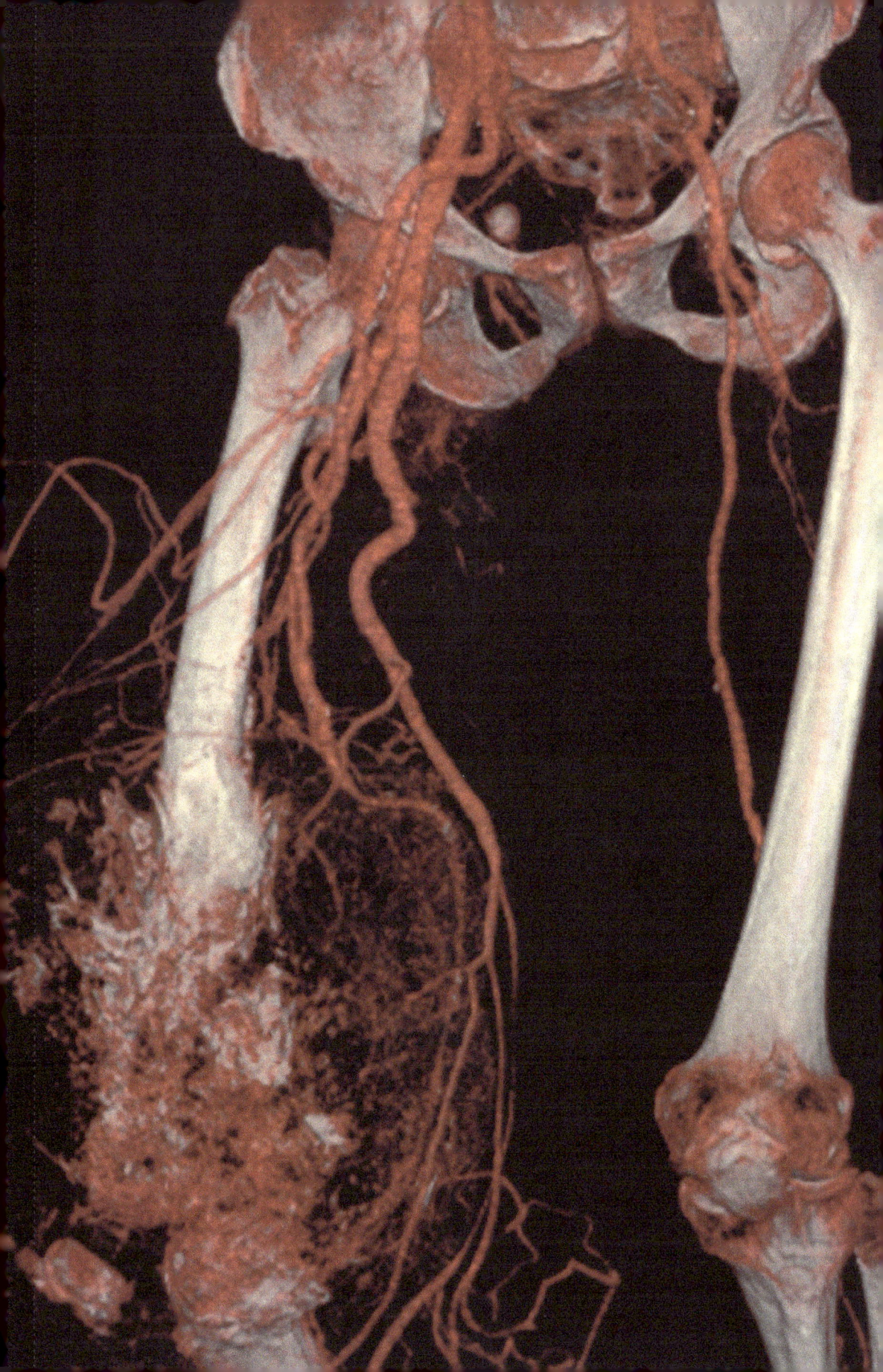

Vascular: Aortic Runoff, Abdominal CTA

Andreas H. Mahnken · Joachim E. Wildberger · Marco Das

Case 1: Follow-Up After Transarterial Embolization of a Liver Metastasis
Case 2: Assessment of Peripheral Artery Disease

With the introduction of multislice spiral computed tomography (MSCT) there has been an exponential increase in computed tomography (CT) angiography. Over the last decade MSCT angiography made up for invasive aortic angiography. Currently, diagnostic catheter angiograms of the visceral and peripheral arteries are gradually replaced by non-invasive imaging techniques such as MSCT. The high spatial resolution along the z-axis and, in particular, the tremendously improved image acquisition rate of MSCT fostered this development. Rapid scanning allows data acquisition during optimal opacification of the visceral as well as the peripheral vessels from a single intravenous injection of contrast material. Simultaneously efficient post-processing tools were introduced in clinical routine.[1] The nearly ubiquitous availability of MSCT scanners, examination speed and the ease of use made MSCT angiography a routine tool that provides high quality vessel imaging during 24-h a day.

When compared with Magnetic Resonance (MR) imaging, this technique is considered advantageous with respect to therapeutic confidence and costs for the initial evaluation of peripheral artery disease.[2] Moreover, MSCT also requires less investment costs for equipment. However, the accuracy of MSCT angiography is limited in heavily calcified vessels.[3]

Radiation exposure is another commonly stated drawback of MSCT angiography. Consequently, there is a strong demand for dose reduction techniques. Nowadays there are dedicated tools for reduction of radiation exposure during MSCT scanning. Nevertheless, the most efficient way to reduce radiation exposure is to limit the scan volume. The use of individually body-weight-adapted examination protocols is another easy way of reducing radiation exposure. Recently automated attenuation-based tube current modulation algorithms have been implemented. Second generation tube current modulation algorithms permit automated adjustment of the tube current in the x-y plane as well as along the patient's z-axis. Several studies have shown an up to 60% dose reduction applying these techniques. Effect of these techniques depends on the anatomical region and the individual patient's physique. Ongoing studies further reduce radiation exposure by decreasing tube voltage. An appreciated side effect of this particular approach is the improved iodine contrast due to optimized attenuation values.

Vascular: Aortic Runoff, Abdominal CTA

Slice-by-slice assessment of the axial source images in CT angiography is inadequate and daunting. The assessment of volumetric MSCT angiography data asks for advanced visualization strategies. With isotropic voxel size in high resolution CT scans, multiplanar reformats (MPR) and maximum intensity projections (MIP) became the methods of choice for routine assessment of the visceral and peripheral arteries from contrast enhanced MSCT datasets. Additional 3D-volume rendering (VRT) provides a helpful overview in the presence of complex or anomalous anatomy. This technique is also helpful for demonstration of vascular pathology to the referring physician. Over the last few years methods for semi-automated and fully automated segmentation of the peripheral arteries were introduced. Vessel tracking, calculation of orthogonal arterial diameters and bone removal became clinical routine. These techniques facilitate data assessment and presentation.

An increasing range of indications have been established for abdominal and peripheral MSCT angio-graphy.[4,5] Most common indications include evaluation of acute and chronic ischemia. Several studies indicated excellent sensitivities and specificities for detecting and grading stenoses including popliteo-crural arteries. From a clinical point of view the assessment of vascular injuries is one of the most relevant indications for MSCT angiography of the abdomen or the peripheral arteries. Indications for MSCT angiography in trauma patients include abnormal distal pulses, signs of hemorrhage, limb ischemia, or a penetrating injury. Post-interventional vascular surveillance is another major indication of MSCT angiography. While Duplex ultrasound is the first line method for postoperative vessel imaging, MSCT is emerging as an alternative that is particularly useful for assessing the entire course of extra-anatomical arterial bypass grafts which may be difficult to evaluate with Duplex ultrasound. Further relevant indications cover assessment of arterial aneurysms, congenital abnormalities, inflammatory conditions and arterial embolism.

Recently, Dual Source Computed Tomography (DSCT) was introduced. This new technology is capable of simultaneously acquiring data with two tube-detector systems with a 90° angular offset between both acquisition systems. By focusing on dual energy imaging and cardiac CT, one often forgets that DSCT scanners also include a high performance 64-slice CT system for state-of-the-art vascular imaging. Combining the power of both x-ray sources offers relevant advantages for vascular imaging in obese patients. Nevertheless, single source scan modes are not obsolete. They offer some inherent advantages like a consistent noise distribution because of homogeneous dose utilization across the full field-of-view.

However, even with the most advanced hardware the key towards a successful CT angiography remains optimization of the scanning procedure in combination with an individually tailored contrast injection protocol. Particular attention has to be paid to the numerous factors which influence bolus geometry and vessel opacification.[6] These factors amount to a wide inter-individual range of the time from the venous injection site to the arterial volume of interest. This is particularly true in patients with cardiac disease. Peripheral artery obstruction as well as dilatative arteriopathy also affect contrast arrival time. Therefore, a fixed scanning delay cannot be recommended for MSCT angiography. For optimal image quality, the individual patient's contrast medium arrival time should be determined using a test bolus or applying a bolus-tracking technique. Another noteworthy fact is that biphasic contrast material injections typically result in more uniform contrast enhancement over time. This is particularly relevant for long scan and injection times. Finally, these considerations should result in an ideal contrast injection protocol, producing a uniform, prolonged arterial contrast enhancement that is perfectly synchronized to the scanning duration.

Attention to proper patient preparation and patient positioning is a matter of course. Optimized image acquisition has to be combined with the best suited post-processing technique to fully utilize the potential of current CT technology. As peripheral MSCT angiography acquisition parameters generally follow those of abdominal MSCT angiography, this chapter summarizes the basic steps on the way to a high quality DSCT angiography of both visceral and peripheral arteries.

Andreas H. Mahnken · Joachim E. Wildberger · Marco Das
University Hospital, RWTH Aachen University
Department of Diagnostic Radiology

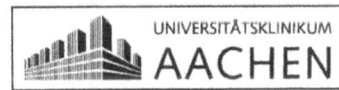

References

[1] Fleischmann D, Hallett RL, Rubin GD. CT angiography of peripheral arterial disease. J Vasc Interv Radiol 2006;17:3–26

[2] Ouwendijk R, de Vries M, Pattynama PM, et al. Imaging peripheral arterial disease: a randomized controlled trial comparing contrast-enhanced MR angiography and multi-detector row CT angiography. Radiology 2005; 236:1094–1103

[3] Willmann JK, Baumert B, Schertler T, et al. Aortoiliac and lower extremity arteries assessed with 16-detector row CT angiography: prospective comparison with digital subtraction angiography.

Radiology 2005;236:1083–1093

[4] Guven K, Acunas B. Multidetector computed tomography angiography of the abdomen. Eur J Radiol 2004;52:44–55

[5] Hiatt MD, Fleischmann D, Hellinger JC, Rubin GD. Angiographic imaging of the lower extremities with multidetector CT. Radiol Clin North Am 2005;43:1119–1127

[6] Cademartiri F, van der Lugt A, Luccichenti G, Pavone P, Krestin GP. Parameters affecting bolus geometry in CTA: a review. J Comput Assist Tomogr 2002;26:598–607

Vascular: Aortic Runoff, Abdominal CTA

Basic considerations

Abdominal and peripheral CTA are robust techniques for elective and emergency indications. Examinations require 10 to 15 minutes of room time. Assessment of small peripheral vessels requires a high spatial resolution. We recommend the acquisition of a thin collimated raw dataset. To achieve optimal and reliable contrast enhancement, biphasic injection protocols are preferred as they result in more uniform attenuation, especially if long scan times are needed. The contrast injection time should be about 10% longer than the scan time in order to ensure sufficient contrast enhancement along the entire scan volume.

Scan Parameters

Scan mode	Single Source, non-gated
Scan area	depending on indication
Scan direction	cranio-caudal
Scan time	depending on indication
Tube voltage	120 kV
Tube current	180 quality ref. mAs
Dose modulation	CARE Dose4D
CTDI$_{vol}$	~13 mGy
Rotation time	0.5 s
Pitch	1.2
Slice collimation	0.6 mm
Acquisition	64 x 0.6 mm
Slice width	0.75 mm
Reconstruction increment	0.4 mm
Reconstruction kernel	B31f

Tricks

Align the patient's legs and feet close to the isocenter of the scanner and keep the FoV as small as possible. In case of suspected arterial occlusion, the use of repeated test-bolus scans (instead of bolus tracking) above and below the level of occlusion may help to optimize contrast timing and avoid outrunning the bolus. Automated tube current modulation should be used to minimize radiation.

Pitfalls

High attenuation objects, e.g. calcifications may mimic stenosis due to blooming artifacts. Window adjustment with window widths up to 1500 HU is most effective to avoid this problem. Editing artifacts like inadvertent vessel removal or inaccurate centerline definition are other relevant pitfalls. These artifacts can be identified with additional views or review of source images.

Contrast Injection Protocol

	Iodine concentration 300 mg I/ml	Iodine concentration 370 mg I/ml
Injection scheme	Biphasic	Biphasic
Iodine delivery rate	1.85 g/s, 1.48 g/s	1.85 g/s, 1.48 g/s
CM volume	scan time x 6.2 ml/s	scan time x 5 ml/s
CM flow rate	6.2 ml/s, 4.9 ml/s	5 ml/s, 4 ml/s
Body weight adaption	no	no
Bolus timing	bolus tracking*	bolus tracking*
Bolus tracking threshold	180 HU	180 HU
ROI position	juxtarenal aorta	juxtarenal aorta
Scan delay	7 s	7 s
Saline flush volume	60 ml	60 ml
Saline injection rate	4.9 ml/s	4 ml/s
Needle size	18 G	18 G
Injection site	antecubital vein	antecubital vein

*Depending on the preference of the individual site, test bolus can be used as an alternative

Case 1 Follow-Up After Transarterial Embolization of a Liver Metastasis

Case history

72-year-old female with a history of uterine leiomyosarcoma and repeated surgery for liver metastases.

Question

Prior to hepatic radiofrequency ablation the extent of residual viable tumor and the status of the hepatic vasculature had to be assessed.

Diagnosis / Differential diagnosis

· Widely necrotic metastasis of a uterine leiomyosarcoma.
· Vascular occlusion (arrows) after embolization therapy.
· Normal anatomy of the hepatic artery without variants.

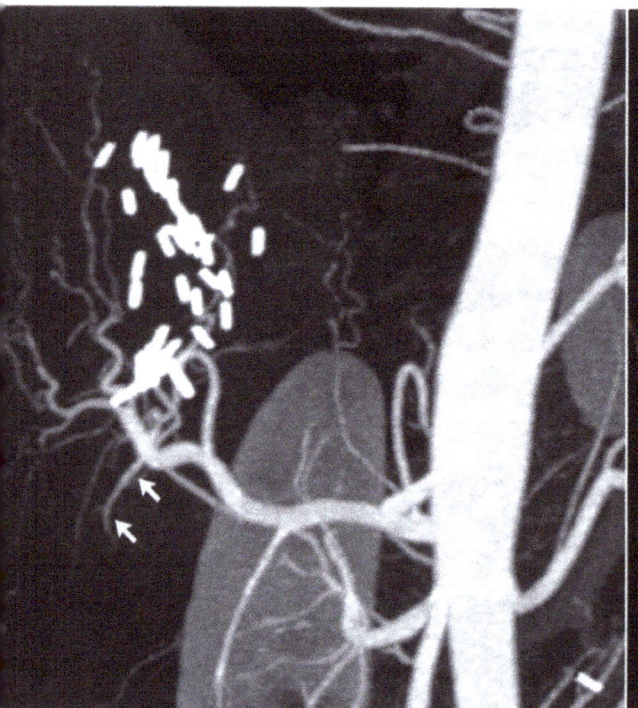 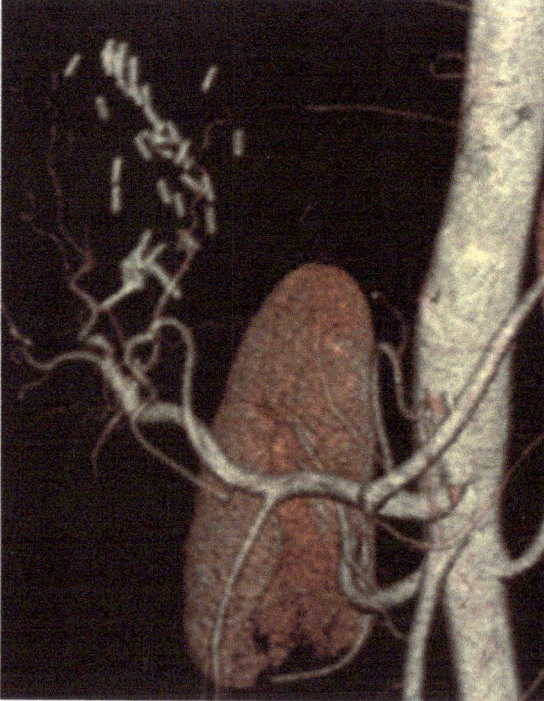

[1] Maximum intensity projection (MIP) computed from the arterial phase CT data shows the embolized segment artery VI (arrows).

[2] 3D-volume rendering (VRT) provides a three-dimensional overview of the hepatic vasculature. After previous surgery multiple clips can be identified.

Findings

Solitary liver metastasis with small areas of viable tumor after transarterial embolization and a normal anatomy of the hepatic artery. The segment VI artery is occluded after embolization. After previous liver surgery multiple clips are present.

Take-home message

Applying a single tube mode, Dual Source CT provides excellent visceral angiography datasets. This technique is suited for the assessment of the visceral arteries as well as the assessment of soft tissue tumors.

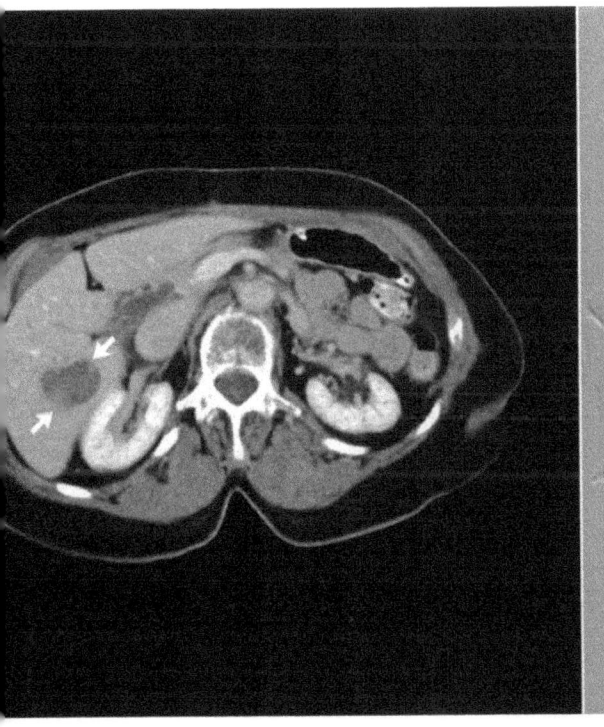

[3] Venous phase image shows small viable parts of the previously embolized metastasis (arrows).

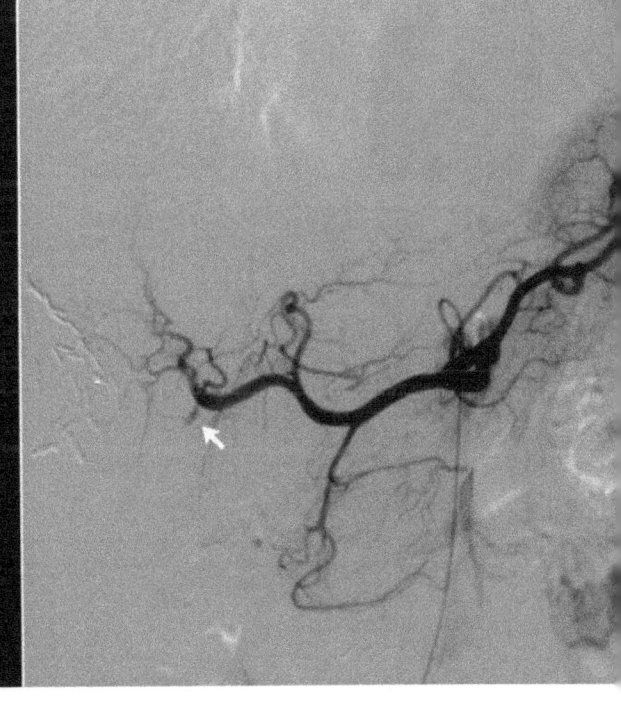

[4] The DSCT findings correlate well with the invasive angiogram. After selective embolization the segment VI artery is occluded (arrow).

Case 2 Assessment of Peripheral Artery Disease

Case history

68-year-old male with a history of peripheral artery disease and aorto-femoral bypass surgery. The patient presented with left sided claudication.

Question

CT angiography was requested to assess bypass patency and to exclude further significant ortho-periphery artery stenosis.

Diagnosis / Differential diagnosis

· Occlusive peripheral artery disease with extensive arterial calcification.
· Patent aorto-femoral bypass graft on the right side (arrows).
· Chronic occlusion of the distal left superficial femoral artery (arrows) with distinct collateral vessels.

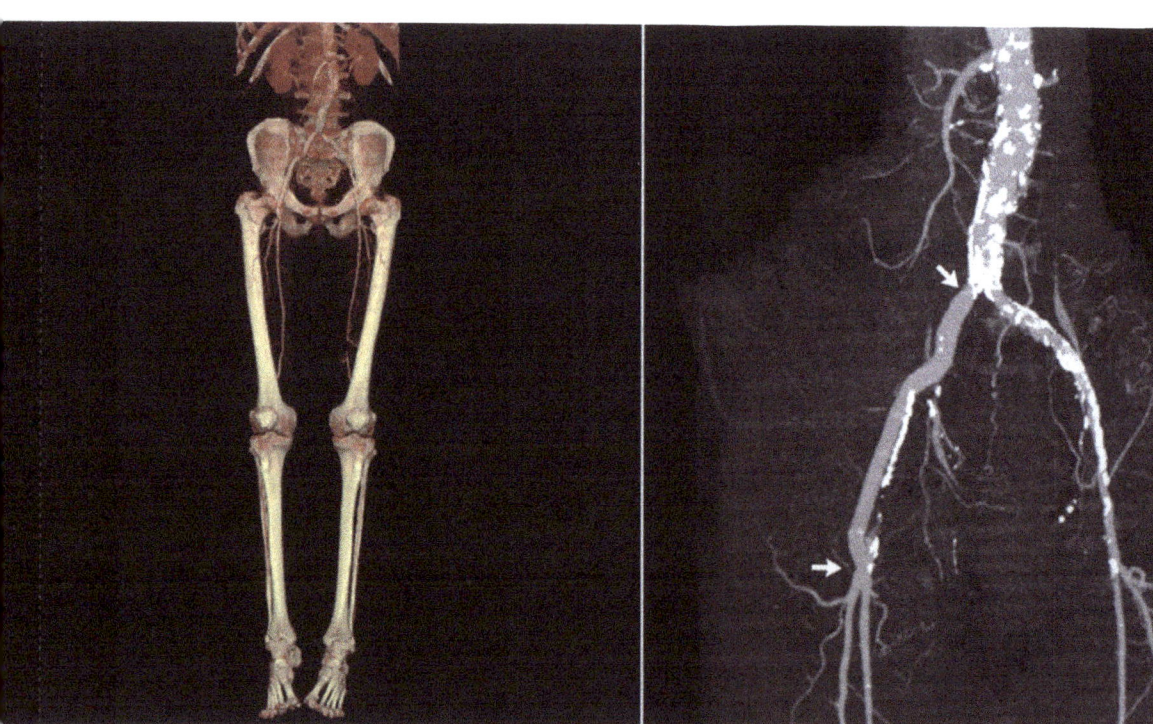

[1] 3D-volume rendering of the abdominal aorta and the peripheral lower limb arteries provides an overview on anatomy and pathology.

[2] After bone removal the course of an aorto-femoral bypass graft is depicted. The proximal as well as the distal anastomosis are patent (arrows).

Findings

CT shows a patent right sided aorto-femoral xenograft with patent anastomoses. The infrarenal aorta as well as the pelvic and lower limb arteries present with calcifications. There is a chronic occlusion of the left superior femoral artery with several collateral vessels.

Take-home message

Utilizing only a single tube-detector system, Dual Source CT is as powerful as 64-slice CT for assessing peripheral artery disease. This technique provides excellent image quality and allows an accurate and reliable assessment of the peripheral arteries of the upper and the lower extremities.

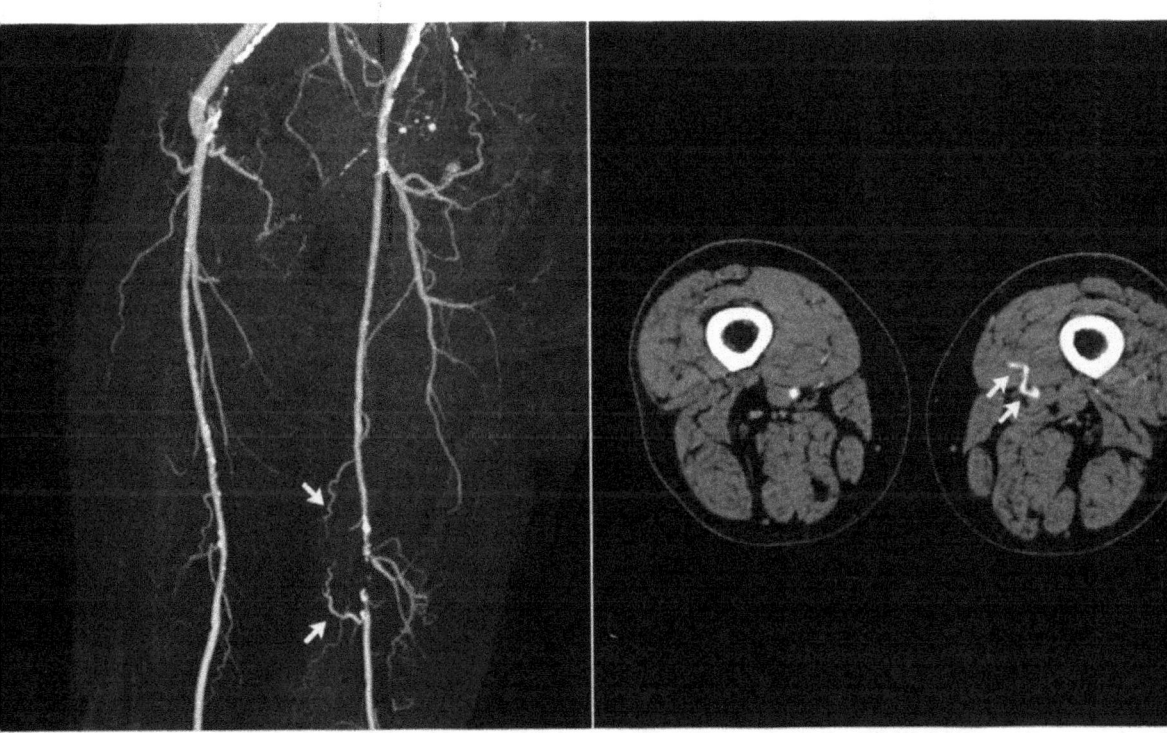

[3] Maximum intensity projection reveals an occlusion of the distal left superior femoral artery. CT also depicts some collateral vessels (arrows).

[4] The axial source image shows the origin of a collateral vessel from the superior femoral artery (arrows).

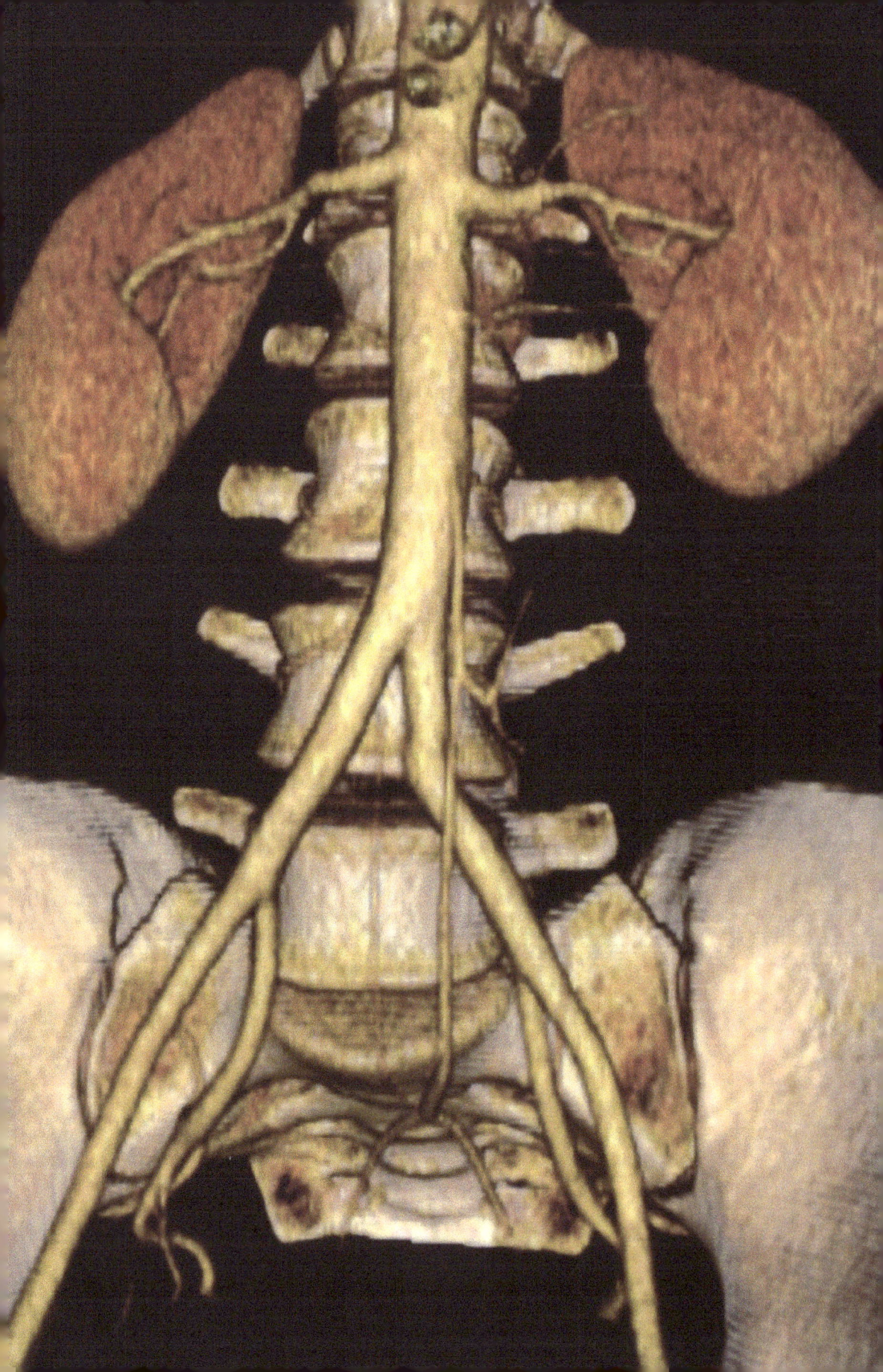

Vascular: Renal CTA

Robert P. Hartman · Terri J. Vrtiska · Cynthia McCollough

Case 1: Renal Artery Dissection

Case 2: Living Renal Donor

Computed tomography angiography (CTA) plays an integral role in the pre-operative evaluation of patients for donor nephrectomies. It can also be useful in the evaluation of patients with hypertension suspected to be caused by renal artery stenosis (RAS). Examinations including plain film intravenous urography for the detection of stones and renal masses combined with catheter-directed conventional angiography for depicting the renal arterial supply were once common in pre-operative evaluations. Recently, protocols including MR angiography (MRA) and CTA have been instituted at many centers. These provide all of the necessary information and are less invasive.

CT renal donor protocols have become particularly useful with advances in scanner technology, including high-speed multi-detector computed tomography (MDCT) which provides contiguous thin-slice axial images. These datasets can then be reconstructed into multiple planes for the evaluation of the kidneys, renal arteries and veins. In addition, the data can be processed to obtain 3-D volume rendered images capable of providing an overall anatomic depiction of the aorta, renal arteries, kidneys and renal veins, which improves pre-operative surgical planning for the removal of the donor kidney. This has become especially useful in recent years as laparoscopic donor nephrectomies are being performed. Given the limited area of visualization during a laparoscopic procedure, the vascular anatomy including tiny accessory arteries and veins need to be identified.[1]

Patients presenting for renal donor evaluation are particularly suited for CT with renal CTA. In general, these patients are younger and in good health. Their kidney function is usually normal without contraindications for the administration of iodinated contrast or particular concern for the development of contrast induced nephropathy. CT for the evaluation of a potential donor is useful given its ability to identify all possible findings related to the kidney itself that may preclude an individual from donation. These include renal malignancy, polycystic kidney disease, and in some institutions, multiple renal stones.

Multi-detector CTA using thin collimation and slice thickness provides datasets with high spatial resolution to depict the aorta and renal arteries.[2] CTA of the renal arteries using a 64-channel MDCT provides a complete evaluation of the abdominal aorta and renal arteries and is performed in less than 10 seconds with sub-millimeter spatial resolution.

Vascular: Renal CTA

Using protocols capable of scanning the entire abdomen in a single breathhold, CTA is adept at the identification of tiny accessory arteries arising anywhere along the course of the aorta from the diaphragm through the proximal iliac arteries. The identification of these accessory renal arteries is important for surgical planning as their presence may exclude one of the two kidneys from explantation.

Abnormalities of the renal arteries themselves including atherosclerotic disease and fibromuscular dysplasia (FMD) are easily depicted. The presence of atherosclerosis and subsequent stenosis of the renal artery can be identified, and in many cases, graded with accuracy.[3] Additionally, the higher spatial resolution of CTA over MRA allows for detection of more mild changes from fibromuscular dysplasia. This ability of CTA provides information to the clinician that may be used either to disqualify the patient as a donor or to initiate pre-transplant therapy such as angioplasty of FMD prior to donation.

As previously mentioned, CTA provides a road map for the surgeon in addition to identifying potential donation problems. This, however, often requires time-consuming post processing in a 3-D lab where the volume rendered models are developed and any additional coronal or sagittal reformatted image series are generated.

CTA can also be used to evaluate hypertension suspected to be secondary to renal artery stenosis. However, CTA is not as widely employed in these instances as other modalities, especially MRA. This is primarily due to a concern of contrast-induced nephropathy resulting from injection of iodinated contrast media. Atherosclerotic disease of the renal arteries is a common cause of renal artery stenosis that can be depicted with CTA. However, many of these patients with atherosclerosis present with concomitant renal insufficiency. This is a known risk factor, along with diabetes, for the development of contrast induced nephropathy. Therefore, many of these patients are selectively evaluated with MRA in hopes of protecting renal function.

CTA of renal arteries with stenoses secondary to atherosclerosis can also be limited by the presence of calcification within the plaque. Although this is useful information if intervention is required, the calcification can be problematic for CTA. The attenuation of the calcification and the iodinated contrast in the lumen of the vessel are often similar. It is therefore difficult in certain instances to separate the calcification from the contrast-filled lumen of the renal artery. This can lead to underestimation of the degree of stenosis.

A subgroup of patients with suspected FMD as the cause of hypertension is ideally suited for CTA. This patient group is usually comprised of younger women without renal insufficiency. CTA in these cases has been shown to detect changes from FMD as well as conventional catheter directed angiography.[4]

Dual energy CT has the potential for providing all of the information currently acquired from CTA of the renal arteries and CT donor protocols while eliminating much of the post processing time, thereby improving overall efficiency.[5] Dual energy CT's ability to differentiate iodine from calcium, and in particular bone, gives dual energy CT the unique ability to perform a rapid bone removal, providing a CT angiogram arterial overview 3D image in a matter of minutes as opposed to hours in a 3D lab.[6] There is also a potential to provide better information regarding the severity of atherosclerotic disease when present through the use of tissue differentiation and subtraction techniques.

Robert P. Hartman · Terri J. Vrtiska · Cynthia McCollough

Mayo Clinic College of Medicine

Department of Radiology

References

[1] Namasivayam S, Kalra MK, Small WC, Torres WE, Mittal PK. Multidetector row computed tomography evaluation of potential living laparoscopic renal donors: the story so far. Curr Probl Diagn Radiol 2006; 35:102-114

[2] Glockner JF, Vrtiska TJ. Renal MR and CT angiography: current concepts. Abdom Imaging 2006;32(3):407-420

[3] Rountas C, et al. Imaging modalities for renal artery stenosis in suspected renovascular hypertension: prospective intraindividual comparison of color Doppler US, CT angiography, GD-enhanced MR angiography, and digital substraction angiography. Ren Fail 2007; 29:295-302

[4] Sabharwal R, Vladica P, Coleman P. Multidetector spiral CT renal angiography in the diagnosis of renal artery fibromuscular dysplasia. Eur J Radiol 2007; 61:520-527

[5] Flohr TG, McCollough CH, Bruder H, et al. First performance evaluation of a dual-source CT (DSCT) system. Eur Radiol 2006; 16:256-268

[6] Johnson TRC, Krauss B, Sedlmair M et al. Material differentiation by dual energy CT: initial experience Eur Radiol. 2007 Jun;17(6):1510-7

Vascular: Renal CTA

Basic considerations

The protocol is identical to that used on SOMATOM Sensation 64 systems for the evaluation of renal arteries. Due to the variability of the renal artery anatomy, scan coverage area should be at least from the diaphragm to the iliac bifurcation to ensure the inclusion of accessory renal arteries. If renal mass is suspected, consider including non-contrast images and/or a delayed venous-phase scan for the accurate assessment of renal enhancement. Delayed excretory-phase images can also be helpful to evaluate the intrarenal collecting system, ureters, and bladder.

Scan Parameters

Scan mode	Single Source, non-gated
Scan area	diaphragm to iliac bifurcation
Scan direction	cranio-caudal
Scan time	~10–15 s
Tube voltage	120 kV
Tube current	240 quality ref. mAs
Dose modulation	CARE Dose4D
CTDI$_{vol}$	~17 mGy
Rotation time	0.5 s
Pitch	0.8 (lower pitch for larger patients)
Slice collimation	0.6 mm
Acquisition	64 x 0.6 mm
Slice width	0.75 mm
Reconstruction increment	0.4 mm
Reconstruction kernel	B31f

Tricks

Reconstruct a smaller FoV just focusing on the kidneys with overlapping reconstructions. Coronal and sagittal multi-planar reformats and 3D reconstructions can provide additional information and are particularly helpful for communicating findings to referring physicians. Use of a smoother kernel (e.g. B20) can further improve quality of 3D reconstruction.

Pitfalls

Test bolus method should not be used to avoid opacification of renal parenchyma prior to CT angiogram. To avoid images that are too noisy, consider increasing the quality ref. mAs in obese patients.

Contrast Injection Protocol

	Iodine concentration 300 mg I/ml	Iodine concentration 370 mg I/ml
Injection scheme	Monophasic	Monophasic
Iodine delivery rate	1.5 g/s	1.5 g/s
CM volume	100 ml	80 ml
CM flow rate	5 ml/s	4.1 ml/s
Body weight adaption	no	no
Bolus timing	bolus tracking	bolus tracking
Bolus tracking threshold	150 HU	150 HU
ROI position	aorta, 2 cm above diaphragm	aorta, 2 cm above diaphragm
Scan delay	4 s	4 s
Saline flush volume	60 ml	60 ml
Saline injection rate	5 ml/s	4.1 ml/s
Needle size	18 G	18 G
Injection site	antecubital vein	antecubital vein

Case 1 Renal Artery Dissection

Case history

50-year-old male presented to the ER with acute onset of left flank pain. CT angiogram was performed to evaluate abnormality in the renal hilum discovered on non-contrast scan.

Question

Is there a vascular abnormality in the left renal hilum to account for findings on the non-contrast scan?

Diagnosis/Differential diagnosis

Renal artery dissection, renal artery aneurysm or arteriovenous malformation may all present as focal abnormalities along the course of the renal artery near the renal hilum. Non-vascular abnormalities including lymph nodes or malignancies are also considerations.

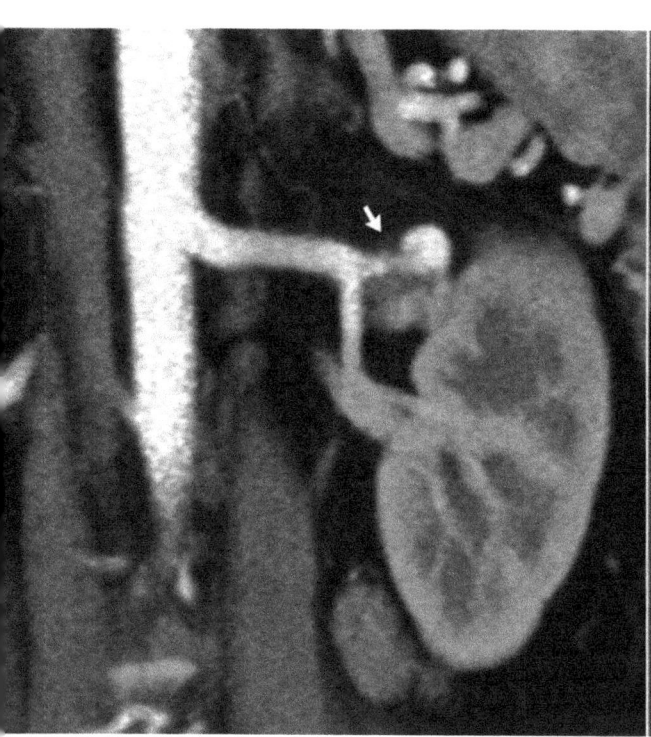

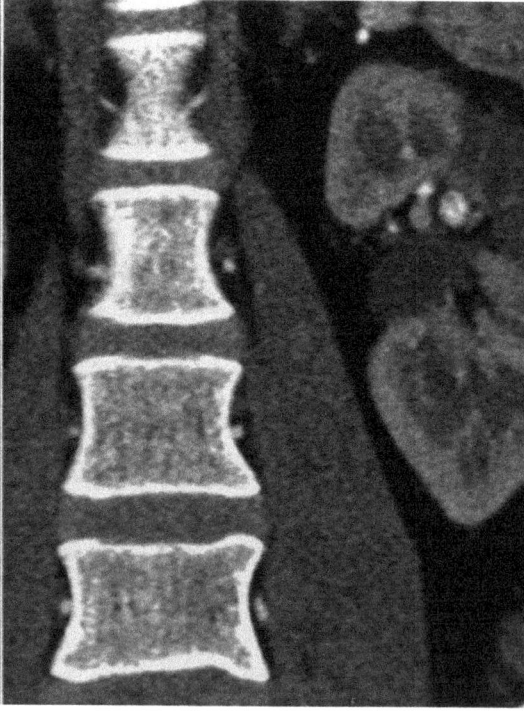

[1] Oblique coronal image through the left renal artery demonstrates a focal dissection (arrow) involving a branch of the artery in the renal hilum.

[2] Coronal image through the left kidney demonstrates a focal area of decreased enhancement in the upper pole consistent with an area of ischemia/infarction.

Findings

A focal dissection of a segmental renal artery was present. This extended into branches within the renal parenchyma. A focal area of ischemia/infarction was present in the upper pole secondary to the dissection.

Take-home message

CT angiography of the renal arteries provides high spatial resolution images allowing for the detection of abnormalities including renal artery stenosis, renal artery dissection, and/or renal artery aneurysms. Non-vascular abnormalities including urolithiasis or renal malignancies can also be identified.

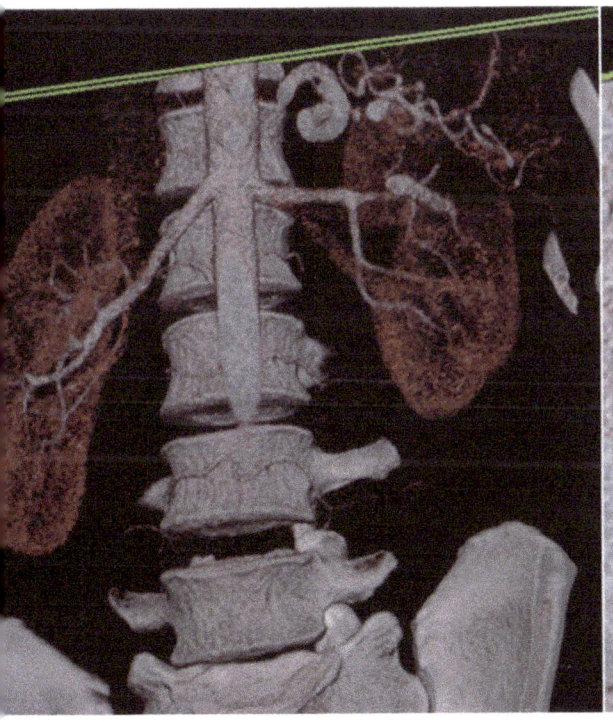
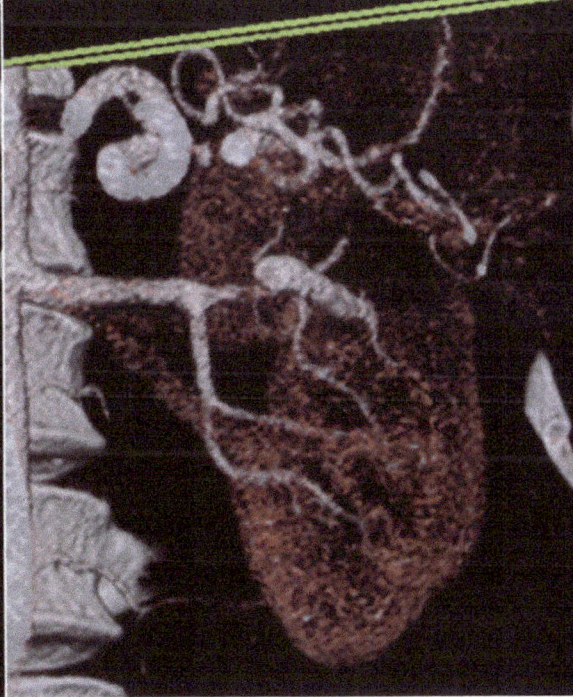

[3] 3D rendering of the aorta and renal arteries demonstrating the dissection in the left renal hilum.

[4] 3D rendering of left kidney magnifying the renal artery dissection.

Case 2 Living Renal Donor

Case history

CTA evaluation of 34-year-old female being considered for living renal donation.

Question

How many renal arteries and veins; what is the branching pattern? Are there venous anatomic variants or other important extravascular findings?

Diagnosis / Differential diagnosis

· Normal living renal donor with single right and two left renal arteries.
· Normal renal parenchyma.
· No renal calculi.
· No renal masses.
· Normal intra-abdominal contents with no unsuspected extraurinary pathology.

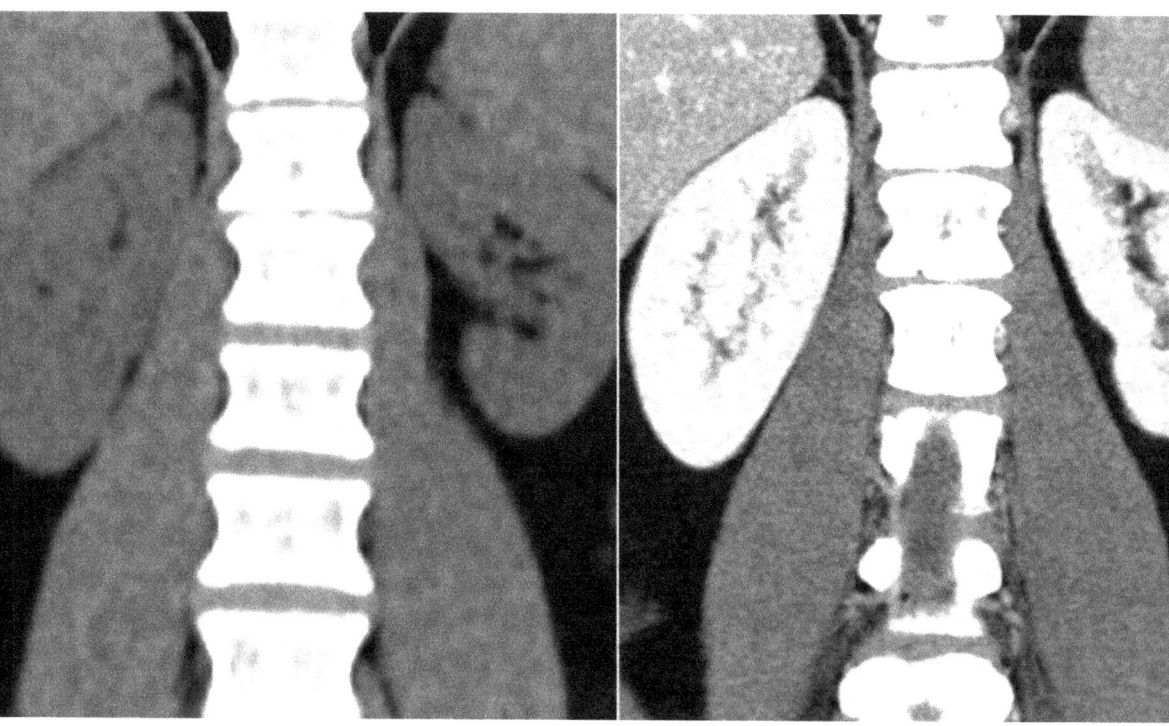

[1] Complete evaluation of the kidneys by CT includes non-contrast images to exclude renal calculi.

[2] Complete evaluation of the kidneys by CT evaluation demonstrates normal renal parenchyma bilaterally and excludes unexpected renal pathology prior to donor nephrectomy.

Findings

Right renal artery bifurcates 25 mm after take-off from abdominal aorta; 3 right renal veins; no urinary calculi; normal renal parenchyma and collecting system; 2 left renal arteries. The more superior and dominant left renal artery branches 13 mm distal to origin from abdominal aorta. The more inferior accessory left renal artery arises 40 mm distal to dominant vessel; 2 left renal veins; postop cholecystectomy.

Take-home message

A CT angiogram, CT venogram and CT urogram can be performed in one diagnostic CT exam for living renal donors. Images can be reconstructed to maximally demonstrate renal anatomy and anatomic variants. Important renal donor CT information includes: renal arterial branching, number of renal arteries/veins, anomalous renal artery and/or venous anatomy, renal parenchymal and extrarenal abnormalities.

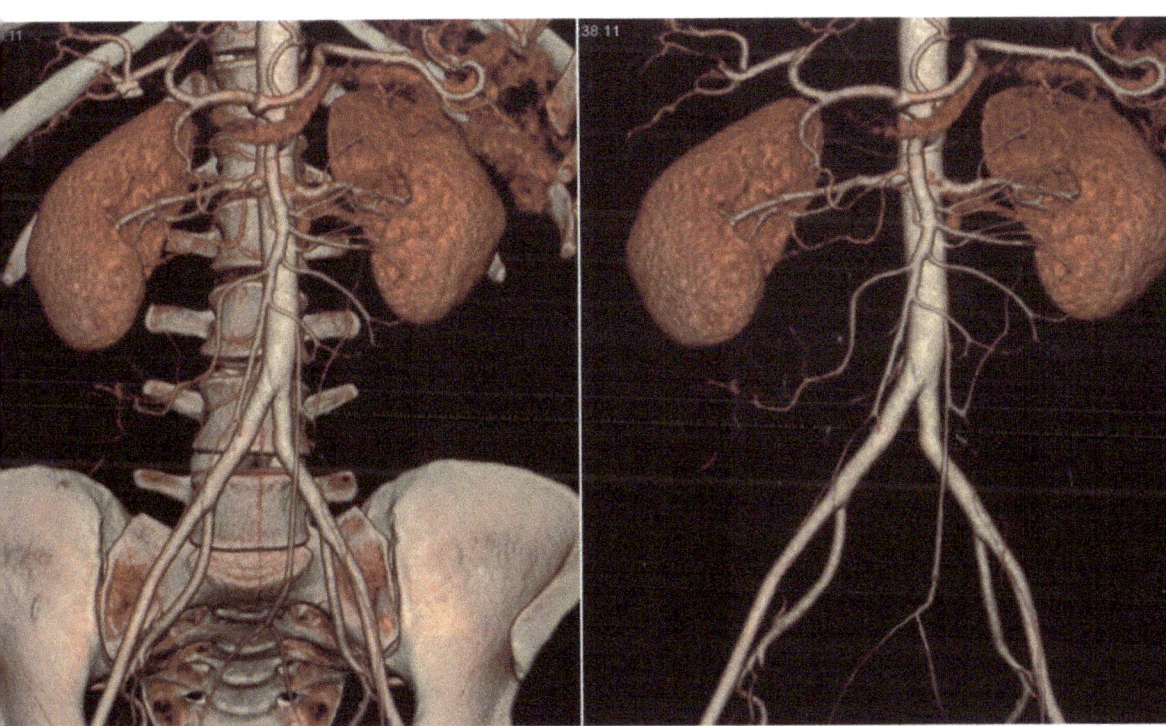

[3] CTA volume-rendered 3D reconstruction shows single right and two left renal arteries. The background bones provide accurate display of anatomic landmarks to the surgeon.

[4] Automatic bone removal provides additional information on the depiction of the arterial anatomic relationship. This is a key workflow consideration.

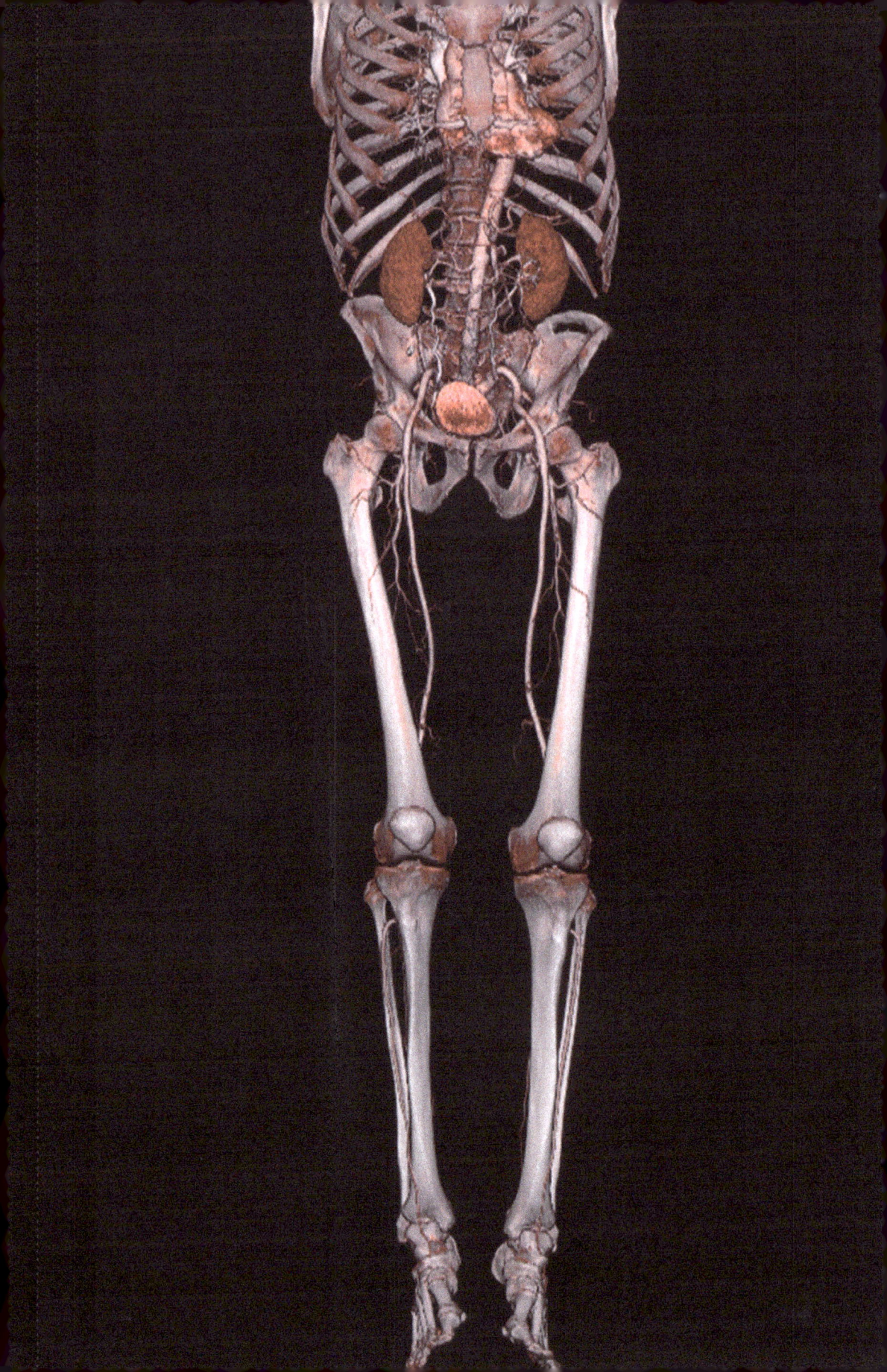

Vascular: Peripheral Runoff

Axel Kuettner · Katharina Anders · Michael Lell

Case 1: Suspicion of Peripheral Occlusive Disease

Case 2: Suspicion of Femoral Artery Stenosis

As the population of the Western world continues to age, there is an increasing prevalence of peripheral arterial disease. At a current rate of approximately 12% in an adult population, the associated morbidity and burden of cost for society is significant. Several treatment options are available such as transluminal and surgical revascularization techniques as well as pharmacologic treatment options, requiring accurate diagnosis of the location and severity of arterial involvement. Conventional digital subtraction angiography (DSA) is still considered the reference standard for assessing aortoiliac and lower extremity arteries, with the advantage of immediate therapeutic interventions is during the examination. Its main disadvantages, however, include its invasive nature, the considerably high costs, patient discomfort, and a complication rate of approximately 1%.[1]

The introduction of multi-detector row CT scanners has substantially improved non-invasive CT angiography for various vascular territories by offering increased volume coverage, decreased contrast medium dose, decreased acquisition time, and improved spatial resolution for assessment of smaller arterial branches, including the aortoiliac and lower extremity arteries. However, because of the limited spatial resolution along the z-axis, early four-detector row CT angiography was limited in the assessment of small vessels, including the internal iliac arteries and the peripheral arteries of the calves. The rate of diagnostic agreement between first generation multislice CT angiography and conventional DSA has been shown to be significantly lower for assessing arterial stenosis of the peripheral arteries of the calves when compared with the assessment of the larger proximal arteries of the thigh. By offering a improved z-axis, the latest generation 64-detector row CT scanners and now the novel generation of Dual Source CT scanners may overcome this limitation of CT angiography and further improve diagnostic accuracy of CT angiography when compared with conventional DSA in patients with peripheral arterial disease.[2]

Contrast medium delivery for computed tomographic (CT) angiography of the lower extremity inflow and runoff arteries is very challenging, particularly in patients with peripheral arterial occlusive disease. It is well known from intra-arterial angiography that coexisting cardiovascular disorders may substantially delay the opacification of the peripheral arterial tree and may make the outcome unpredictable. With fast multi-detector row CT scanners and DSCT scanners, it might thus be possible

Vascular: Peripheral Runoff

for scanning to outpace the contrast medium bolus despite correct timing of the scanning delay at the level of the abdominal aorta, with subsequent inadequate opacification of distal arterial branches. On the other hand, as the CT data acquisition follows the bolus down through the aorta and the peripheral arterial tree, it might be possible to use an injection duration that is shorter than the total CT acquisition time and thus to save contrast medium. An indispensable parameter for optimizing contrast medium injection protocols for patients with PAOD is the speed at which an intravenously injected bolus of contrast medium propagates through the peripheral arterial tree. To adequately predict the CM bolus transit time, Fleischman et al. performed a study in patients with PAOD to prospectively determine the range of aortopopliteal bolus transit times in patients with moderate to severe PAOD, as a guideline for developing injection strategies for peripheral arterial CT angiography.[3] The results showed that it is virtually impossible to accurately predict the CM transit time for any individual patient, as the bolus transit time may not correlate with the severity of the disease at all. Thus, a double test bolus at both levels – the beginning and end of the scan range – is warranted.[3]

The analysis of peripheral arteries has yet to overcome another challenge. Most exams are interpreted in coronal or sagittal fashion. The existing osseous structures thus obscure the arteries when using MIPs. Bone removal algorithms are capable of discriminating arterial from osseous structures. However, when both structures are close together (e.g. in the lower limb), the algorithms may accidentally remove vascular structures and thus causing a pseudo total occlusion.[4] The differentiation of material in computed tomography (CT) is based on their x-ray attenuation as quantified in Hounsfield units and displayed in shades of gray at different window levels in normal CT scans. Attenuation is caused by absorption and scattering of radiation by the material under investigation. By its natural principle, CT is not able to differentiate between different highly dense material such as iodine in vessels and adjacent bone when using a single energy spectrum. Spiral dual energy CT may overcome this limitation in a unique way. The two main mechanisms responsible for attenuation in the photon energy range used in CT are the Compton scatter and the photo effect. The contribution of these two processes to the attenuation of different materials varies and also depends on the energy of the x-ray photons. Thus, materials can be differentiated further by applying different x-ray spectra and analyzing the differences in attenuation. This works especially well in materials with large atomic numbers due to the photo effect. One of these materials is iodine, which is generally known to have stronger enhancement at low tube voltage settings. This effect makes it beneficial to use the spectral information to differentiate iodine from other materials that do not show this behavior such as calcium.[5] With the two tubes and detectors mounted orthogonally in Dual Source CT, both spiral acquisitions run simultaneously, which largely excludes changes in contrast enhancement or patient movement between the acquisitions. Thus the purpose of iodine differentiation in imaging can be to display contrast enhanced vessels without any calcium containing structures such as bone to correctly assess the lumen. Using the same underlying principle, calcified plaque material, prone to obscure the lumen by blooming artifacts, may also be overcome using the spiral dual energy approach.[6] This chapter displays the technique of Dual Source CT for peripheral runoff imaging using the conventional monospectral 120 kV approach. It also demonstrates the limitation of monospectral imaging. A separate chapter in this book is dedicated for the technique of spectral dual energy peripheral runoff imaging.

Axel Kuettner · Katharina Anders · Michael Lell

University of Erlangen-Nuremberg

Department of Diagnostic Radiology

Universitätsklinikum
Erlangen

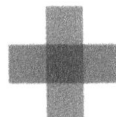

References

[1] Ota H, Takase K, Igarashi K, Chiba Y, Haga K, Saito H, Takahashi S. MDCT compared with digital subtraction angiography for assessment of lower extremity arterial occlusive disease: importance of reviewing cross-sectional images. AJR Am J Roentgenol. 2004 Jan;182(1):201-9

[2] Willmann JK, Baumert B, Schertler T et. al. Aortoiliac and lower extremity arteries assessed with 16-detector row CT angiography: prospective comparison with digital subtraction angiography. Radiology. 2005 Sep;236(3):1083-93

[3] Fleischmann D, Rubin GD Quantification of intravenously administered contrast medium transit through the peripheral arteries: implications for CT angiography Radiology. 2005 Sep;236(3):1076-82

[4] Meyer BC, Ribbe C, Kruschewski M, Wolf KJ, Albrecht T 16-row multidetector CT angiography of the aortoiliac system and lower extremity arteries: contrast enhancement and image quality using a standarized examination protocol Rofo. 2005 Nov;177(11):1562-70

[5] Boll DT, Hoffmann MH, Huber N, Bossert AS, Aschoff AJ, Fleiter TR Spectral coronary multidetector computed tomography angiography: dual benefit by facilitating plaque characterization and enhancing lumen depiction J Comput Assist Tomogr. 2006 Sep-Oct;30(5):804-11

[6] Johnson TRC, Krauss B, Sedlmair M et al. Material differentiation by dual energy CT: initial experience Eur Radiol. 2007 Jun;17(6):1510-7

Vascular: Peripheral Runoff

Basic considerations

The peripheral artery examination is challenging, because optimal contrast timing is needed to achieve optimal image quality. Since the contrast transit time in the peripheral artery system is different and unpredictable for different patients, the main challenge of this protocol is the contrast timing. Use two separate test boli, one at the proximal begin of the scan range usually cranial to the ostia of the renal arteries (10 ml) and the second in the popliteal artery (20 ml). The difference between both is the contrast transit time and should be taken as scan time. Choose pitch to match that time.

Scan Parameters

Scan mode	Single Source, non-gated
Scan area	renal artery (aortic arch) to feet
Scan direction	cranio-caudal
Scan time	determined by double test bolus
Tube voltage	120 kV
Tube current	130 quality ref. mAs
Dose modulation	CARE Dose 4D
$CTDI_{vol}$	~9 mGy
Rotation time	0.5 s
Pitch	0.7–1.1 (depending on contrast transit time)
Slice collimation	0.6 mm
Acquisition	64 x 0.6 mm
Slice width	1 mm
Reconstruction increment	0.8 mm
Reconstruction kernel	B25f or B41f

Tricks

· Keep legs together (tape).
· Place second test bolus (20 ml) in the popliteal artery.
· For long scan ranges, reverse the patient's positioning to "feet first" position. A flat head rest (on which the feet are placed) can be inserted to extend the scan range.

Pitfalls

· Be aware that using full scan speed one might outrun the CM bolus.
· Clinical parameters such als cardiac output or presence/absence of stenoses do NOT predict the bolus transit time reliably.
· For the second test bolus make sure that the initial start delay is prolonged and that enough scan repetitions are programmed.

Contrast Injection Protocol

	Iodine concentration 300 mg I/ml	Iodine concentration 370 mg I/ml
Injection scheme	Monophasic	Monophasic
Iodine delivery rate	1.48 g/s	1.48 g/s
CM volume	148 ml	120 ml
CM flow rate	4.9 ml/s	4 ml/s
Body weight adaption	no	no
Bolus timing	double test bolus	double test bolus
Bolus tracking threshold	n.a.	n.a.
ROI position	juxtarenal aorta/poplitea artery	juxtarenal aorta/poplitea artery
Scan delay	max. enhancement plus 2 s	max. enhancement plus 2 s
Saline flush volume	120 ml	120 ml
Saline injection rate	4.9 ml/s	4 ml/s
Needle size	18 G	18 G
Injection site	antecubital vein	antecubital vein

Case 1 Suspicion of Peripheral Occlusive Disease

Case history

53-year-old male, ex-smoker, hypercholesteremia, hypertension and family history of myocardial infarction presents with fatigue in both legs while exercising.

Question

Are there signs for severe stenosis of the peripheral arteries (PAOD) with known underlying risk factors for atherosclerotic disease?

Diagnosis / Differential diagnosis

In this particular patient multiple risk factors are known so that POAD is one differential diagnosis. Of course, all other causes of walking pain need to be need assessed such as simple soreness due to lack of exercise.

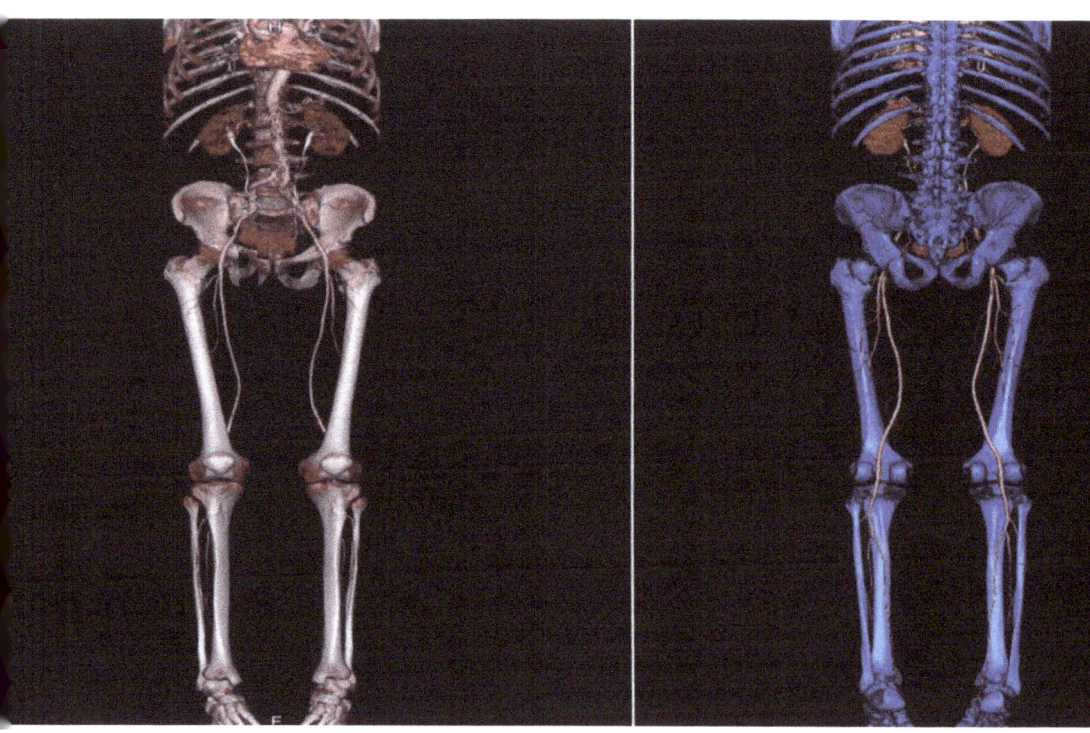

[1] VRT image of the peripheral runoff. Excellent detail depiction of all vascular and osseous structures.

[2] A bone removal algorithm has detected all osseous structures. The blue color facilitates quick verification of the results and correction if necessary.

Findings

Absence of POAD. Atherosclerotic changes of
the abdominal aorta with mild calcifications,
no major plaque burden. Distal of the trifurcation
the anterior tibial artery and the fibular artery
are a small vessel bilaterally, the posterior tibial
artery is the main vessel feeding the plantar arch.

Take-home message

This patient demonstrates that CT imaging
of the peripheral vasculature is feasible and
that bone removal tools help to visualize the
arterial tree. The chosen contrast media injection
parameters as well as scan parameters allowed
to adequately depict the small vessels. Vessels
close to osseous structures can be reliably
segmented as the corresponding images
with/without bone demonstrate.

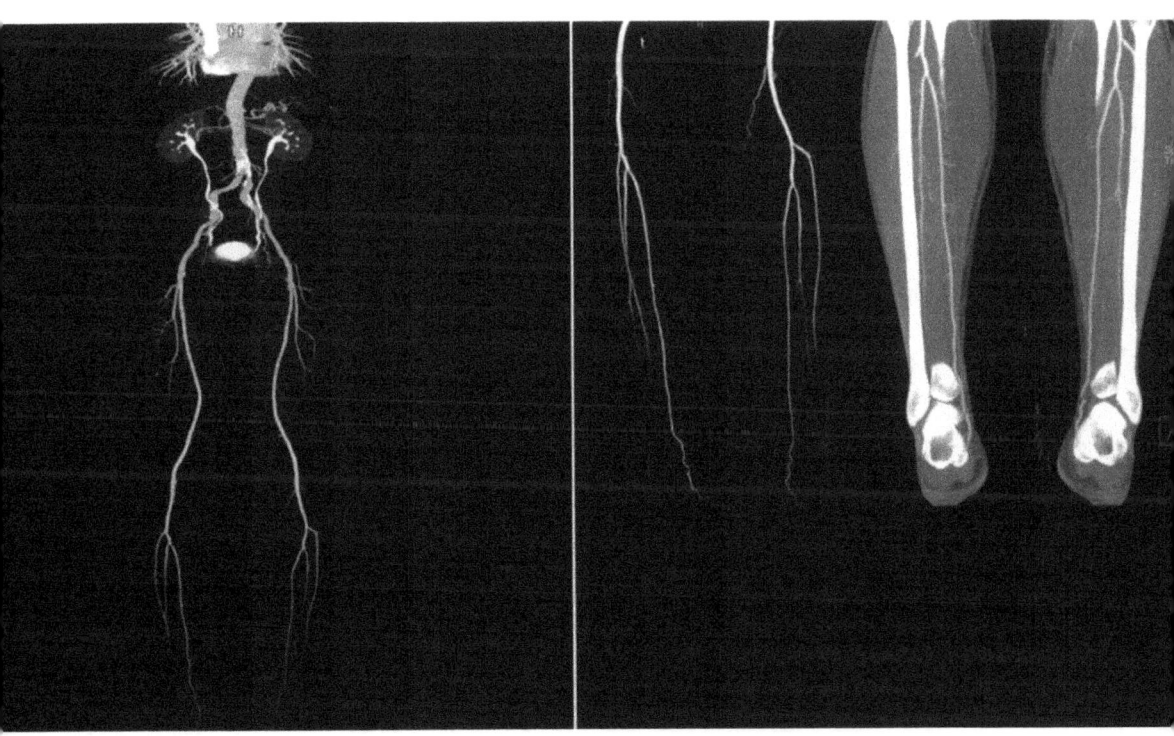

[3] Whole body MIP after bone removal. Note the excellent
display of the distal arteries. The plantar arch is mainly formed
by the posterior tibial artery.

[4] Detailed view of the lower limb arterial tree with and
without bone removal. The small fibular artery close to
the fibula is reliably depicted and not removed by the bone
removal algorithm.

Case 2 Suspicion of Femoral Artery Stenosis

Case history

64-year-old male, prior myocardial infarction and anterior spondylolisthesis presents with difficulties walking. Arterial canulation for cardiac catheterization was impossible over the right femoral artery.

Question

Are there signs for severe stenosis in the right femoral artery or peripheral arteries with a known underlying arteriosclerotic disease (PAOD)?

Diagnosis / Differential diagnosis

In this particular patient, atherosclerosis (prior MI) is known, so that POAD is one differential diagnosis. Of course all other causes of walking pain need to be need assessed such as tumors and neuroforaminal impairment/disc herniation due to the severe anterior spondylolisthesis in the past.

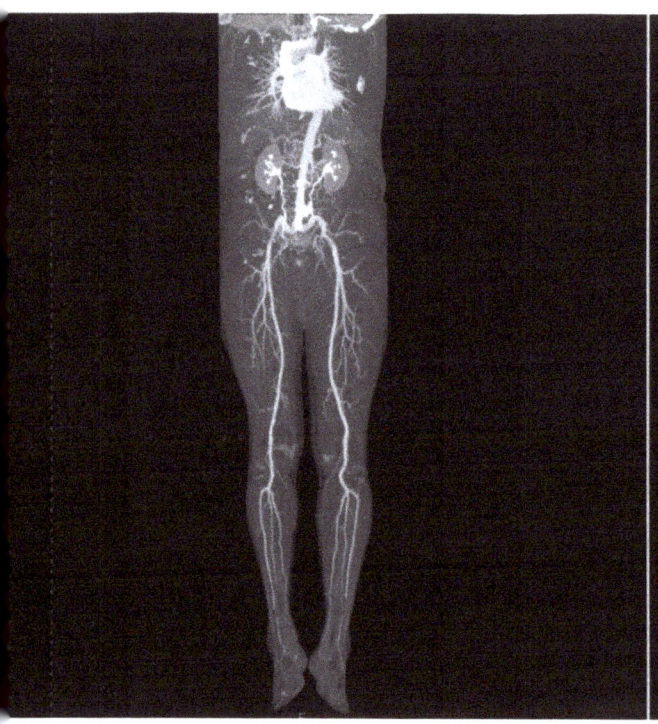

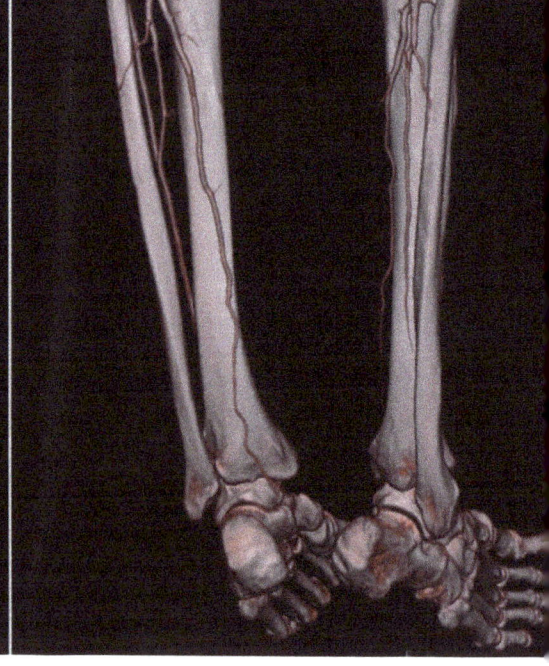

[1] Whole body MIP after bone removal. Note the excellent display of the distal arteries. However, parts of the distal anterior popliteal arteries seem to be highly stenosed.

[2] VRT image of the lower limbs. All vessels are displayed, no sign of PAOD. In correlation to the MIP the "pseudo occlusions" are revealed.

Findings

Absence of POAD. Atherosclerotic changes of the abdominal aorta with a mild aneurism and calcifications; no major plaque burden. Kinking of the common iliac arteries due to the anterior listhesis of vertebra L5/S1 and consecutive shortening of the upper trunk. Osteosynthesis material remaining in the lumbar spine and the sacrum. Severe degenerative changes of the lumbar spine without neuroforaminal impairment.

Take-home message

This case demonstrates that Dual Source CT can perform peripheral runoffs for very long scan ranges. Bone removal can be performed and allows for vessel imaging. However, small vessels close to osseous structures may be accidentally removed requiring a correlation with axial or VRT images. Moreover, this case demonstrates that CT offers global diagnostic capacities to assess multiple differential diagnostics.

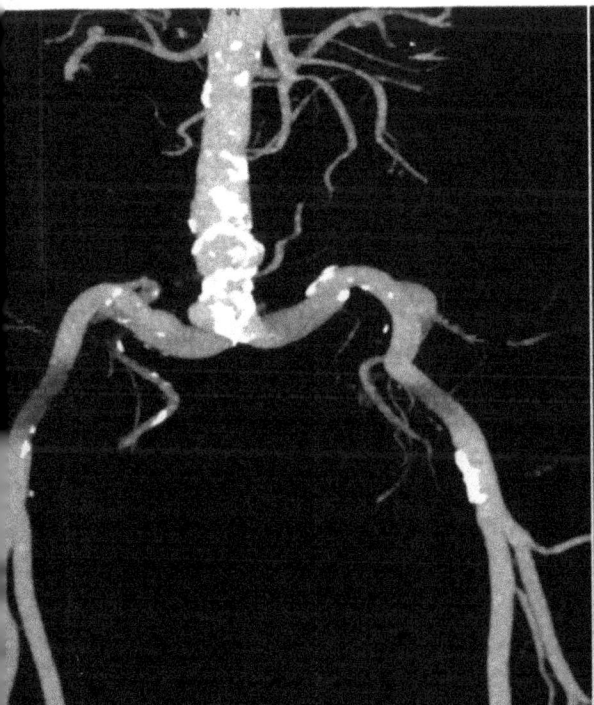
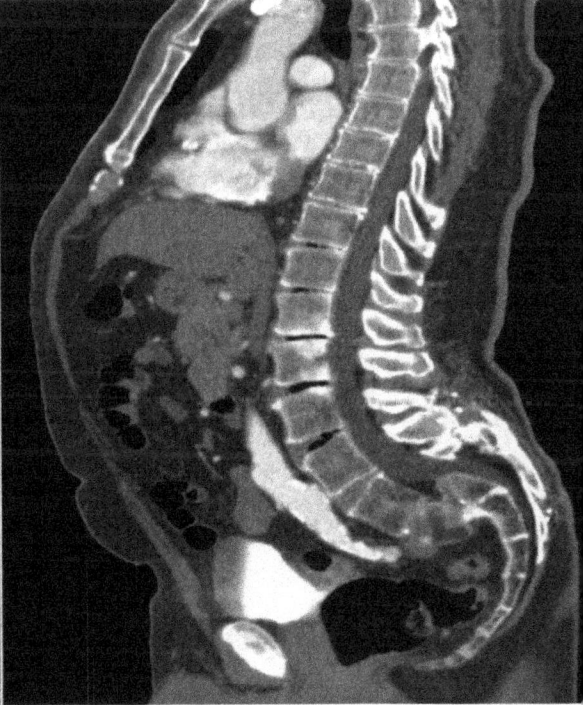

[3] The common iliac arteries are severely kinked. No signs of stenosing atherosclerotic disease. A mild aneurysm of the peripheral aorta is noted.

[4] Lumbar spine of patient. Severe antelistesis of the 5th lumbar vertebra and surgical stabilization. The upper trunk is shortened. Mild aneurysm of the abdominal aorta.

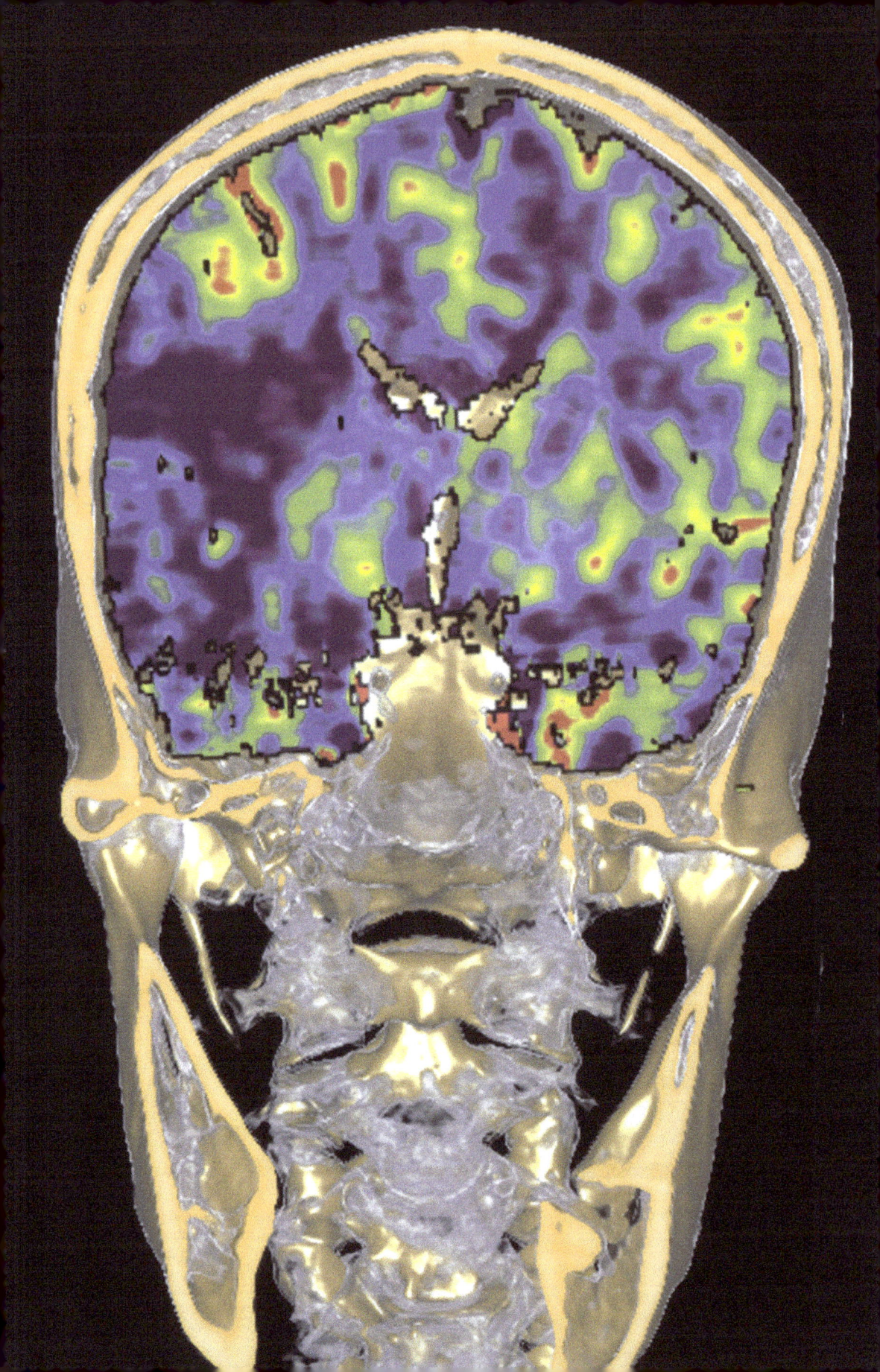

Vascular: Brain Perfusion

Harald Seifarth · Tobias Fischer · Roman Fischbach · Stephan P. Kloska

Case 1: PBV Delineates the Whole Volume of Cerebral Infarction in Hyperacute Phase

Case 2: PBV Shows Small Infarction Missed in Perfusion CT

In western countries, the incidence of acute stroke is about 200/100,000 per year and represents the third most common cause of death. Cerebral ischemia, caused by an occlusion of a cerebral artery, is the usual cause of stroke (85%) and has to be differentiated from intracranial hemorrhage (15%), typically occurring in the region of the basal ganglia. While therapy for intracranial hemorrhage focuses on the control of the space-occupying effect, an acute or hyperacute ischemic stroke offers the chance to recanalize the occluded vessel and to restore the neurological deficits at least to a certain extent. Due to the very limited tolerance of brain tissue to hypoxia, the patient benefits most if appropriate therapy starts immediately – "Time is brain". While interventional endovascular treatment such as local chemical intra-arterial thrombolysis or mechanical thrombolysis is limited to certain specialized centers and is typically not available around the clock, intravenous chemical thrombolysis (e.g. with rt-PA) offers a viable option to treat hyperacute ischemic strokes. However, the time frame available for intravenous thrombolysis is limited: Currently, therapy is restricted to the first 3 hours after the onset of symptoms. Furthermore, the extent of the cerebral infarction limits the use of intravenous thrombolysis due to an increased risk of secondary bleeding in large territorial infarctions. An expansion of the therapeutic time window is desirable to offer this option to more patients suffering from ischemic stroke.[1]

Fast and reliable diagnosis is important in patients with suspected hyperacute stroke before thrombolytic therapy can be started. Hence, modern neuroimaging has to offer more than simply differentiating between ischemia and hemorrhage. Imaging in acute stroke must allow the physician to determine the location and extension of the ischemic event and should further provide hemodynamic parameters for the estimation of regional blood perfusion. In summary, stroke imaging has to pave the way for individualized, sophisticated therapy. It should also help to predict the patient's outcome and improve patient management.

Today, both CT and MRI are established technologies for acute stroke imaging. Both modalities have minor advantages and disadvantages regarding contraindications, patient management and diagnostic validity.[2] Nevertheless, CT remains the most frequently used diagnostic tool for diagnosing acute stroke due to its wide availability.

Vascular: Brain Perfusion

Non-Enhanced CT (NECT) is still the primary modality in suspected acute stroke. NECT is used to exclude intracranial hemorrhage and to visualize early signs of brain infarction. However, in the initial state of ischemic stroke these early signs can be delineated only in a portion of patients. To meet the requirements of stroke imaging, multimodal CT concepts including NECT, CT angiography (CTA) and perfusion CT (PCT) are necessary. Multimodal stroke CT doubles the detection rate of cerebral infarction in the early stages compared to NECT alone.[3] It also offers delineation of the extra- and intracranial vessels (CTA) and provides insight into cerebral hemodynamics (PCT).

Perfusion CT allows the calculation of the cerebral blood flow (CBF), the cerebral blood volume (CBV) and the time to peak enhancement (TTP), which serves as a surrogate for cerebral perfusion. PCT is a contrast enhanced, dynamic examination and results in color-coded maps of CBF, CBV and TTP. PCT maps allow for detailed evaluation of cerebral perfusion disturbances and thus the differentiation of the infarct core (irreversibly damaged brain tissue) from the potentially salvageable tissue (penumbra). The perfusion defect in the CBV-map represents the infarct core, the area of mismatch between CBV and CBF represents the penumbra.[4] In contrast to diffusion weighted MRI or MRI perfusion measurement (MR-mismatch), PCT evaluation is restricted to a subvolume of the brain due to the limited width of the CT detector. Therefore, an ischemic area may only be partially covered; smaller infarctions outside of the preselected PCT scan level may be missed altogether.

By contrast, calculation of "perfused blood volume" maps (PBV) offers fast three-dimensional display of the perfusion of the entire brain. PBV-imaging is a post processing step based on routine NECT and CTA scans. Therefore, it can be seamlessly integrated into established multimodal CT stroke protocols without any additional scanning.

The fundamentals of PBV-imaging are already described by Hunter et al.[5] Brain tissue and cerebral vessels are segmented from routine CTA and NECT images. Dedicated subtraction algorithms allow the calculation of the enhancement of the brain tissue itself. The resulting enhancement values are correlated to a predefined color scale, coding for the cerebral blood volume. Enhancement in a venous vessel, selected semiautomatically during PBV calculation, serves as an individual standard of reference. Thus, the calculation results in a three-dimensional dataset of the whole brain, displaying the local blood perfusion in correlation to the cerebral blood volume. Recent evaluations showed a good correlation between areas with reduced perfusion in the PBV-maps to the infarct size in NECT follow up images in patients with hyperacute stroke after successful thrombolytic therapy.[6] Moreover, PBV seems to match well to CBV maps in PCT, so PBV might be a good predictor of the extent of the infarct core, but further evaluations are necessary.[6] However, PBV imaging cannot visualize the penumbra of an infarction. This is reserved to the dynamic PCT examination with the calculation of different perfusion parameters.

In summary, PBV can increase sensitivity of CT stroke imaging due to the coverage of the whole brain and provide further information about the entire extent of the infarct core.

Harald Seifarth · Tobias Fischer · Roman Fischbach · Stephan P. Kloska
University of Münster
Department of Clinical Radiology

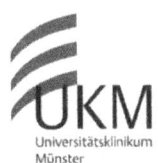

References

1 Khaja AM, Grotta JC. Established treatments of acute ischemic stroke. Lancet. 2007;369:319-30

2 Sirinivasan A, Goyal M, Al Azri F, Lum C. State-of-the-art imaging of acute stroke. Radiographics. 2006;26:S75-S95

3 Kloska SP, Nabavi DG, Gaus C, et al. Acute stroke assessment with CT: do we need multimodal evaluation? Radiology. 2004;233(1):79-86

4 Murphy BD, Fox AJ, Lee DH, et al. Identification of penumbra and infarct in acute ischemic stroke using computed tomography perfusion-derived blood flow and blood volume measurements. Stroke. 2006;37(7):1771-1777

5 Hunter GJ, Hamberg LM, Ponzo JA, et al. Assessment of cerebral perfusion and arterial anatomy in hyperacute stroke with three-dimensional functional CT: early clinical results. AJNR Am J Neuroradiol. 1998;19(1):29-37

6 Kloska SP, Fischer T, Nabavi DG, et al. Color-coded perfused blood volume imaging using multidetector CT: initial results of whole-brain perfusion analysis in acute cerebral ischemia. Eur Radiol. 2007;17(9):2352-2358

Vascular: Brain Perfusion

Basic considerations

PBV imaging is based on a subtraction of NECT and CTA data. Therefore, the same field of view and identical reconstruction parameters are required for both examinations. Although the software can correct to some extent for patient movement between the two scans, movement of the head should be strictly avoided. To calculate of the PBV, a CTA scan with sufficient parenchymal and venous enhancement is required. Therefore the cerebral transit time (5 – 6 s) has to be added to the CM arrival time in the cerebral arteries if a test-bolus technique is used to determine the scan delay.

Scan Parameters

Scan mode	Single Source, non-gated
Scan area	aortic arch to superior sagittal sinus
Scan direction	caudo-cranial
Scan time	~7 – 10 s
Tube voltage	120 kV
Tube current	130 eff. mAs
Dose modulation	no
$CTDI_{vol}$	17.5 mGy
Rotation time	0.5 s
Pitch	0.8
Slice collimation	0.6 mm
Acquisition	64 x 0.6 mm
Slice width	1 mm
Reconstruction increment	0.7 mm
Reconstruction kernel	H22f

Tricks

If a perfusion CT is required, it should be done before the cerebral CTA. The scan delay for the CTA can also be determined from the dynamic perfusion scan. Select the time to peak enhancement in the superior sagittal sinus as scan delay. In this case, no additional delay time is required to account for cerebral transit time.

Pitfalls

· Do not forget to add the start delay of the PCT scan when determining the CTA delay from an arterial vessel in the PCT scan.
· If the CTA scan that is to be used to calculate the PBV is started too early, it results in overestimation of the infarction.

Contrast Injection Protocol

	Iodine concentration 300 mg I/ml	Iodine concentration 370 mg I/ml
Injection scheme	Monophasic	Monophasic
Iodine delivery rate	1.48 g/s	1.48 g/s
CM volume	100 ml	80 ml
CM flow rate	4.9 ml/s	4 ml/s
Body weight adaption	no	no
Bolus timing	test bolus*	test bolus*
Bolus tracking threshold	n.a.	n.a.
ROI position	basilar artery	basilar artery
Scan delay	peak time plus 6 s	peak time plus 6 s
Saline flush volume	60 ml	60 ml
Saline injection rate	4.9 ml/s	4 ml/s
Needle size	18 G	18 G
Injection site	antecubital vein	antecubital vein

* Depending on the preference of the individual site, bolus tracking can be used as an alternative

Case 1 PBV Delineates the Whole Volume of Cerebral Infarction in Hyperacute Phase

Case history

80-year-old male presenting with left-sided hemiparesis and neglect; onset 2 hours ago.

Question

Exclusion of intracerebral hemorrhage. Demarcation of ischemic brain tissue, location and extent of cerebral infarction.

Diagnosis / Differential diagnosis

· The patient suffers from a right-sided ischemic infarction following thromboembolic occlusion of a M2 branch of the middle cerebral artery.
· In addition, frontotemporal atrophy is present.

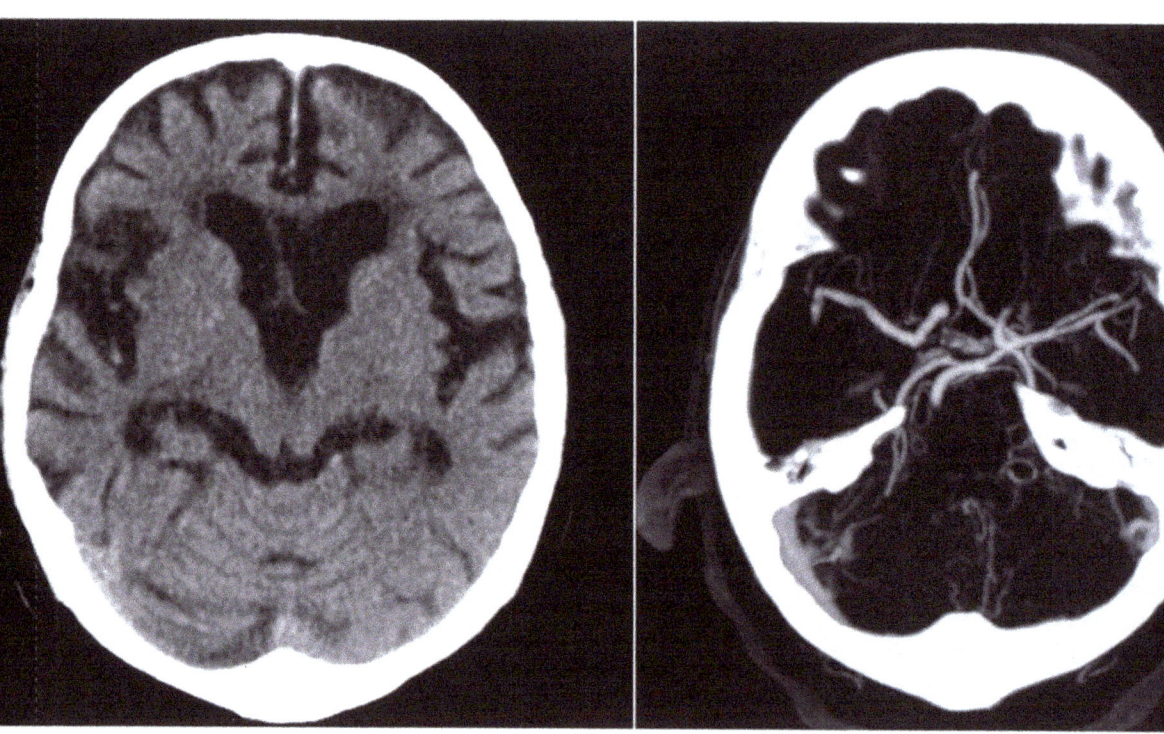

[1] NECT Image.

[2] MIP reformation of CTA.

Findings

Slight fading of the basal ganglia on the right.
Note the hyperdense MCA branches in the insular
cistern on the right. The CTA shows a proximal M2
branch occlusion. PCT shows a perfusion deficit in
the frontotemporal parenchyma and the insular
ribbon on the right side. The whole extent of the
perfusion deficit can be seen on reformations of
the PBV data.

Take-home message

PBV depicts the perfusion deficit correlating to
the CBV in axial slices in the hyperacute phase
of an ischemic infarction. The three-dimensional
extent of the perfusion deficit can be seen in
sagittal and coronal reformation of the PBV
dataset.

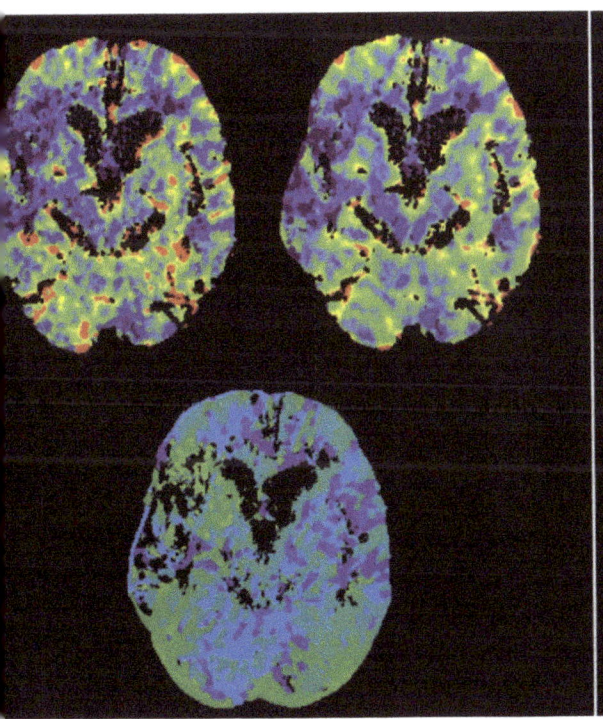

[3] PCT images: CBF (upper left), CBV (upper right) and time to
peak (TTP).

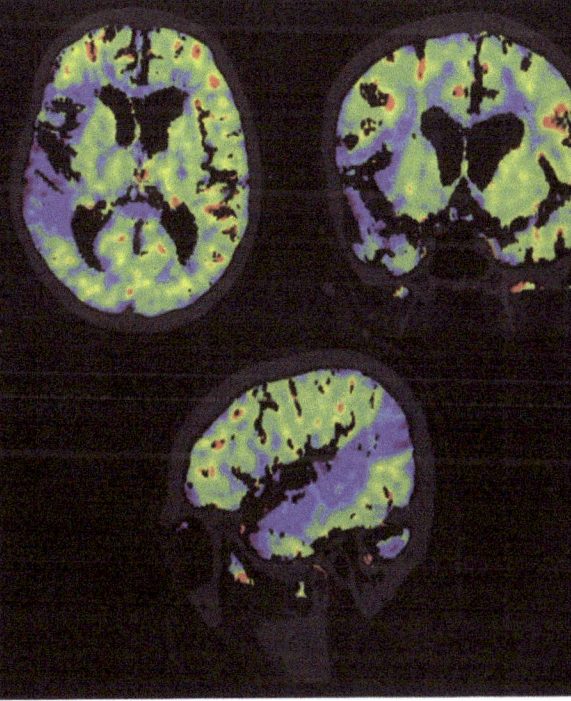

[4] Reformations of PBV dataset: axial (upper left), coronal
(upper right) and parasagittal.

Case 2 PBV Shows Small Infarction Missed in Perfusion CT

Case history

81-year-old male, right-sided, predominantly brachiofacial hemiparesis, onset 3 hours ago, known atrial fibrillation.

Question

Exclusion of intracerebral hemorrhage. Demarcation of ischemic brain tissue, location and extent of cerebral infarction.

Diagnosis / Differential diagnosis

· The patient suffered from a left-sided, peripheral thromboembolic MCA branch occlusion, leading to a small ischemic infarction in the left precentral region.

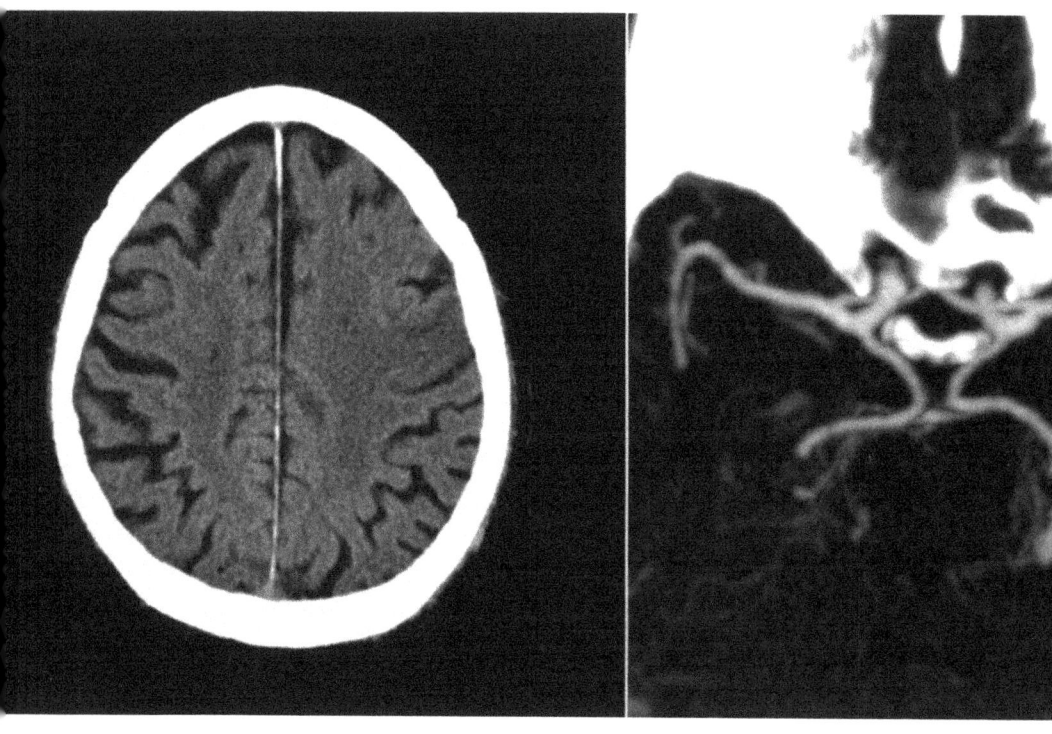

[1] NECT Image.

[2] Axial MIP reformation of CTA.

Findings

The NECT images show subtle early signs of infarction with a loss of corticomedullar contrast in the left precentral region. PCT images show symmetrical brain perfusion without any perfusion deficit. The PBV images depict a small perfusion deficit in the precentral region.

Take-home message

Due to the limited coverage of the axial PCT scan, small infarctions might be missed. Because of the coverage of the entire brain, even these small perfusion deficits can be delineated using PBV.

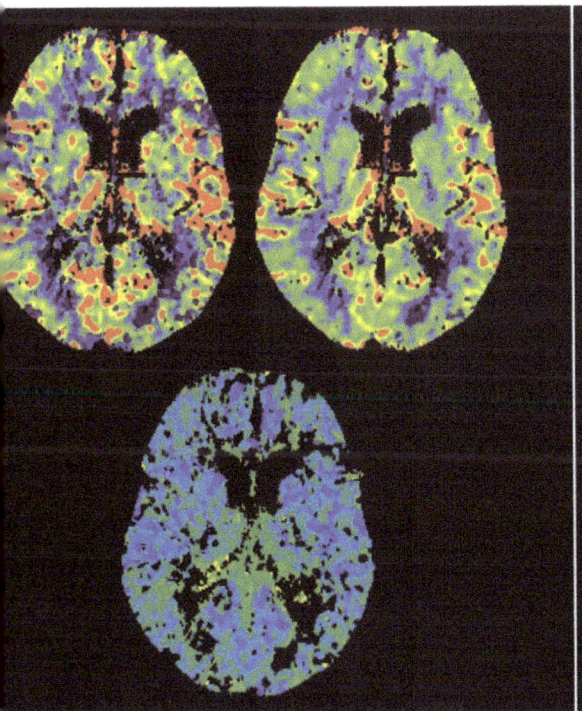

[3] PCT images: CBF (upper left), CBV (upper right) and time to peak (TTP).

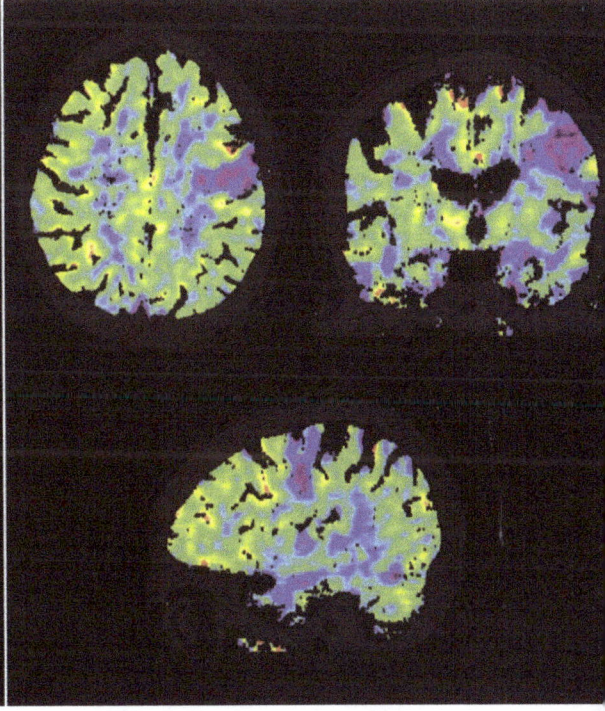

[4] Reformations of PBV dataset: axial (upper left), coronal (upper right) and parasagittal.

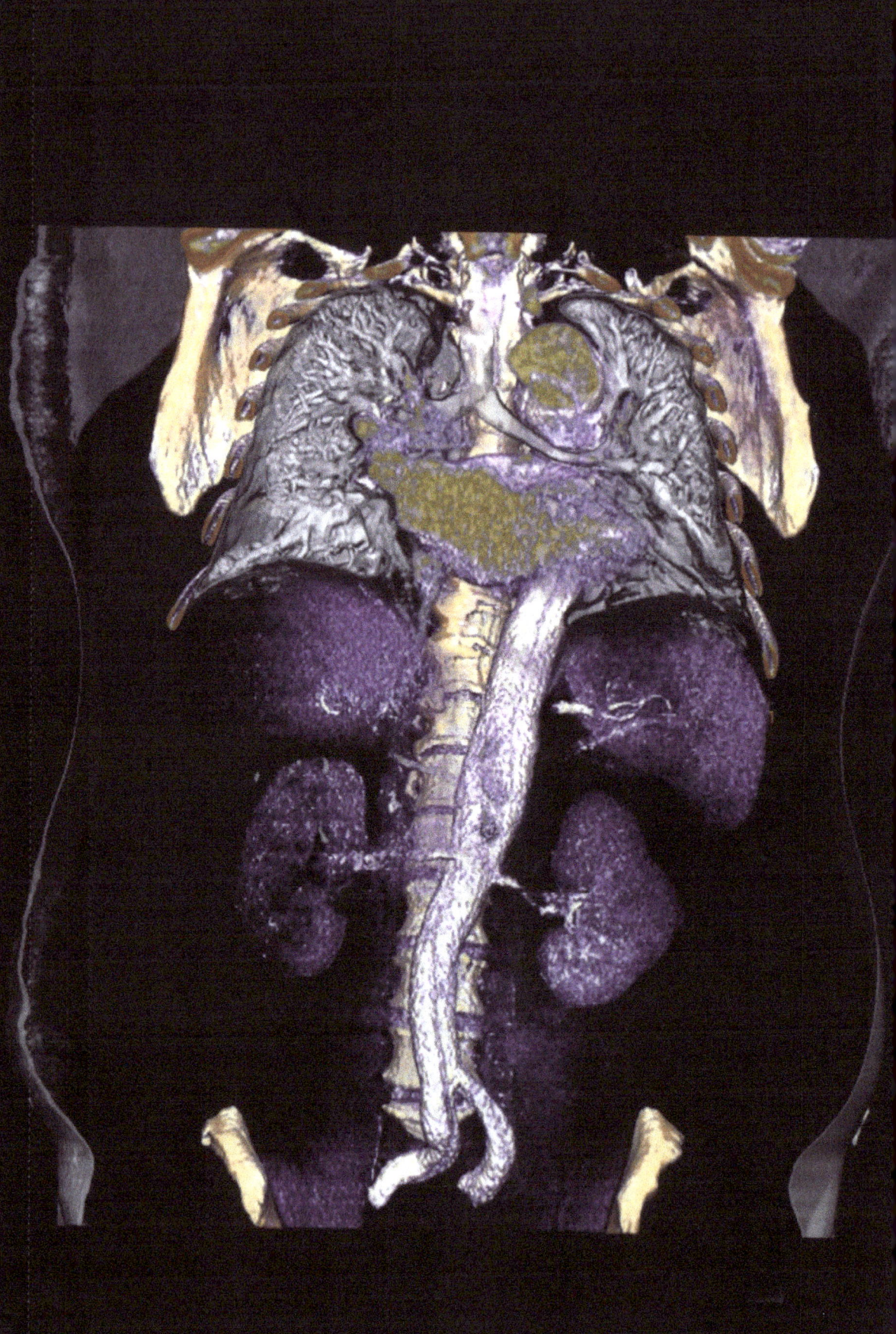

Body: Obese Mode

Elizabeth McDonald · Robert P. Hartman · Cynthia McCollough

Case 1: Aortic Dissection in 183 kg Male

Case 2: Abdominal Abscess in 206 kg Male

The prevalence of obesity in the United States has been increasing at an alarming rate over the past twenty years. According to the 2003–2004 National Health and Nutrition Examination Survey (NHANES), approximately 66 percent of U.S. adults are either overweight or obese. This has a dramatic effect on health care providers, who must equip their facilities with larger beds, larger wheelchairs and procedure tables capable of supporting weights approaching 1000 lbs (450 kg).

This high occurrence of obese patients, coupled with the increasing use of bariatric surgery, has resulted in a higher demand for medical imaging techniques and products specifically suited for obese patients. This has presented many challenges to medical personnel in the radiology department.[1, 2] Due to their increased girth, x-rays in the energy range used in diagnostic imaging have difficulty penetrating the patient's body, resulting in images of very poor or even non-diagnostic quality. In many cases, the weight capacity limitations of the patient table (typically 350 lbs [159 kg]) or the size of the opening (approximately 45 cm) makes many obese patients ineligible for fluoroscopic imaging. For patients who can be imaged, the images generally have degraded image quality.

Manufacturers of medical imaging devices have responded to the increasing numbers of obese patients by increasing both the weight capacity of their patient tables and the dimensions of the opening into which the patient must fit. For CT, weight limits of 500–600 lbs (227–272 kg), or more, are now commercially available and gantry openings up to 100 cm have been manufactured, although most high-end diagnostic CT systems have a maximum gantry opening of 70–80 cm. Within Siemens SOMATOM CT systems, the SOMATOM Sensation Open offers the largest gantry opening diameter of 82cm, with a maximum patient weight of 615 lbs (280 kg). The SOMATOM Definition has a gantry opening diameter of 78 cm, with a maximum patient weight of 485 lbs (220 kg).

If the CT scanner can accommodate a patient, modifications to the typical scanning protocols must be made to provide adequate image quality. Typical adjustments include increasing the x-ray tube potential to 140 kV and increasing the quality reference effective mAs as high as the scanner will allow. The use of automatic exposure control systems is recommended, as the tube current can be

Body: Obese Mode

decreased for some thinner projections, which may allow higher values to be used for the thicker projections.[3] As in the shoulder and pelvis regions in normal-size patients, the use of automatic exposure systems such as CARE Dose4D can decrease streak artifacts due to photon starvation and better equalize the noise texture of the resultant image.[4]

Methods of reducing noise in images of obese patients include making use of thick image section widths (5–10 mm), longer gantry rotation times or sequential scan acquisition modes. While this may decrease image noise, partial volume averaging or motion artifacts are increased and volumetric spiral imaging, such as is needed for high quality CT angiography or cardiac CT examinations, is either unable to be performed or results in less than desirable results. In spiral imaging, the use of lower pitch values allows for the accumulation of dose for any given tissue location and hence decreases image noise. However, this can result in unacceptably long scan times as might the use of longer gantry rotation times.

Another option to reduce image noise in photon-limited situations is to use smoother reconstruction kernels. On the Siemens systems, the number associated with the kernel indicates the relative smoothness or sharpness of the resultant image: B10 being the smoothest (lowest noise) and B80 the sharpest (highest image noise) reconstruction kernels for body imaging. Again, the user must trade off competing image quality metrics – spatial resolution or image noise.

When the number of photons reaching the detector is very low, the electronic noise of the detection system can begin to exponentially increase image noise. At these low signal levels, some signal averaging is performed to reduce streak artifacts. Both of these factors can degrade image quality in a manner that cannot be recovered using smoother reconstruction kernels, often producing ring artifacts or subtle non-uniformities within the image. To address this, a special kernel was created on Siemens' systems that more effectively reacts to these signal imperfections, known as B18. The use of B18 is recommended if ring artifacts appear when B10 or B20 is used, as it will substantially decrease such rings. When no ring artifacts are present, B18 should not be used, because it may create artifacts.

Finally, to avoid these very low detector-level signals, the use of wider detector collimations is recommended. On 40-, 64- and Dual Source CT systems, the 1.2 mm collimation is preferable to the 0.6 mm collimation. It is extremely unlikely that reconstructed image widths less than 1 mm would be desired on obese patients. Thus the avoidance of sub-mm collimation presents no practical disadvantage, increases the signal brightness at the detector and decreases the overall scan time due to the wider total beam width.

The development of Dual Source CT enables a unique mechanism by which to improve image quality in obese patients: That is, both x-ray sources may be simultaneously energized using the same x-ray tube potential, and the resultant data may be appropriately summed prior to image reconstruction.[5] This effectively doubles the x-ray tube power available for the scan, which allows scans to be performed with higher pitch values (shorter scan times), higher effective mAs values (lower image noise), narrower image section widths, or some combination of these. Interestingly, even though the tube-current time product may increase by as much as a factor of two, the radiation risk to the patient does not increase to the same degree. This is because the layers of adipose tissue surrounding the internal radiosensitive tissues attenuate the incoming x-ray beam prior to reaching the sensitive tissues.[6]

Elizabeth McDonald · Robert P. Hartman · Cynthia McCollough
Mayo Clinic College of Medicine
Department of Radiology

References

[1] Uppot RN, Sahani DV, Hahn PF, Gervais D, Mueller PR. Impact of obesity on medical imaging and image-guided intervention. AJR Am J Roentgenol 2007; 188:433-440

[2] Uppot RN, Sahani DV, Hahn PF, Kalra MK, Saini SS, Mueller PR. Effect of obesity on image quality: fifteen-year longitudinal study for evaluation of dictated radiology reports. Radiology 2006; 240:435-439

[3] McCollough CH, Bruesewitz MR, Kofler JM, Jr. CT dose reduction and dose management tools: overview of available options. Radiographics 2006; 26:503-512

[4] Gies M, Kalender WA, Wolf H, Suess C, Madsen M. Dose reduction in CT by anatomically adapted tube current modulation: Simulation studies. Medical Physics 1999; 26:2235-2247

[5] Flohr TG, McCollough CH, Bruder H, et al. First performance evaluation of a dual-source CT (DSCT) system. Eur Radiol 2006; 16:256-268

[6] Schmidt B, Kalendar WA. A fast voxel-based Monte Carlo method for scanner- and patient-specific dose calculations in computed tomography. In: Guerra AD, ed. Physica Medica. Erlangen, Germany: European Journal of Medical Physics, 2002; 43-53

Body: Obese Mode

Basic considerations

Dual Source CT provides the ability to simultaneously operate both x-ray tubes at the same tube voltage, essentially doubling the available x-ray power. This provides the needed x-ray photons to adequately image even morbidly obese patients without the need to compromise the exam quality by decreasing pitch, which increases the scan time.

Operators must use appropriate caution with regard to table weight limits and gantry opening dimension. Employing tube current modulation adapted to individual patient anatomy (CARE Dose4D) is especially important to reduce radiation dose in this patient population.

Scan Parameters (exemplified for abdominal CT)

Scan mode	Dual Source, non-gated
Scan area	diaphragm to iliac crests or symphysis
Scan direction	cranio-caudal
Scan time	~7 s
Tube voltage	120 kV
Tube current	350 quality ref. mAs
Dose modulation	CARE Dose4D
$CTDI_{vol}$	23 mGy, depending on patient size
Rotation time	0.5 s
Pitch	0.85
Slice collimation	1.2 mm
Acquisition	24 x 1.2 mm
Slice width	5 mm
Reconstruction increment	5 mm
Reconstruction kernel	B30f / B18f

Tricks

· Use extended FOV reconstruction to avoid artifacts that occur when all patient tissue does not fit into a 50 cm FOV.

· Use B18 kernel if ring artifacts occur. Do not use B18 if there are no ring artifacts.

· Wrapping the patient in balloon silk or applying a wide belt across the abdomen may help fit the patient into the gantry's dimensions.

Pitfalls

· Use of 64 x 0.6 collimation in morbidly obese patients can result in artifacts in the pelvis from detector-level signal averaging, so 24 x 1.2 mm collimation is highly recommended.

· An increase in image noise can be observed outside the central 26 cm FoV.

Contrast Injection Protocol

	Iodine concentration 300 mg I/ml	Iodine concentration 370 mg I/ml
Injection scheme	Monophasic	Monophasic
Iodine delivery rate	1.5 g/s	1.5 g/s
CM volume	225 ml	180 ml
CM flow rate	5 ml/s	4.1 ml/s
Body weight adaption	yes	yes
Bolus timing	–	–
Bolus tracking threshold	–	–
ROI position	–	–
Scan delay	80 s	80 s
Saline flush volume	60 ml	60 ml
Saline injection rate	5 ml/s	4.1 ml/s
Needle size	18 G	18 G
Injection site	antecubital vein	antecubital vein

Case 1 Aortic Dissection in 183 kg Male

Case history

45-year-old obese male (183 kg / 402 lbs;
BMI=49.3 kg/m^2) post surgical repair of his
ascending aorta for an acute aortic dissection
presents with increasing shortness of breath
and chest discomfort.

Question

Evaluation of a proximal descending thoracic
aortic aneurysm associated with a chronic aortic
dissection.

Diagnosis / Differential diagnosis

This CT was needed to evaluate whether an obese
patient with a known aortic aneurysm and past
aortic dissection repair would need emergent
surgery for type-A aortic dissection or expansion
of the known aneurysm.

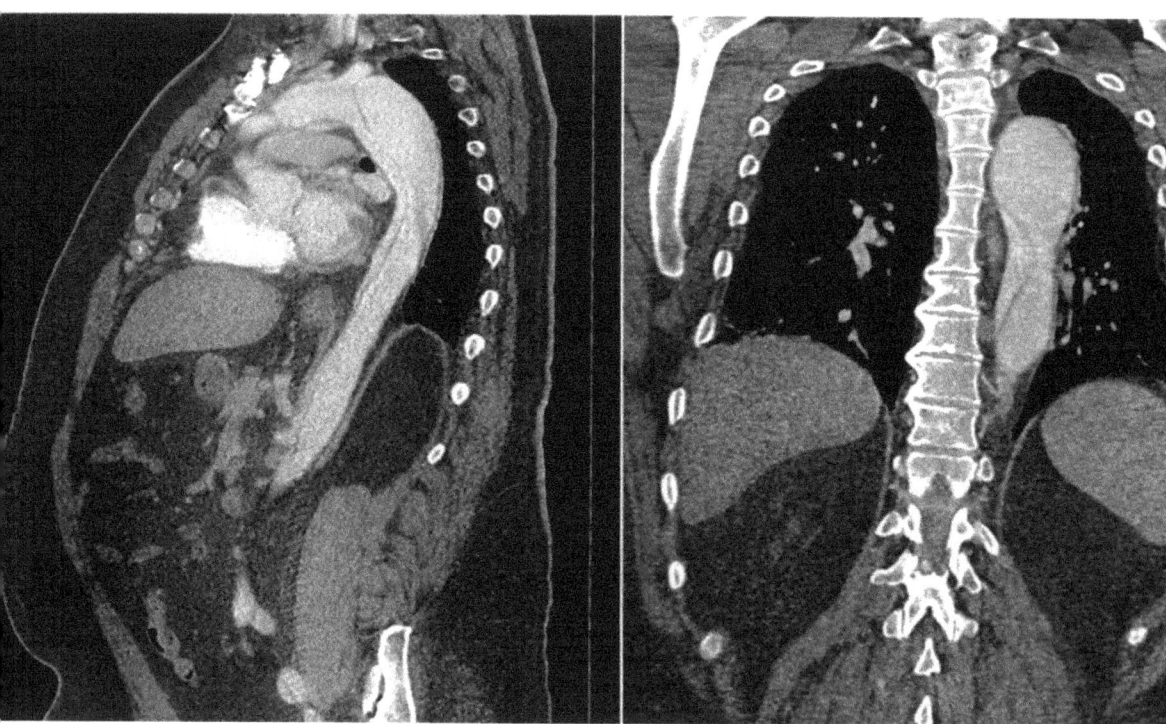

[1] Contrast enhanced sagittal image shows the dissection flap
extending from the aortic arch through the mid-abdomen. The
celiac axis and SMA arise from the true lumen.

[2] Contrast enhanced coronal image shows focal aneurysmal
dilatation of the proximal aorta with a dissection flap seen
distally.

Findings

Type-A aortic dissection with postoperative changes of ascending aorta repair. Focal 6 cm diameter aneurysmal dilatation of proximal descending thoracic aorta. There are large fenestrations present on the dissection flap, both proximally and distally. The dissection flap extends into both common iliac arteries. Celiac, SMA, IMA, and right renal artery are from the true lumen. Left renal artery is from the false lumen.

Take-home message

Type-A aortic dissection with focal aneurysmal dilatation of the proximal descending thoracic aorta. This was surgically repaired the next day. In obese patients, high spatial resolution CT angiographic images of the chest, abdomen, and pelvis can be successfully obtained.

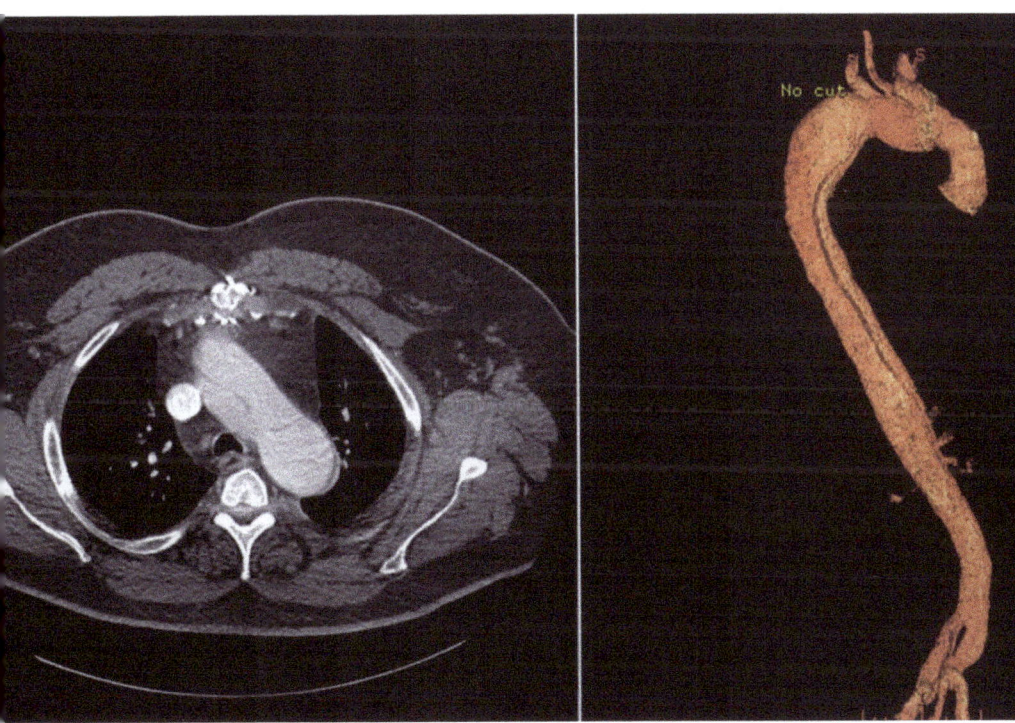

[3] Contrast enhanced axial image of the dissection flap nicely demonstrates a fenestration.

[4] Three-dimensional rendering of the type-A aortic dissection extending from the aortic arch to the common iliac arteries.

Case 2 Abdominal Abscess in 206 kg Male

Case history

57-year-old diabetic morbidly obese male (206 kg/452 lbs; BMI=66.7 kg/m²) presents with recurrent staphylococcal septicemias for the last three years.

Question

Is there an abdominal abscess as the source for these repeated infections?

Diagnosis/Differential diagnosis

This CT was needed to find the source of recurrent sepsis. The differential diagnosis included an abdominal abscess, immunosuppression or occult malignancy.

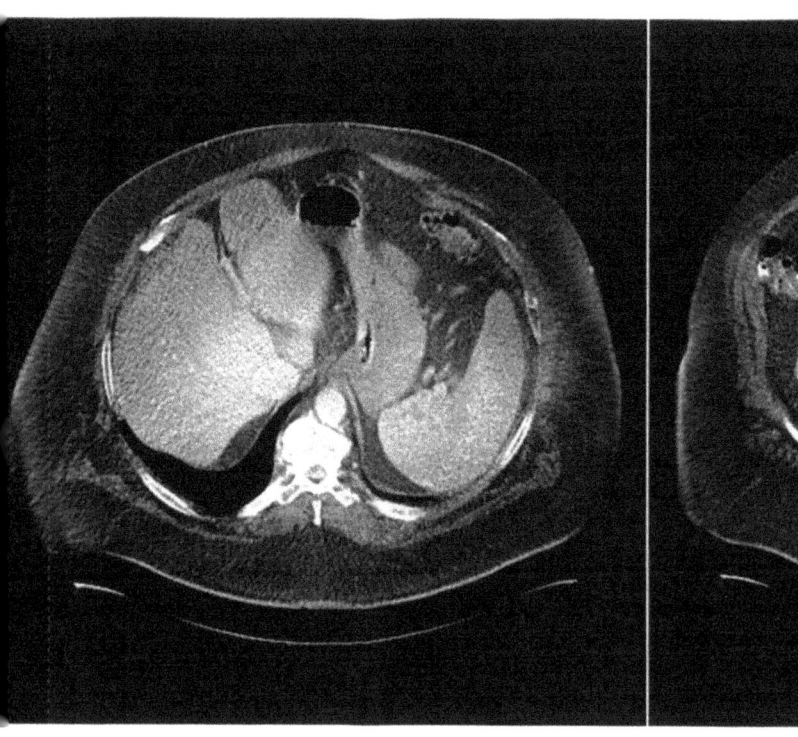
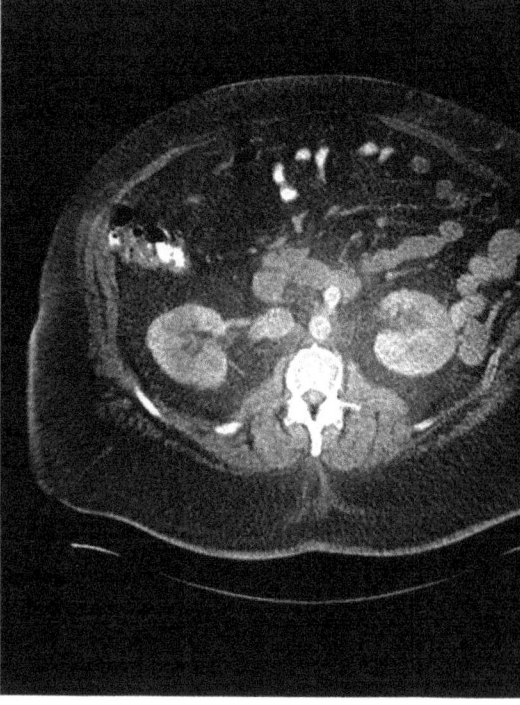

[1] Contrast enhanced axial image demonstrates cirrhotic configuration of the liver.

[2] Contrast enhanced axial image demonstrates multiple splenic varices.

Findings

Cirrhotic configuration of the liver with evidence for portal venous hypertension including multiple splenic varices and a large caliber spontaneous splenorenal shunt. The spleen is normal in size. No evidence of intra-abdominal abscess. No additional findings.

Take-home message

Dual Source CT allows sufficient x-ray power to acquire diagnostic, 3D reformatted images of morbidly obese patients.

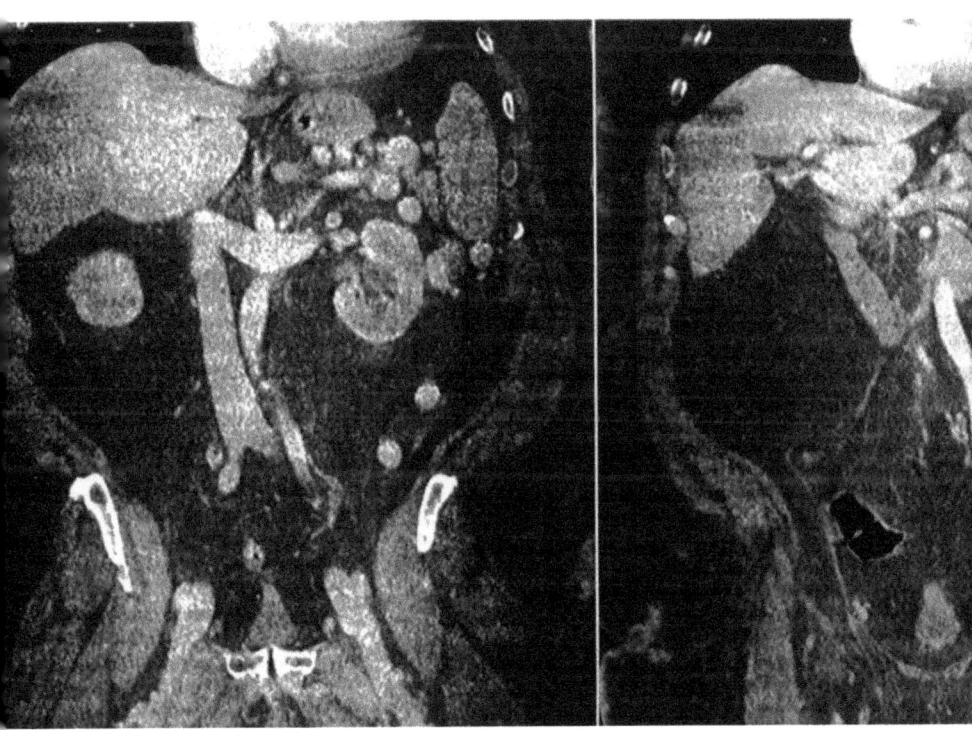

[3] Contrast enhanced coronal image demonstrates multiple splenic varices.

[4] Contrast enhanced coronal image shows a large caliber splenorenal shunt which courses deep into the left upper pelvis before ascending to the left renal vein.

Dual Energy CT Applications

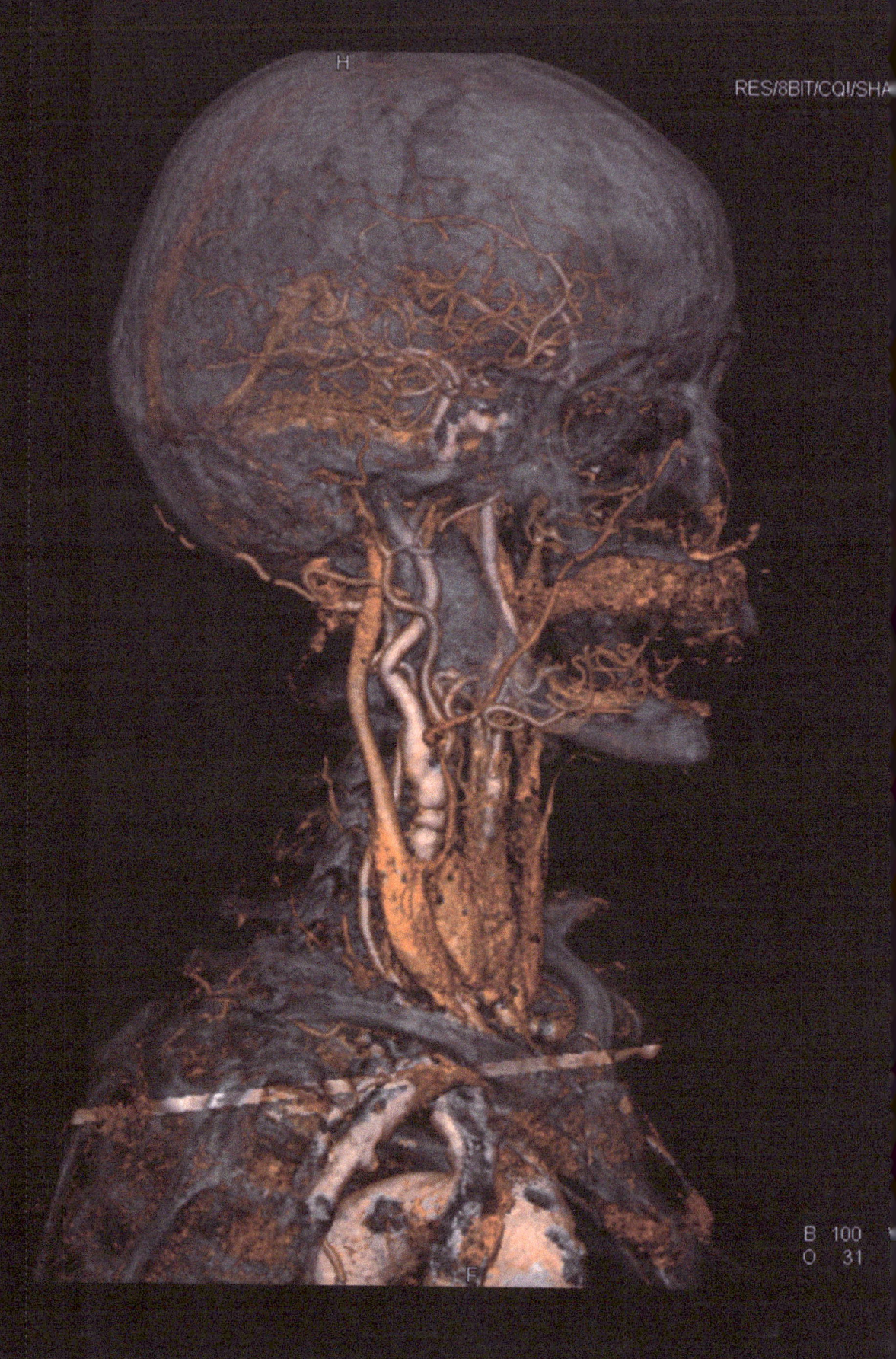

Dual Energy: CTA of Head and Neck

Dominik Morhard · Thorsten R. C. Johnson · Christoph R. Becker

Case 1: Multi-segmental Stenosis of all Cervical Vessels and Intracranial Aneurysm

Case 2: Stenosis of Internal Carotid Artery

Recent technical developments in multislice computed tomography (CT) have opened new perspectives in the non-invasive investigation of supra-aortic extracranial and intracranial vessels. Simultaneous acquisition of 64 slices at 0.33 seconds rotation times has made long scan ranges at high spatial resolution feasible. With the introduction of Dual Source CT in 2006, in which two tubes and detectors are mounted orthogonally, it is now possible to acquire one axial image by a gantry rotation of 90° instead the 180° needed in single-source scanners. This cuts acquisition time by half, which is an important factor especially in cardiac imaging. It is also possible to run the two tubes at different voltages – the so-called spiral dual energy CT mode (e.g. 140 and 80 kV) – in order to obtain different attenuations for material decomposition. Multiple dual-energy applications are currently under evaluation: material differentiation, bone removal, iodine quantification, perfusion mapping and plaque imaging to name a few.[1-6]

Although innovations in magnet resonance imaging (MRI) like parallel acquisitions techniques and higher magnetic fields strength have significantly shortened acquisition time, and despite the fact, that the use of diffusion-weighted-imaging (DWI) and MR perfusion is considered to be the most accurate modality in evaluation of stroke, computed tomography remains the most frequently used and most widespread modality in the triage and classification of patients with acute ischemic and hemorrhagic stroke. Specialized CT protocols for the evaluation of stroke – known as "Stroke-protocols" – consist of a non-enhanced CT scan (NECT) of the cerebrum, a supraaortic CT angiography (CTA) and a dynamic sequence CT-perfusion scan (CTP). CTP is very useful in cases of early stroke (3–6 h) when hemorrhage has been ruled out and morphologic signs of ischemia are absent or subtle. Territorial differences in contrast transit time (mean transit time (MTT) or time to peak (TTP)) indicate impaired supratentorial perfusion in the area supplied by a specific major cerebral artery or its branches. CTA findings in this situation include internal carotid artery stenosis or occlusion, dissection and thromboembolism causing obstruction of intracranial vessels. In cases of acute (< 8 h) vertebro-basilar deficits, CTA can be performed – without perfusion CTA – in order to assess the patency of the extra- and intracranial vertebral arteries and the basilar artery. CTA may provide clues as to thromboembolism as the principle mechanism of artery obstruction or recognize pre-existing stenosis with subsequent appositional thrombus. It is also possible to perform CTP during neurosurgical

Dual Energy: CTA of Head and Neck

aneurysm clipping procedures to ensure sufficient blood perfusion peripheral to temporal aneurysm clips before possible infarction occurs. Special CT installations, for example, CT-scanners with a sliding gantry, are mandatory for this.

To evaluate hemorrhagic stroke, a NECT and an intracranial CTA are used to rule out vascular pathologies like intracranial aneurysm, vascular malformations or thrombosis of the cerebral veins and sinuses. Recent studies correlating CTA to DSA in cases of subarachnoidal hemorrhage (SAH) show excellent sensitivity and specificity for the detection of intracranial aneurysm of a minimum size of 3 mm on the basis of multislice CTA. The sensitivity only drops dramatically when in cases of very small aneurysm (< 3 mm) correlated to DSA as a gold standard. In SAH as well as in other indications, the delineation of vasculature in close vicinity to bony structure, such as the base of skull, is limited in MDCT angiography compared with MRA and DSA. To cope this limitation, there are different approaches for to remove bone from the CTA datasets such as region-growing algorithm or section-by-section digital subtraction. These algorithms often lead to insufficient results. With dual-energy material-differentiation (bone and iodine), it is now possible to perform reliable bone and calcified-plaque subtraction out of CTA volume data. Translocations between the two parallel scans are extremely rare with the two-tube setup. This is a clear benefit compared with single-energy bone subtraction techniques, which often suffer from translocations between the two sequence scans (NECT CTA). After bone subtraction, more convenient reconstructions like thick maximum intensity projections (MIP) and the volume rendering technique (VRT) can be used and reading time can be significantly reduced. Further investigations will have to prove if bone-removal can increase the sensitivity of detecting very small aneurysms. On the other hand, by visualizing bony structures and intracranial vasculature at one time, CTA can provide information to surgeons for therapy planning.

For the evaluation of stenosis of the supraaortic arteries – mainly common and internal carotid arteries, but also vertebral and basilar arteries – CTA is a robust and non-invasive modality. Specialized post-processing software enables swift, semi-automatic 2D- and 3D-reconstructions, such as stretched multiplanar reformations (MPR) and MIP for reliable morphology-based stenosis quantification providing relative and absolute diameter and area information. CTA as a modality for follow-up examinations after stent angioplasty has a clear benefit over MRA because of lower susceptibility artifacts and it provides reliable information about stent patency even in stents with a lumen diameter of 3 mm (e.g. in the vertebral or basilar artery).

All together, modern neurovascular CT angiography as a non-invasive imaging modality is replacing conventional diagnostic DSA and MRA more and more because of it is less time consuming and less susceptible to motion artifacts in critically ill patients as well in clinical routine.

Dominik Morhard · Thorsten R. C. Johnson · Christoph R. Becker

University of Munich-Grosshadern

Department of Clinical Radiology

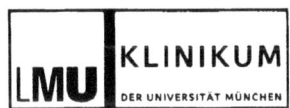

References

1 Johnson TRC, Krauß B, Sedlmair M, Grasruck M, Bruder H, Morhard D, Fink C, Weckbach S, Lenhard M, Schmidt B, Flohr T, Reiser MF, Becker CR. (2007) Material differentiation by dual energy CT: initial experience. Eur Radiol 17(6):1510-1517

2 Farkas J, Xavier A, Prestigiacomo CJ (2004) Advanced imaging application for acute ischemic stroke. Emergency radiology 11:77-82

3 Tomandl BF, Hammen T, Klotz E, Ditt H, Stemper B, Lell M (2006) Bone-subtraction CT angiography for the evaluation of intracranial aneurysms. Ajnr 27:55-59

4 Zhang Z, Berg M, Ikonen A, Kononen M, Kalviainen R, Manninen H, Vanninen R (2005) Carotid stenosis degree in CT angiography: assessment based on luminal area versus luminal diameter measurements. Eur Radiol 15:2359-2365

5 Hollingworth W, Nathens AB, Kanne JP, Crandall ML, Crummy TA, Hallam DK, Wang MC, Jarvik JG (2003) The diagnostic accuracy of computed tomography angiography for traumatic or atherosclerotic lesions of the carotid and vertebral arteries: a systematic review. European journal

6 Lell MM, Anders K, Uder M, Klotz E, Ditt H, Vega-Higuera F, Boskamp T, Bautz WA, Tomandl BF (2006) New Techniques in CT Angiography. Radiographics 26 Suppl 1:S45-62

Dual Energy: CTA of Head and Neck

Basic considerations

Good image quality always depends on good pre-scan preparations: A comfortable headrest position for compliant and a effective fixation of non-compliant patients in emergency conditions is mandatory to avoid motion artifacts, even at a high pitch and 0.33 s gantry rotation time. Dental implants tend to cause severe beam hardening artifacts. Individual head positioning with the adjustable head rest can avoid artifacts over the carotid bulb, one of the regions with the highest clinical impact.

Depending on the indication, good enhancement of arteries (only) or arteries and veins has to be achieved. Start delay has to be adjusted depending on desired contrast-phase.

Scan Parameters

Scan mode	Spiral dual energy with Dual Source
Scan area	all supra-aortic vessels or intracranial
Scan direction	caudo-cranial
Scan time	~ _ ~7 s
Tube voltage A/B	140 kV/80 kV
Tube current A/B	55 quality ref. mAs / 234 quality ref. mAs
Dose modulation	CARE Dose 4D
CTDI$_{vol}$	~10 mGy
Rotation time	0.33 s
Pitch	0.7
Slice collimation	0.6 mm
Acquisition	64 x 0.6 mm
Slice width	0.75 mm
Reconstruction increment	0.5 mm
Reconstruction kernel	D20f

Tricks

Timing of contrast agent injection can be adjusted to achieve pure arterial enhancement to evaluate arteries with less venous overlay. To get the best enhancement to evaluate all intracranial vasculature, delay can be set between 30 and 35 seconds (e.g. to rule out venous thrombosis). Dual topograms in anterior-posterior and lateral projection help positioning.

Pitfalls

Missing contrast bolus by placing monitoring ROI outside the aorta. Using cranio-caudal scan direction for early arterial phase scanning (long range table movement may waste valuable seconds). Removed calcified plaque may result in irregularities of the vessel wall mimicking a more complex aneurysm architecture with lobulations and "baby-aneurysm".

Contrast Injection Protocol

	Iodine concentration 300 mg I/ml	Iodine concentration 370 mg I/ml
Injection scheme	Monophasic	Monophasic
Iodine delivery rate	2.2 g/s	2.2 g/s
CM volume	100 ml	80 ml
CM flow rate	7.3 ml/s	6 ml/s
Body weight adaption	yes	yes
Bolus timing	bolus tracking*	bolus tracking*
Bolus tracking threshold	200 HU	200 HU
ROI position	ascending aorta	ascending aorta
Scan delay	4 s for pure arterial 25 s for arteries and venous	4 s for pure arterial 25 s for arteries and venous
Saline flush volume	100 ml	100 ml
Saline injection rate	7.3 ml/s	6 ml/s
Needle size	18 G	18 G
Injection site	antecubital vein	antecubital vein

*Depending on the preference of the individual site, test bolus can be used as an alternative

Case 1 Multi-segmental Stenosis of all Cervical Vessels and Intracranial Aneurysm

Case history

This patient presented with a long history of arterial hypertension and known stenosis of the carotid arteries. Controversial findings in duplex. Multiple small ischemic lesions at the right hemisphere.

Question

Extent of supra-aortic atherosclerosis and stenosis? Other vascular pathologies?

Diagnosis / Differential diagnosis

Severe atherosclerosis changes of the supraaortic vessels with multiple bilateral stenosis of the common carotid arteries and internal carotid arteries, as well as an infraophthalmic aneurysm of the right internal carotid artery.

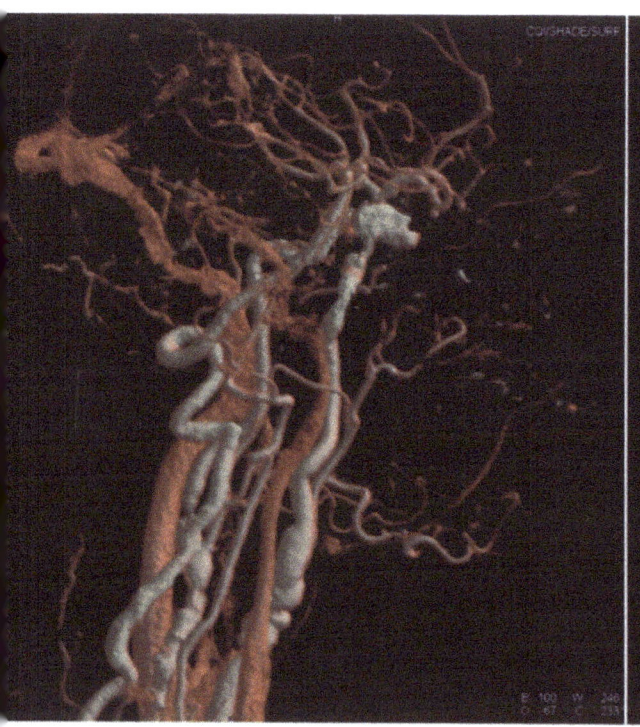

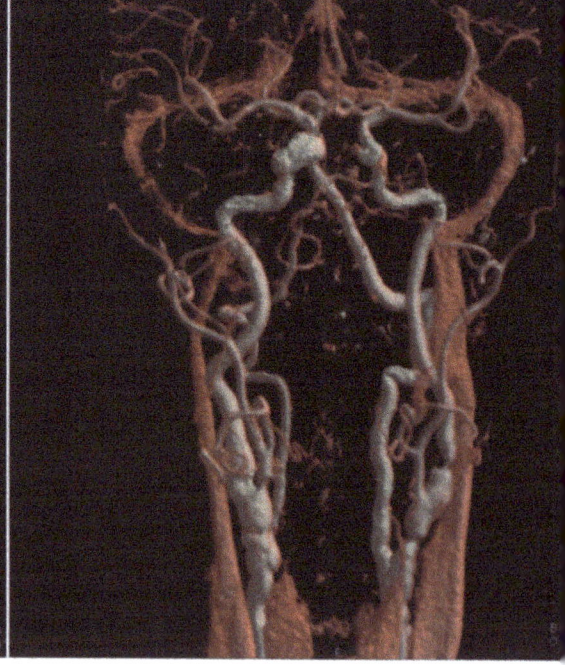

[1] VRT reconstruction of supra-aortic spiral dual energy bone removal CTA showing multiple high-grade stenosis of the carotid arteries.

[2] A more lateral view shows the anterior orientation of the infraophthalmic ICA aneurysm on the right as well as the stenosis inferior of the aneurysmal neck.

Findings

Selective, dual-energy based bone removal offers excellent motion-artifact-free results but note that the subtraction of calcified plaque can mimic irregularities of the aneurysm wall on the VRT reconstruction. Compare the real stenosis adjacent with the aneurysm neck.

Take-home message

In case of irregularities of aneurysm wall on subtracted images, always keep in mind that this might be a result of subtracting calcified plaque components and re-check/correlate to unsubtracted CTA images.

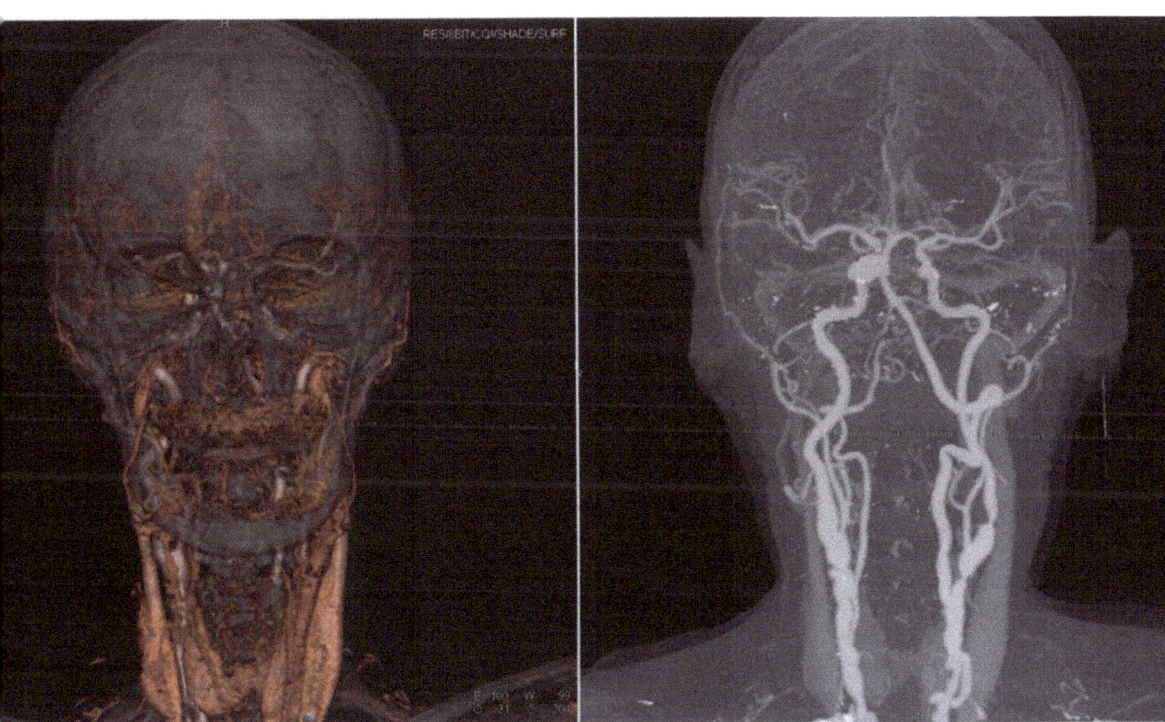

[3] VRT reconstruction using selective mapping of a dataset consisting of only iodine-enhanced supraaortic vessels (red color map) and a second dataset of bony data (grey).

[4] Bone removal allows thick MIP reconstruction giving an excellent, MRA-like overview of all supraaortic vessels.

Case 2 Stenosis of Internal Carotid Artery

Case history

72-year-old female with known peripheral atherosclerotic disease admitted to the ER with an episode of transient right sided hemiplegia.

Question

Atherosclerotic chances of the brain feeding arteries like stenosis or occlusions of the carotid or vertebral arteries.

Diagnosis / Differential diagnosis

High-grade stenosis at the proximal internal carotid artery on the left side due to mixed plaque. Differential diagnosis: Short ranged dissection of the arterial wall resulting in a high-grade stenosis of the vessel lumen.

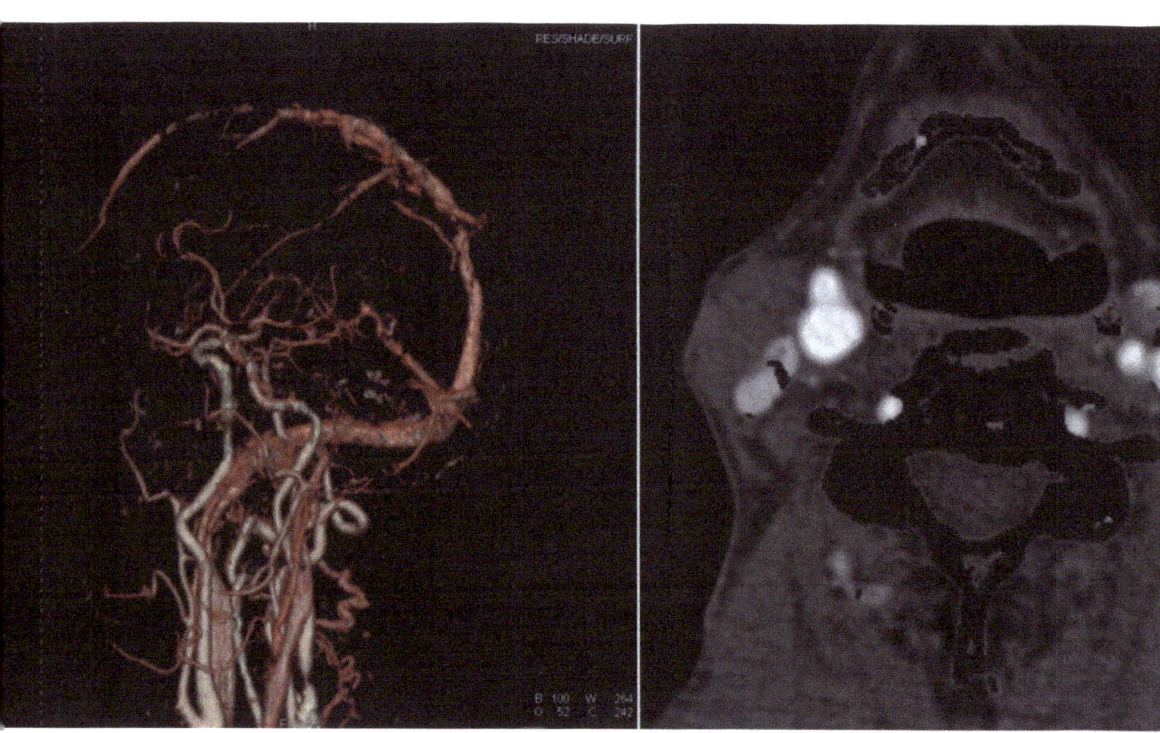

[1] VRT reconstruction of the bone-subtracted dual energy CTA dataset showing the high-grade stenosis of the proximal left internal carotid artery.

[2] Axial MPR. All calcified areas of the mixed plaque have been removed by the bone-removal algorithm. (Image taken just below the maximum extends of the lumen narrowing.)

Findings

A mixed plaque (soft and calcified compounds) next to the carotid bulb results in an 85–90% area stenosis of the internal carotid artery. Distal to the stenosis, the vessel lumen appears quite normal and good contrasted, an indirect hint for a stenosis grade under 98%.

Take-home message

Bone subtraction can simplify stenosis quantification, especially when using semi-automatic vessel analysis tools. Using area measurements instead of only diameter measurements results in more accurate and realistic stenosis quantifications.

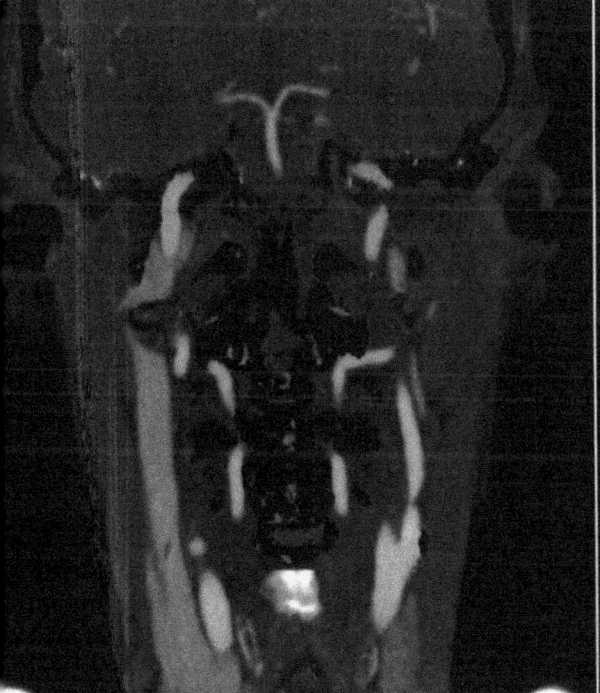 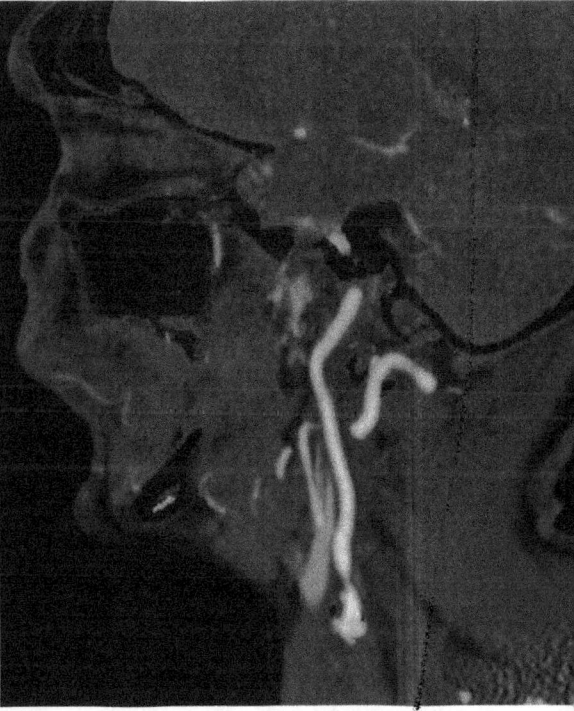

[3] Coronal MIP reconstructions show the excellent results of the spiral dual energy bone removal as well as the stenosis and the intracavernous segments of both ICA.

[4] Sagittal MIP shows removed calcified plaque and non-calcified (not removed) plaque components at the stenosis.

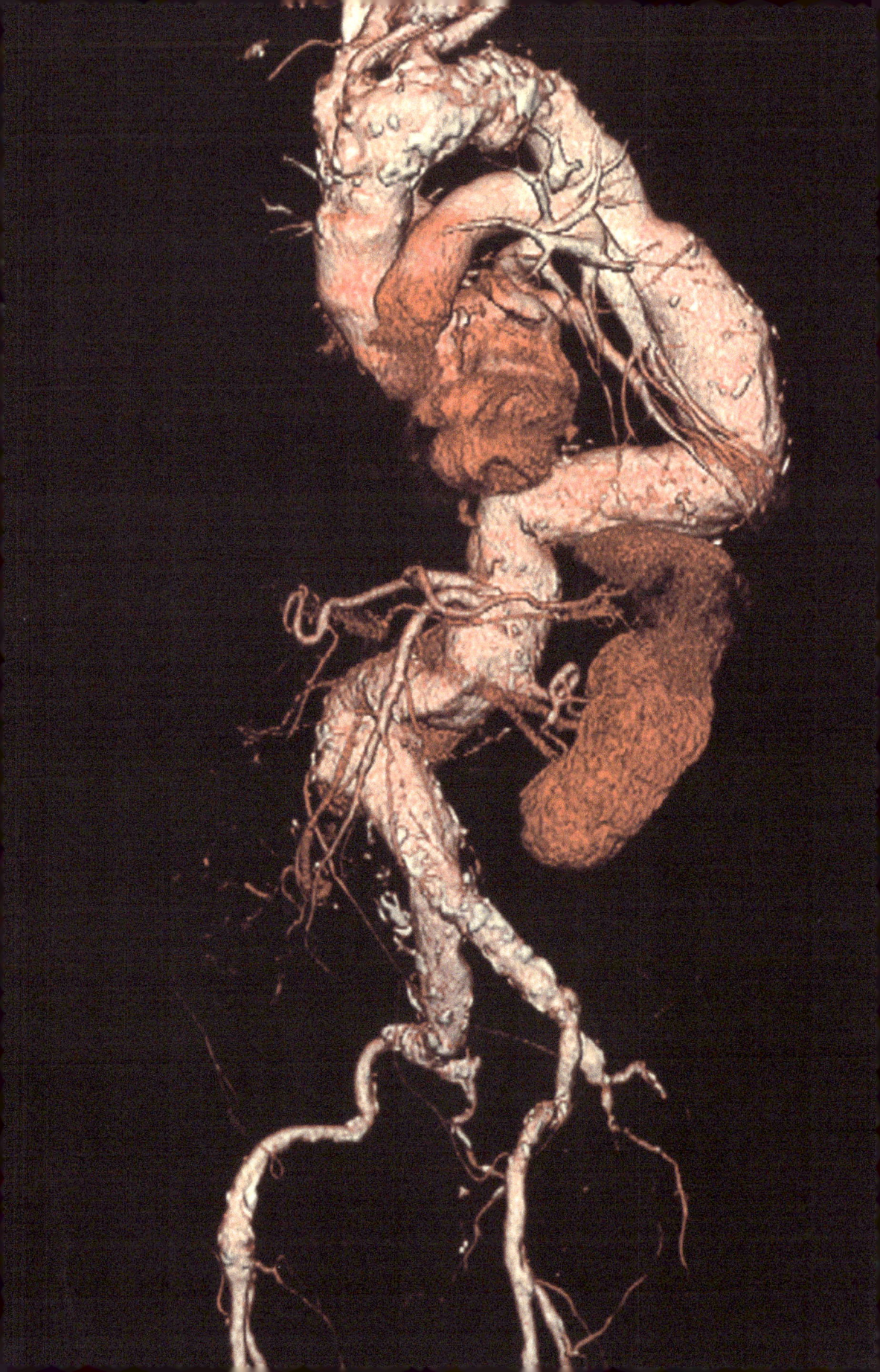

Dual Energy: CTA Aorta

Marco Das · Andreas H. Mahnken · Joachim E. Wildberger

Case 1: Abdominal Aortic Aneurysm and Interventional Stent Placement

Case 2: Prosthesis Infection After Surgical Abdominal Aortic Prosthesis

Aortic aneurysms are a common pathology, with the potential risk of rupture.[1] Aneurysms can be differentiated into true aneurysms, which involve all three layers of the vessel wall (intima, media and adventitia), false aneurysms (pseudoaneurysms), where a collection of blood communicates with the arterial lumen but is not surrounded by normal vessel wall, and dissecting aneurysms, in which the blood is between the normal vessel lumen and the intima. Initially, a tear in the intimal layer of the aorta occurs. As high pressure exists in the aorta, blood enters the media. The force of the blood entering the media causes the tear to extend. It may extend proximally or, distally or both. As a result of the extending tear the blood will move through the media, creating a false lumen separated by a layer of intimal tissue (intimal flap).

The vast majority of aortic dissections originate with an intimal tear in either the ascending aorta (65%), the aortic arch (10%) or distal to the ligamentum arteriosum in the descending thoracic aorta (20%).[2] Most patients (> 90%) with aortic dissection present with severe sudden onset of pain. It may be described as a tearing stabbing or sharp pain. About 15% of individuals will feel the pain migrate as the dissection extends down the aorta. The location of pain is associated with the location of the dissection. Pericarditis and heart attack must be ruled out, especially if pain is felt in the anterior thorax.

According to epidemiological studies, 9% of all patients over 65 do have an abdominal aortic aneurysm (AAA). Interestingly, AAA is uncommon in individuals of African, African American, Asian and Hispanic descent. The physiological infrarenal diameter varies between 1–3 cm. Larger diameters of 3 cm are considered to be aneurysms, but the risk of rupture is still low. Aneurysms larger than 5 cm, growing aneurysms or symptomatic aneurysms require therapy. Male patients are more frequently affected than women. The main underlying disease is hypertension. Patients with a ruptured AAA usually present with low back, flank or abdominal pain. Often bleeding leads to a hypovolemic shock with hypotension, tachycardia, cyanosis and altered mental status. Mortality is high (75–90%) – most patients die before arriving at the hospital. Less frequently, the aorta is affected by inflammatory changes (e.g. drug abuse, lues) or congenital diseases like Marfan's syndrome. Basically aortic aneurysm may occur in any segment of the aorta. Thoracic-abdominal

Dual Energy: CTA Aorta

aneurysms are less frequent as >92% of aneurysms are located infrarenal. Because about 7% of all emergency patients present with chest pain, aortic dissection may be the cause of acute thoracic pain. In emergencies, pulmonary embolism, acute heart attack and aortic dissection need to be ruled out. Depending on the entrance into the vessel wall, dissecting aneurysm are classified using Stanford's classification. Entrance of the bleeding in the ascending aorta is referred to as Stanford A, while entrance of the bleeding in the descending aorta is referred to as Stanford B. As the coronary arteries might be involved in Stanford A aortic dissection, these patients need immediate surgical therapy. The therapeutical options for Stanford B dissections depend on how far the membrane extends, and whether the visceral arteries origin ate from the real or the false lumen of the aorta. Endovascular aortic repair (EVAR) has gained attention over the last year, showing promising results.[3,4] The interdisciplinary patient management between interventional radiologists and vascular surgeons will further increase the acceptance of this method. This less invasive procedure should be considered, especially in patients with few co-morbidities. EVAR also represents a secure option in patients with covered ruptured aortic aneurysm, providing a fast method to prevent the aorta from further rupture and to allow definite repair.

Multislice spiral CT (MSCT) has replaced digital subtraction angiography (DSA) in the assessment of the aorta in the emergency room and mostly in routine practice. Compared with DSA, MSCT can be considered a minimally invasive procedure without potential complications of patient bleeding or discomfort after intervention. Additionally, MSCT enables visualization of the aorta beyond the vessel wall, also showing, for example, intramural thrombi or periaortic infections.[5,6] MSCT allows you to scan the aorta from the aortic root to the pelvis within a few seconds and as well as quick 3D reconstruction (volume rendering technique or VRT) multiplanar reformats (MPR) or maximum intensity projections (MIP) in any direction with the same image quality as the axial images. Its high spatial resolution has made MSCT the first-line modality in the emergency room where it is available 24/7 for pathologies of the aorta like aortic aneurysm and consecutive aortic rupture, aortic dissection, leriche syndrome, aortic infection, ulcers and potentially extra aortic causes of symptoms. Furthermore, as EVAR in the aorta has shown promising results, MSCT is the perfect tool for individual pre-interventional assessment for optimal stent dimensions, as every stent has to be manufactured individually for each patient. MSCT after EVAR is also the perfect tool to evaluate therapy success and to evaluate potential endoleakage.

The latest technical evolution of MSCT to DSCT further increased spatial and temporal resolution of aortic examinations. Facilitating the use of two different tube voltages allows direct bone removal for direct visualization of the aorta and branching vessels. In this respect, optimal contrast bolus timing is essential to achieve high quality images with optimal contrast enhancement of the aorta. This chapter shall provide parameters and protocols to achieve excellent image quality of the aorta and thereby optimize examinations.

Marco Das · Andreas H. Mahnken · Joachim E. Wildberger
RWTH Aachen University
Department of Diagnostic Radiology

References

1. Yu T, Zhu X, Tang L, Wang D, Saad N. Review of CT Angiography of Aorta. Radiol Clin North Am. 2007 May;45(3):461-83
2. Siegal EM. Acute aortic dissection. J Hosp Med. 2006 Mar;1(2):94-105.
3. Piffaretti G, Tozzi M, Lomazzi C, Rivolta N, Caronno R, Castelli P. Endovascular repair of abdominal infrarenal penetrating aortic ulcers: a prospective observational study. Int J Surg. 2007 Jun;5(3):172-5 Epub 2006 Jul 12
4. Saratzis NA, Saratzis AN, Melas N, Ginis G, Lioupis A, Lykopoulos D, Lazaridis J, Dimitrios K. Endovascular repair of traumatic rupture of the thoracic aorta: single-center experience. Cardiovasc Intervent Radiol. 2007 May-Jun;30(3):370-5
5. Hagspiel KD, Turba UC, Bozlar U, Harthun NL, Cherry KJ, Ahmed H, Bickston SJ, Angle JF. Diagnosis of aortoenteric fistulas with CT angiography. J Vasc Interv Radiol. 2007 Apr;18(4):497-504
6. Rakita D, Newatia A, Hines JJ, Siegel DN, Friedman B. Spectrum of CT findings in rupture and impending rupture of abdominal aortic aneurysms. Radiographics. 2007 Mar-Apr;27(2):497-507

Dual Energy: CTA Aorta

Basic considerations

The patient is placed into the gantry in a supine position. In most cases, the complete aorta from the aortic root to the inguinal arteries should be imaged to be able to rule out aortic dissection, which may extend into the thorax or originate from the thorax. No ECG-gating is necessary for the abdominal aorta. The examination should start with a non-enhanced scan for the whole scan field to be able to rule out intramural haematoma and to allow for differentiation of calcifications from bleeding. In the future, a virtual non-contrast reconstruction based on DE may take the place of the initial non-contrast scan. The bolus tracking region of interest (ROI) is placed on the descending aorta and the scan is started with a scan delay of seven seconds.

Scan Parameters

Scan mode	Spiral dual energy with Dual Source
Scan area	thorax/abdomen
Scan direction	cranio-caudal
Scan time	~6.5–25 s
Tube voltage A/B	140 kV/80 kV
Tube current A/B	70 quality ref. mAs/297 quality ref. mAs
Dose modulation	CARE Dose4D
CTDI$_{vol}$	~12 mGy
Rotation time	0.5 s
Pitch	0.8
Slice collimation	1.2 mm
Acquisition	14 x 1.2 mm
Slice width	1.5 mm
Reconstruction increment	1 mm
Reconstruction kernel	D30f

Tricks

Placing a large bore i.v. line (e.g. 18 G) is essential for optimal bolus administration, which is a prerequisite for high quality CTA, especially with use of DE. For CTA in general, not the iodine concentration of the contrast media is not essential but rather the iodine delivery rate (mg I/s) is the main determinant for optimal enhancement.

Pitfalls

Currently, a non-contrast enhanced scan is recommended to identify intramural haematoma, and to allow differentiation of calcifications, which may have an appearance like arterial bleeding. A late phase scan is recommended especially after endovascular stent placement to rule out endoleakage.

Contrast Injection Protocol

	Iodine concentration 300 mg I/ml	Iodine concentration 370 mg I/ml
Injection scheme	Monophasic	Monophasic
Iodine delivery rate	1.48 g/s	1.48 g/s
CM volume	148 ml	120 ml
CM flow rate	4.9 ml/s	4 ml/s
Body weight adaption	no	no
Bolus timing	bolus tracking*	bolus tracking*
Bolus tracking threshold	150 HU	150 HU
ROI position	descending aorta	descending aorta
Scan delay	7 s	7 s
Saline flush volume	60 ml	60 ml
Saline injection rate	4.9 ml/s	4 ml/s
Needle size	18 G	18 G
Injection site	antecubital vein	antecubital vein

* Depending on the preference of the individual site, test bolus can be used as an alternative

Case 1 Abdominal Aortic Aneurysm and Interventional Stent Placement

Case history

80-year old male presented with suspicion of abdominal aortic aneurysm after a pulsating tumor was palpable in his abdomen during a routine examination.

Question

To exclude a malignant tumor in the abdomen and to evaluate a potential aortic aneurysm.

Diagnosis/Differential diagnosis

The first differential diagnosis in a pulsating tumor includes abdominal aortic aneurysm. This can be a true aneurysm or a false aneurysm, which often occurs after intervention (e.g. coronary intervention). Secondly, an intraabdominal tumor must be excluded. Acute bleeding can be ruled out as well.

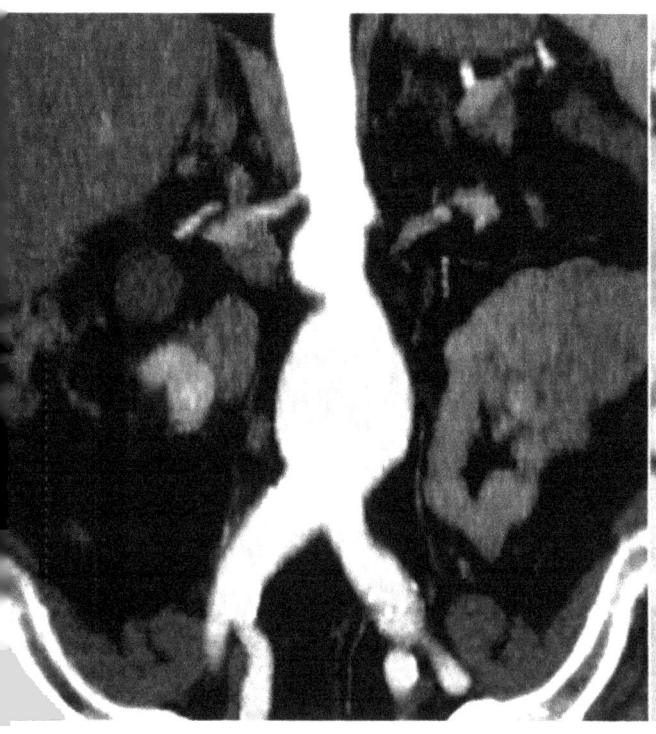

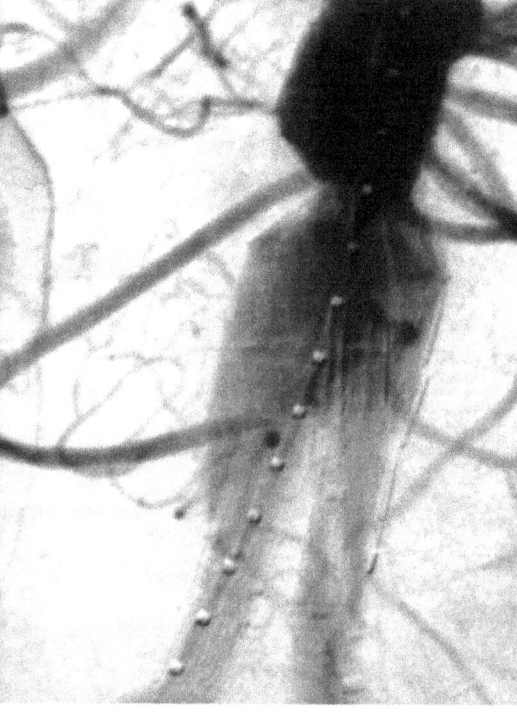

[1] CT of the aorta shows infrarenal abdominal aneurysm. As the size of the aneurysm includes potential rupture, interventional stent placement was planned using MPRs.

[2] Angiography shows excellent stent position where the aneurysm could be excluded.

Findings

An abdominal aortic aneurysm was found originating caudal of the renal arteries, extending to the common iliac arteries. The maximum axial aortic diameter was 6 cm, and the cranio-caudal extent was 9 cm. As no relevant additional diagnosis could be found, this patient was referred to interventional aortic stent placement.

Take-home message

With optimal bolus timing, a high quality CT Angiography of the abdominal aorta was achieved. The use of MPRs allowed optimal stent planning. Stent placement showed optimal results eliminating the aneurysm. DSCT was utilized for direct visualization of the aortic aneurysm.

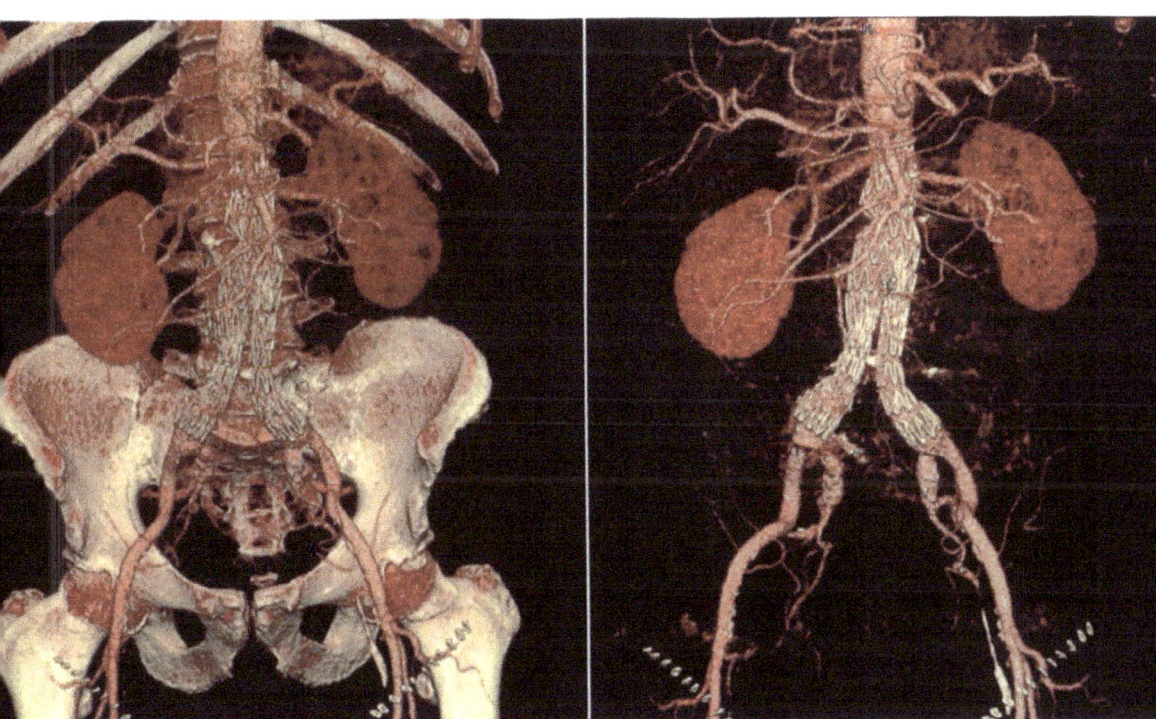

[3] 3D view of the prosthesis shows excellent result with full exclusion of the aneurysm and no signs of endoleakage.

[4] With automated bone removal, even better visualization of the aorta can be achieved, showing optimal stent positioning after EVAR.

Case 2 Prosthesis Infection After Surgical Abdominal Aortic Prosthesis

Case history

68-year old male with a history of surgical aortic repair after aortic rupture. Patient showed elevated infectious parameters.

Question

CT angiography of the abdominal aorta was performed to rule out an intraabdominal focus or prosthesis infection.

Diagnosis / Differential diagnosis

First differential diagnosis in this patient would be an intraabdominal focus like abscess formation as pulmonary infection was ruled out earlier. Potential bleeding after surgery needs to be ruled out. In rare cases, prosthesis infection occurs. Additionally prosthesis insufficiency or endoleak needs to be ruled out.

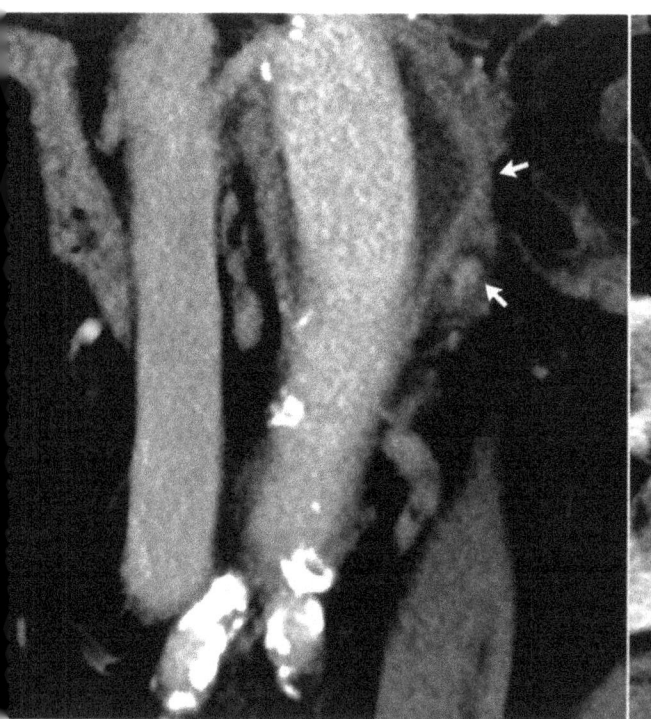

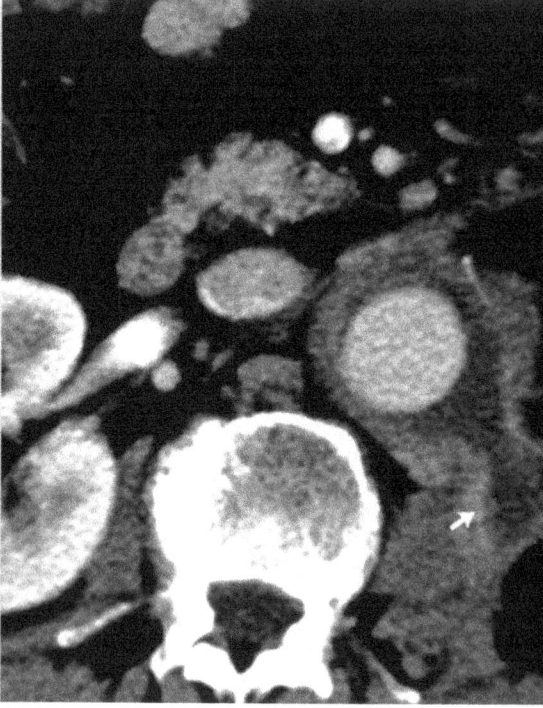

[1] Coronal MPR shows large fluid collection originating from the aorta.

[2] Axial image shows the large fluid collection and also shows fluid around the aorta and enhancement of the aortic vessel wall.

Findings

Fluid around the aortic prosthesis is found. The aortic wall shows significant enhancement and oedematous fluid in the surrounding fat, as a sign of infection. The patient underwent nephrectomy on the left side.

Take-home message

The use of MSCT/DSCT allows optimal visualization not only of the aorta itself like in DSA, but also allows visualization beyond the vessel wall. The use of multiplanar reformats offers visualization in any dimension with the same high image quality.

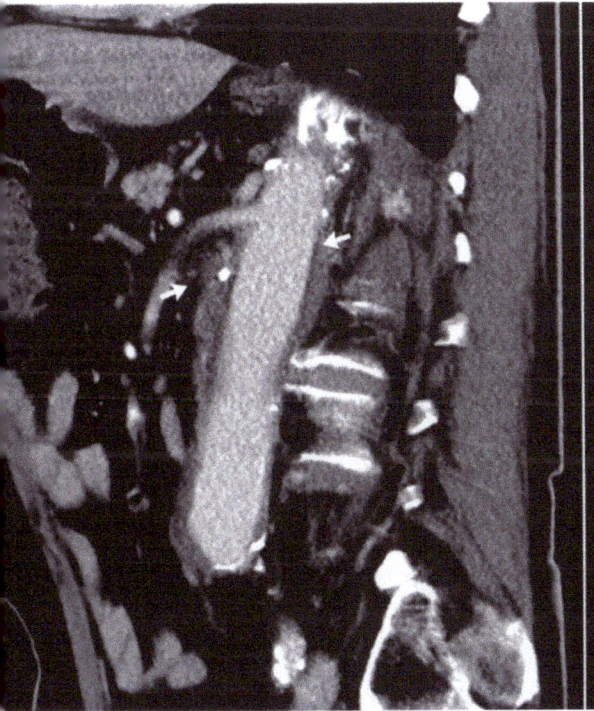
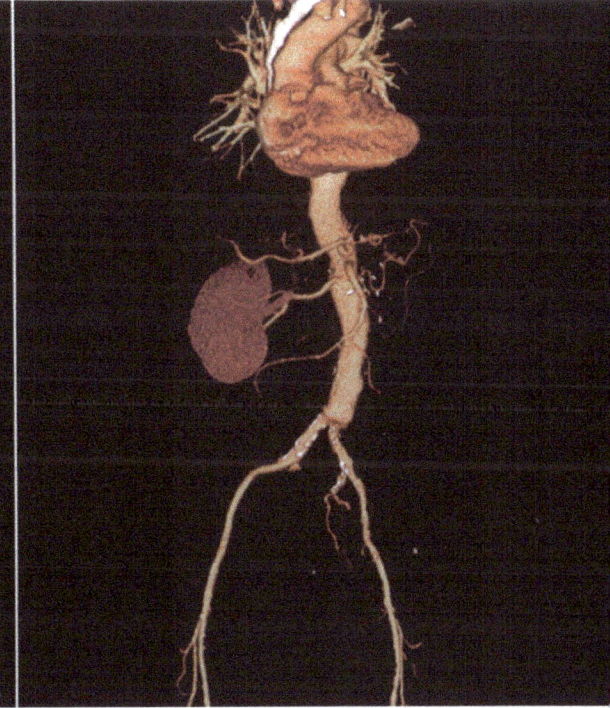

[3] Sagittal image shows fluid around the prosthesis in cranio-caudal extent.

[4] 3D VRT delineates the aortic prosthesis. Due to the threshold settings, the fluid collection cannot be delineated.

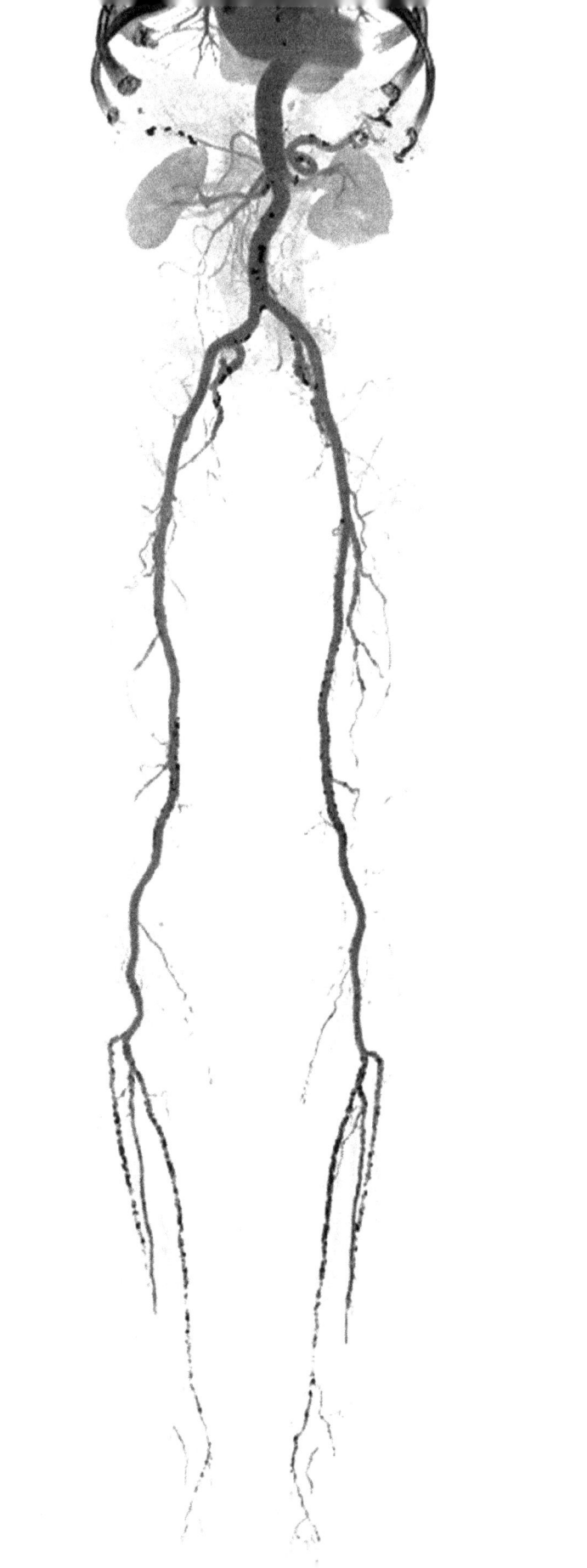

Dual Energy: CTA Runoff

Andrew Misselt · Cynthia McCollough · Eric Williamson

Case 1: Diabetic Female with Bilateral Calf Pain

Case 2: Elderly Hypertensive Male with Severe Leg Pain

Basis of spiral dual energy CT

A unique function of the SOMATOM Definition Dual Source CT system is its capacity to operate each x-ray tube at different kV and mA settings. While dual-energy CT was originally developed and evaluated 20 years ago, technical limitations of the CT scanners and post processing software at that time prevented the development of routine clinical applications.[1]

Today, the SOMATOM Definition Dual Source CT system provides the ability to simultaneously acquire spiral CT data at two different x-ray tube potentials (kV settings). The scanner then reconstructs images from each tube and then uses the dual-energy attenuation data in automated post processing techniques to identify and remove voxels of specific material composition, such as bone or iodine.

Image data are typically acquired with one source utilizing low energy (e.g. 80 kV) and the other high energy (e.g. 140 kV) settings. In Dual Source CT, the data are acquired simultaneously with subsecond gantry rotation times. By using different kV settings, distinct photon energy spectra are produced from each tube. Since x-ray absorption is energy-dependent, the same material will produce different attenuation values for tube A and tube B. However, the relative attenuation differences between different materials will change with tube voltage. For example, as x-ray tube voltage decreases, there is a much larger relative increase in the attenuation value of iodine than is seen with bone. This effect is the basis for iodine-bone separation using dual-energy imaging.[2]

Spiral dual energy CT for Peripheral Runoff

Since the widespread introduction of multi-detector row CT (MDCT) technology in the early part of this decade, CT angiography of the peripheral vasculature has rapidly gained acceptance.[4] The inherent advantages of MDCT angiography over conventional digital subtraction angiography (DSA) are numerous. Notably, MDCT angiography provides a more comprehensive imaging display. The potential for cross-sectional, multiplanar, and 3D evaluations by MDCT angiography far exceeds that of projectional data produced by conventional DSA.[3] Furthermore, MDCT allows imaging of a larger coverage area using only a single intravenous injection of contrast, as opposed to the relatively narrow scope provided by the more invasive intra-arterial catheter based techniques of DSA

Dual Energy: CTA Runoff

(which image only the vessel lumens distal to the catheter tip). With a single intravenous contrast injection, MDCT angiography provides a comprehensive evaluation of the peripheral vasculature bed with inclusion of collateral pathways originating far proximal to the area of disease, all at a lower cost and with greater safety for the patient. Indeed, the initial resistance to this newer imaging technique has given way as studies have shown that MDCT angiography provides excellent image quality which is often equivalent to DSA in diagnosis and treatment planning.[5]

Of note, one commonly expressed drawback to MDCT angiography is the time, expertise, and access to sophisticated software, which are required for post-processing production of useful 3D or bone-subtracted images. In the context of runoff examinations, a major utility of dual-energy scanning is the semi-automated removal of calcium from the field of view. Thus, by exploiting the inherent attenuation differences of iodine and calcium in the dual-energy mode, the SOMATOM Definition Dual Source CT system has the potential to further refine and streamline the powerful technique of MDCT angiography.

While the primary benefit of dual-energy for peripheral MDCT angiography currently involves semi-automatic removal of boney structures to allow direct visualization of vascular anatomy, calcium removal also has the potential to remove calcified "hard" plaques from images to facilitate visualization of the patency or stenosis of vessel lumens.[1] However, the Definition system offers the hope for more. By using spiral dual energy scanning techniques, material-specific differences in attenuation may allow CT classification of tissue type. As such, the dual-energy technique may facilitate characterization of atherosclerotic plaque, improve visualization of in-stent restenosis or provide perfusion maps of various tissues based on iodine concentration.[2]

Challenges of Runoff CT using Definition

Successful use of the Dual Source CT system requires new strategies in bolus timing, bolus duration, and patient positioning. In comparison to initial experiences with 4-channel MDCT, the innate imaging speed of the Definition DSCT is striking. With 4-, 8-, and even 16-channel MDCT systems, bolus propagation more or less paralleled the scanner speed. However, with DSCT the speed of the scanner may simply out-run the propagation of the bolus through the arterial system. Thus, runoff examinations using the DSCT system require more sophisticated bolus triggering and timing techniques such as automated injection delays and the use of a saline bolus chaser. Additionally, many operators of the DSCT system will find it prudent to prepare in advance for immediate delayed scanning of the distal extremities in cases where the scanner has out-run the bolus. Another consideration unique to the SOMATOM Definition is the need to position the patient centrally within the bore of the gantry. Because post-processing of spiral dual energy CT requires the combination of data acquired simultaneously from both A and B tubes, central positioning of the anatomy to be imaged is key to ensure that the target anatomy is completely covered.

In summary, peripheral runoff MDCT angiography performed using spiral dual energy DSCT further refines this proven technique for peripheral vascular imaging.

Andrew Misselt · Cynthia McCollough · Eric Williamson
Mayo Clinic College of Medicine
Department of Radiology

References

[1] Flohr TG, McCollough CH, Bruder H, et al. First performance evaluation of a dual-source CT (DSCT) system. Eur Radiol 2006; 16(2):256-268

[2] Johnson TRC, Krauss B, Sedlmair M et al. Material differentiation by dual energy CT: initial experience Eur Radiol. 2007 Jun;17(6):1510-7

[3] Rubin GD, et al. Multi-detector row CT angiography of lower extremity arterial inflow and runoff: initial experience. Radiology 2001; 221(1):146-158

[4] Willmann JK, Mayer D, Banyai M, et al. Evaluation of Peripheral Arterial Bypass Grafts with Multi-Detector Row CT Angiography: Comparison with Duplex US and Digital Subtraction Angiography. Radiology 2003; 229(1):464-474

[5] Catalano C, Fraioli F, Laghi A, et al. Infrarenal Aortic and Lower-Extremity Arterial Disease: Diagnostic Performance of Multi-Detector Row CT Angiography. Radiology 2004; 231(2): 555-563

Dual Energy: CTA Runoff

Basic considerations

For the examinations of peripheral vessels, a slice width less than 1.5 mm is typically desired. Hence, the 64 x 0.6 mm collimation is preferred. This allows reconstruction of thin images, which decrease partial volume averaging and increase spatial resolution. Thin images are particularly important for 3-D image displays. If thin images are not required, the 14 x 1.2 mm collimation is recommended. For large patients, the use of the 14 x 1.2 mm collimation is strongly recommended. CARE Dose4D should be used to modulate the tube current as the patient attenuation varies along the z-axis.

When scanning obese patients, using 14 x 1.2 mm is beneficial in order to reduce image noise.

Scan Parameters

Scan mode	Spiral dual energy with Dual Source
Scan area	thoracic or abdominal aorta to feet
Scan direction	cranio-caudal
Scan time	~41 s
Tube voltage A/B	140 kV/80 kV
Tube current A/B	70 quality ref. mAs/297 quality ref. mAs
Dose modulation	CARE Dose4D
CTDI$_{vol}$	~13 mGy
Rotation time	0.5 s
Pitch	0.7
Slice collimation	0.6 mm (1.2 mm)
Acquisition	64 x 0.6 mm (14 x 1.2 mm)
Slice width	1.5 mm
Reconstruction increment	1 mm
Reconstruction kernel	D30f

Tricks

Centering the patient is very important. Put a cushion under the legs to keep them at the same height above the table top as the torso. The aorta and legs/feet must all be located in the central 26 cm FOV. Tie both knees and ankles together.

Pitfalls

In the presence of severe disease with poor arterial inflow it may be possible to outrun the arterial contrast bolus. Therefore consider planning a second phase of the calf. This phase should be cancelled if symmetric arterial enhancement is seen.

Contrast Injection Protocol

	Iodine concentration 300 mg I/ml	Iodine concentration 370 mg I/ml
Injection scheme	Monophasic	Monophasic
Iodine delivery rate	1.48 g/s	1.48 g/s
CM volume	180 ml	145 ml
CM flow rate	4.9 ml/s	4 ml/s
Body weight adaption	yes	yes
Bolus timing	bolus tracking*	bolus tracking*
Bolus tracking threshold	150 HU	150 HU
ROI position	ascending aorta or juxtarenal aorta	ascending aorta or juxtarenal aorta
Scan delay	10 s; 5 s if chest included	10 s; 5 s if chest included
Saline flush volume	60 ml	60 ml
Saline injection rate	4.9 ml/s	4 ml/s
Needle size	18 G	18 G
Injection site	antecubital vein	antecubital vein

*Depending on the preference of the individual site, test bolus can be used as an alternative

Case 1 Diabetic Female with Bilateral Calf Pain

Case history

66-year-old female with diabetes, dyslipidemia and coronary artery disease presents with bilateral calf and foot pain. Symptoms occur at rest and worsen with exercise.

Question

What is the cause of the patient's bilateral lower extremity pain? Will medical, endovascular or surgical management be indicated?

Diagnosis / Differential diagnosis

Given the patient's diabetes and dyslipidemia with known atherosclerosis in the coronary arteries, the lower extremity pain is likely vascular in origin. Rest pain with claudication suggests severe multilevel atherosclerosis in the pelvis and lower extremities. Alternatively, the history of diabetes may indicate a degree of neuropathic pain.

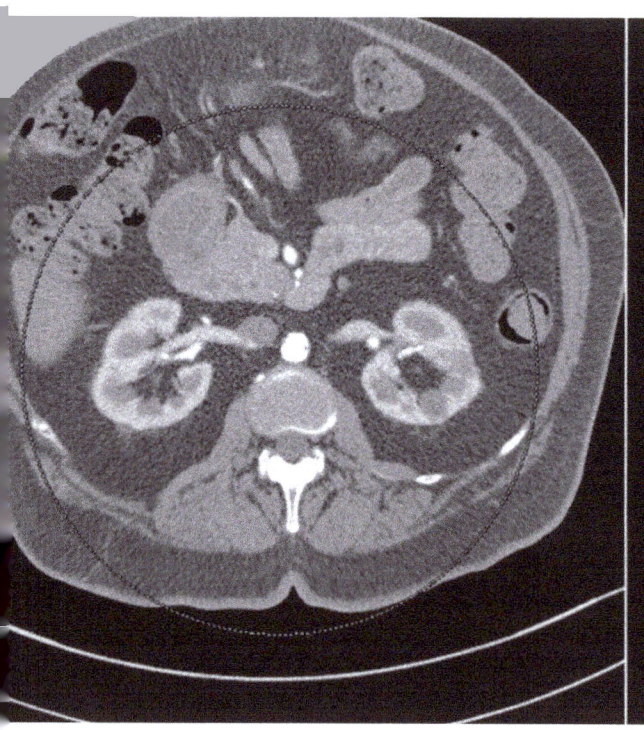

[1] Axial source image from spiral dual energy runoff.

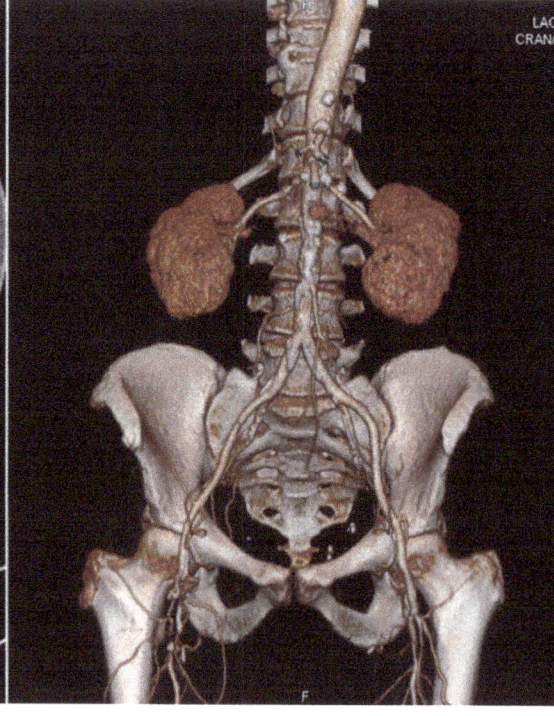

[2] 3D image from spiral dual energy runoff, bones included.

Findings

Aortoiliac atherosclerotic changes with mild stenosis of the distal aorta and both common iliac arteries. Occlusion of both superficial femoral arteries and the right profunda femoral artery. Moderate stenosis of the left profunda femoral artery. Occlusion of the right popliteal artery. Severe stenosis of left popliteal artery. Heavily calcified crural arteries. Occlusion of the right anterior tibial artery.

Take-home message

Spiral dual energy CT acquisition and post processing allows automated removal of bone to quickly demonstrate vascular anatomy.

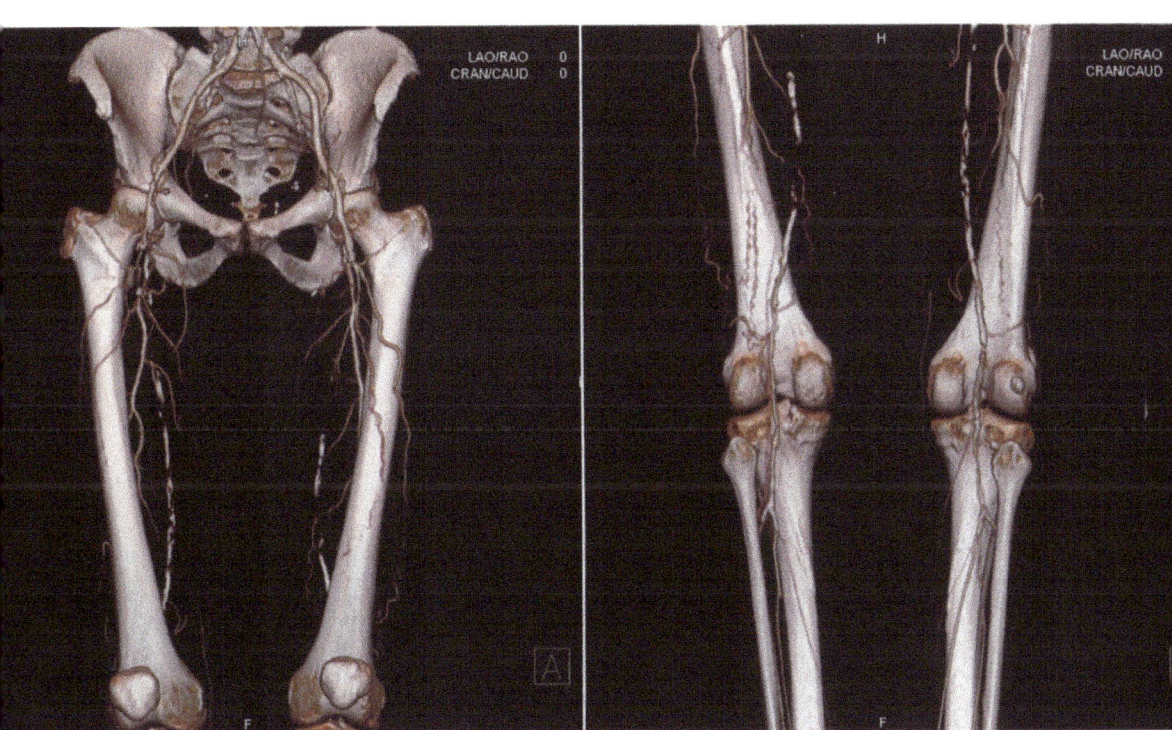

[3] 3D image from spiral dual energy runoff, bones included.

[4] 3D image from spiral dual energy runoff, bones included.

Case 2 Elderly Hypertensive Male with Severe Leg Pain

Case history

79-year-old male with known hypertension presented with severe exertional thigh and calf pain.

Question

Is the patient's exertional thigh and calf pain due to underlying vascular disease?

Diagnosis / Differential diagnosis

Thigh and calf pain precipitated by exertion may occur as a result of claudication. Alternatively, the patients exertional pain may musculoskeletal or neuropathic in origin such as degenerative joint or disc disease, deconditioning or nonischemic myopathy.

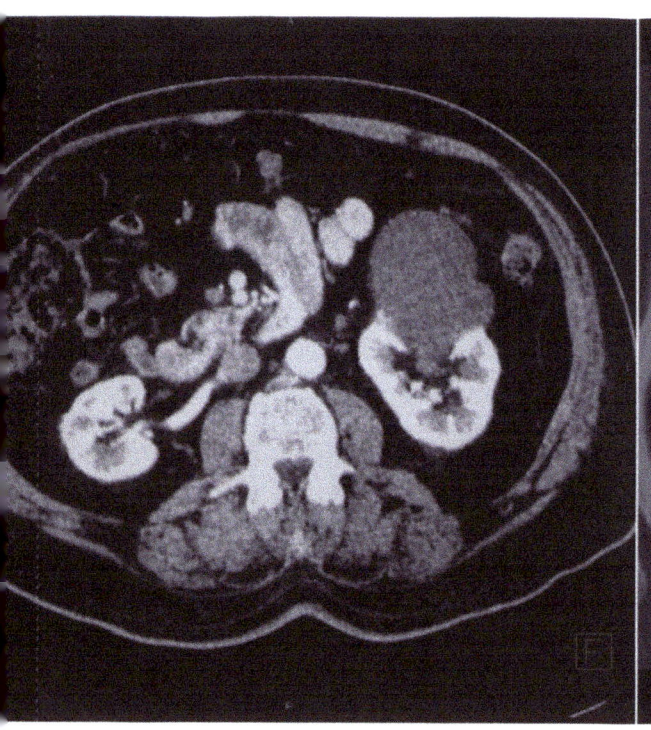

[1] Spiral dual energy axial CT image of abdomen. Large exophytic left renal cyst.

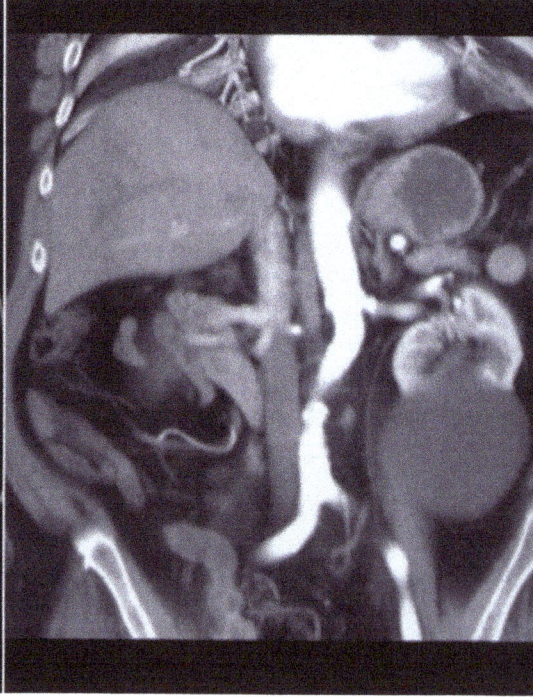

[2] Spiral dual energy coronal MIP image of abdomen. Ectatic nonaneurysmal abdominal aorta. Large exophytic left renal cyst.

Findings

Normal caliber abdominal aorta. Mild dilatation of the left internal iliac artery (1.2 cm). Scattered, nonstenotic atherosclerotic changes in the common femoral, superficial femoral, profunda femoral and popliteal arteries bilaterally. Occluded right anterior and posterior tibial arteries. Occluded left posterior tibial artery. Heavily diseased left anterior tibial artery.

Take-home message

Dual Source CT quickly and accurately identifies the atherosclerotic disease burden in cases suspicious for claudication. CT imaging may also provide or exclude alternative explanations for a patient's pain in cases where atherosclerosis has not been implicated.

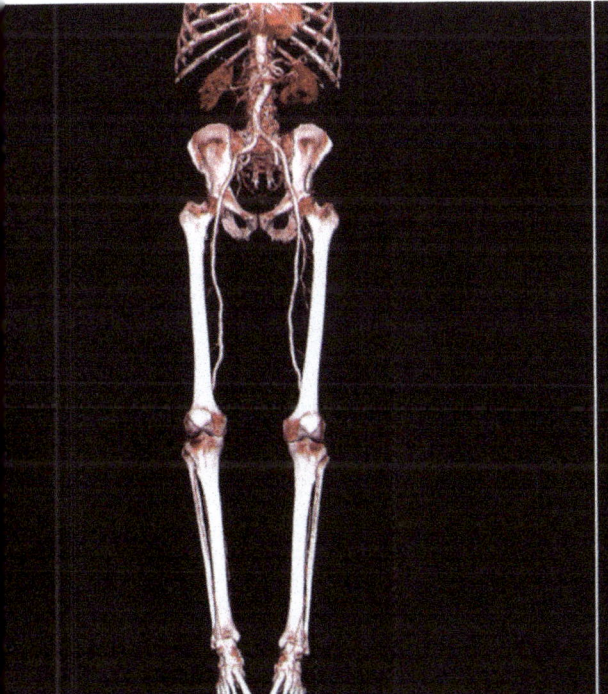

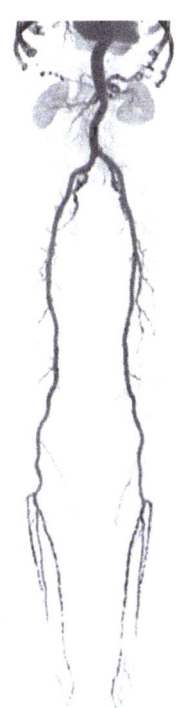

[3] Spiral dual energy CTA image of abdomen, pelvis and lower extremities prior to bone subtraction.

[4] Spiral dual energy CTA image of abdomen, pelvis and lower extremities with automatic dual energy bone subtraction technique.

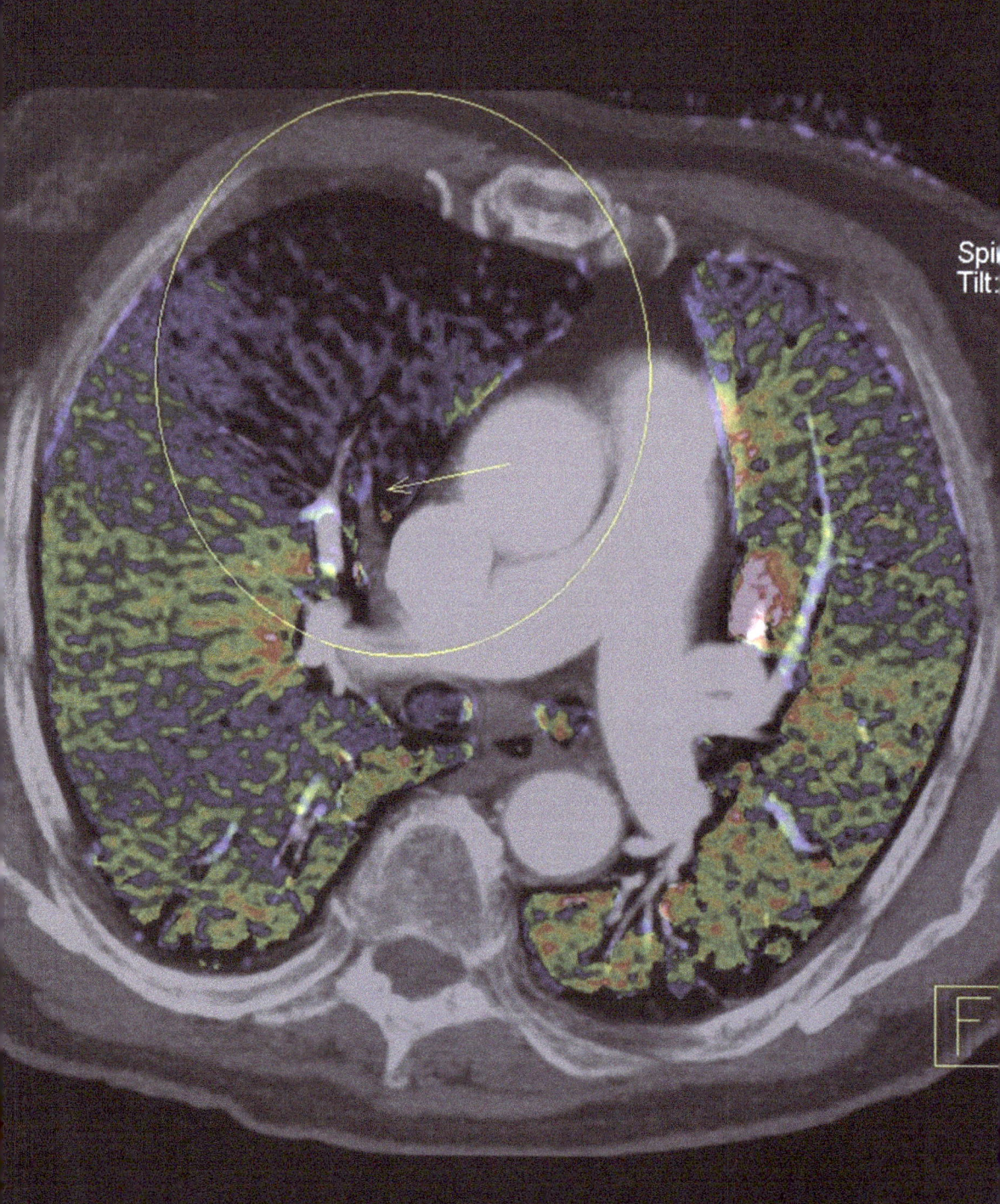

Dual Energy: CTA Lung Perfusion (PE)

Thorsten R. C. Johnson · Christian Fink · Christoph R. Becker

Case 1: Acute Pulmonary Embolism

Case 2: Pulmonary Hypertension Due to Chronic Recurrent Pulmonary Embolism

CT angiography has emerged as the diagnostic standard for detecting pulmonary embolism. It has been shown that pulmonary emboli can be detected with high reliability even at segmental and subsegmental levels.[1, 2]

Both acute and chronic pulmonary emboli are identified as intraluminal filling defects that show a sharp interface with contrast material. In 1980, the detection of pulmonary embolism on contrast enhanced CT was first described.[3] Since then, this noninvasive technique has produced a paradigm shift that has raised the standard of care for patients with this disease. In 1990, the large Prospective Investigation of Pulmonary Embolism Diagnosis (PIOPED) study results were published, which compared ventilation-perfusion (V/Q) scintigraphy with pulmonary angiography and established the diagnostic characteristics of pulmonary embolism on V/Q scintigraphy. The sensitivity of V/Q scintigraphy was found to be 98%, with a specificity of only 10%. The potential of CT pulmonary angiography has now been realized at most institutions and it has become the test of choice and thus the standard of care. Recent studies have shown the sensitivity of CTA to be 90–100% and the specificity to be 89–94% for the detection of pulmonary emboli to the level of the subsegmental arteries, with pulmonary angiography as the standard of reference. The PIOPED II study, which used a composite gold standard, has been published recently and showed that CTA has a sensitivity of 83% with a specificity of 96% for the detection of pulmonary embolism.

With regard to massive pulmonary embolism, one of the most severe complications is acute right heart failure. Right ventricular strain or failure is optimally monitored on echocardiography, but scores based on morphological CT criteria have also been developed to predict cor pulmonale and short-term outcome in patients with pulmonary embolism. In addition, we know that pulmonary hypertension is frequently caused by chronic recurrent pulmonary embolism, constituting secondary pulmonary hypertension, which takes a chronic, unfavorable course in many patients. The relevance of smaller singular pulmonary emboli detected in CT remains somewhat unclear. On the other hand, embolism cannot be found in many symptomatic patients, and the reason may be that the emboli are just too small. Then again, the condition of many patients with large emboli is surprisingly good, and this seems to be especially true for non-occlusive thrombi that are surrounded by contrast material.

Dual Energy: CTA Lung Perfusion (PE)

Altogether, it seems that there is some discrepancy between the clinical relevance and the size or location of pulmonary embolism. Even very small occlusive emboli may be more relevant for blood oxygenation than large central but non-occlusive emboli. Also, chronic thromboembolic pulmonary hypertension is a progressive disease with a poor prognosis, and identifying chronic thromboembolic pulmonary disease as a cause of pulmonary hypertension has major clinical implications as these patients could be potentially offered a surgical cure.[4, 6]

Therefore, perfusion imaging may add relevant information, even though the initial, fast diagnosis is usually made with CT angiography. So far, this was the domain of pulmonary perfusion scintigraphy, in which technetium-marked small albumin spheres are trapped in capillary vessels and thus map pulmonary perfusion.[5] However, spiral dual energy CT angiography also provides the opportunity to assess pulmonary perfusion based on a three-material decomposition for iodine, air and soft tissue. After contrast material administration, perfused and ventilated lung parenchyma will contain all three components. The iodine distribution can be mapped to visualize perfusion. This gives a new, functional aspect to CT, because even perfusion defects caused by small peripheral emboli can be detected, and the hemodynamic significance of larger emboli can be assessed.

To evaluate this technique, we examined 24 patients with suspected pulmonary embolism in an initial study. Exams were performed with a single acquisition, spiral dual energy CT angiography protocol on a Siemens SOMATOM Definition. Voxels containing iodine and air were color-coded by the dual-energy evaluation software. Lung perfusion was assessed by two blinded radiologists. Perfusion defects were classified as being consistent or non-consistent with pulmonary embolism (e.g. caused by artifacts). Subjective image quality of the perfusion maps and CT angiography were rated using a 5-point score. The peak attenuation of the pulmonary arteries, normal lung parenchyma and perfusion defects was assessed. Finally, the CT angiography data alone was assessed for pulmonary embolism by an independent third reader.

Perfusion defects consistent with pulmonary embolism were identified in four patients. In all these cases, pulmonary emboli were visible in the segmental arteries and were also confirmed by the third independent reader. Perfusion defects rated as non-consistent with pulmonary embolism were most frequently caused by streak artifacts from very dense contrast material in the great mediastinal vessels or heart, which can be addressed with optimized contrast material injection protocols. Other reasons included atelectasis or pulmonary edema. Ten pulmonary emboli were regarded as non-occlusive in CT angiography, and there were no perfusion defects detected for these emboli. The median score for the image quality of both the perfusion maps and CT angiography was two. The median quantified iodine-related attenuation of pulmonary arteries, normal lung parenchyma, and perfusion defects was 453 HU, 56 HU, and 18 HU, respectively.

In conclusion, spiral dual energy CT angiography of pulmonary embolism is feasible and simultaneously provides a high-resolution angiography of the pulmonary arteries and the possibility to assess perfusion defects caused by pulmonary embolism.

Thus, spiral dual energy CT of pulmonary perfusion offers the possibility to assess the functional relevance of pulmonary emboli without additional dose, contrast application or examination time.

Thorsten R. C. Johnson · Christian Fink · Christoph R. Becker
University of Munich-Grosshadern
Department of Clinical Radiology

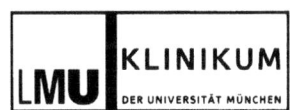

References

[1] Wittram C. (2007) How I do it: CT pulmonary angiography. AJR Am J Roentgenol. 188(5):1255-61

[2] Ghaye B. (2007) Peripheral pulmonary embolism on multidetector CT pulmonary angiography. JBR-BTR 90(2):100-8

[3] Tunariu N, Gibbs SJ, Win Z, Gin-Sing W, Graham A, Gishen P, Al-Nahhas A. (2007) Ventilation-perfusion scintigraphy is more sensitive than multi-detector CTPA in detecting chronic thromboembolic pulmonary disease as a treatable cause of pulmonary hypertension. J Nucl Med. 48(5):680-4

[4] Araoz PA, Gotway MB, Harrington JR, Harmsen WS, Mandrekar JN. (2007) Pulmonary embolism: prognostic CT findings. Radiology 242(3):889-97

[5] Engelke C, Rummeny EJ, Marten K. (2006) Acute pulmonary embolism on MDCT of the chest: prediction of cor pulmonale and short-term patient survival from morphologic embolus burden. AJR Am J Roentgenol. 186(5):1265-71

[6] Tunariu N, Gibbs SJ, Win Z, et al. (2007) Ventilation-perfusion scintigraphy is more sensitive than multidetector CTPA in detecting chronic thromboembolic pulmonary disease as a treatable cause of pulmonary hypertension. J Nucl Med. 48(5):680-4

Dual Energy: CTA Lung Perfusion (PE)

Basic considerations

Central positioning of the patient in the isocenter of the gantry is essential to include the peripheral lung in the field of view. The protocol is aimed to display both the pulmonary arteries and pulmonary perfusion. Therefore, a dense bolus is required and the delay should be a little longer to allow the contrast material to pass into the lung parenchyma. This can be achieved with high-concentration contrast agent at a flow rate of 4.0 ml/s, followed by a saline chaser bolus at the same injection rate.

Bolus tracking should be used for timing with the trigger-region of interest placed in the pulmonary artery.

Scan Parameters

Scan mode	Spiral dual energy with Dual Source
Scan area	diaphragm to lung apex
Scan direction	caudo-cranial
Scan time	~10 s
Tube voltage A/B	140 kV / 80 kV
Tube current A/B	50 quality ref. mAs / 213 quality ref. mAs
Dose modulation	CARE Dose4D
$CTDI_{vol}$	~9 mGy
Rotation time	0.33 s
Pitch	0.7
Slice collimation	1.2 mm
Acquisition	14 x 1.2 mm
Slice width	3 mm
Reconstruction increment	2.5 mm
Reconstruction kernel	D30f

Tricks

The scan direction should be caudo-cranial, because dense contrast material will affect the perfusion mapping due to beam hardening. If the scan starts at the diaphragm, the chaser bolus has washed out the superior vena cava by the time the region is scanned. The patient should be instructed to hold his breath at mild inspiration to avoid excessive influx of non-enhanced blood from the IVC.

Pitfalls

Dense opacification in the SVC and right heart may result in streak artifacts in the lung parenchyma mimicking perfusion defects. Therefore, the recommended injection rate of 4.0 ml/s is rather low to avoid these artifacts. Lung fibrosis may mimic perfusion defects.

Contrast Injection Protocol

	Iodine concentration 300 mg I/ml	Iodine concentration 370 mg I/ml
Injection scheme	Monophasic	Monophasic
Iodine delivery rate	1.48 g/s	1.48 g/s
CM volume	100 ml	80 ml
CM flow rate	4.9 ml/s	4 ml/s
Body weight adaption	yes	yes
Bolus timing	bolus tracking*	bolus tracking*
Bolus tracking threshold	100 HU	100 HU
ROI position	pulmonary trunk	pulmonary trunk
Scan delay	7 s	7 s
Saline flush volume	100 ml	100 ml
Saline injection rate	4.9 ml/s	4 ml/s
Needle size	18 G	18 G
Injection site	antecubital vein	antecubital vein

* Depending on the preference of the individual site, test bolus can be used as an alternative

Case 1 Acute Pulmonary Embolism

Case history

67-year-old female with severe dyspnea and positive D-dimer test is referred for CT angiography to confirm or rule out pulmonary embolism.

Question

The primary clinical concern is pulmonary embolism, and other questions include infarction and right heart dilatation.

Diagnosis / Differential diagnosis

Apart from acute pulmonary embolism, differential diagnoses include right heart failure, pulmonary hypertension, congestive heart failure, coronary artery disease, pneumonia and pneumothorax.

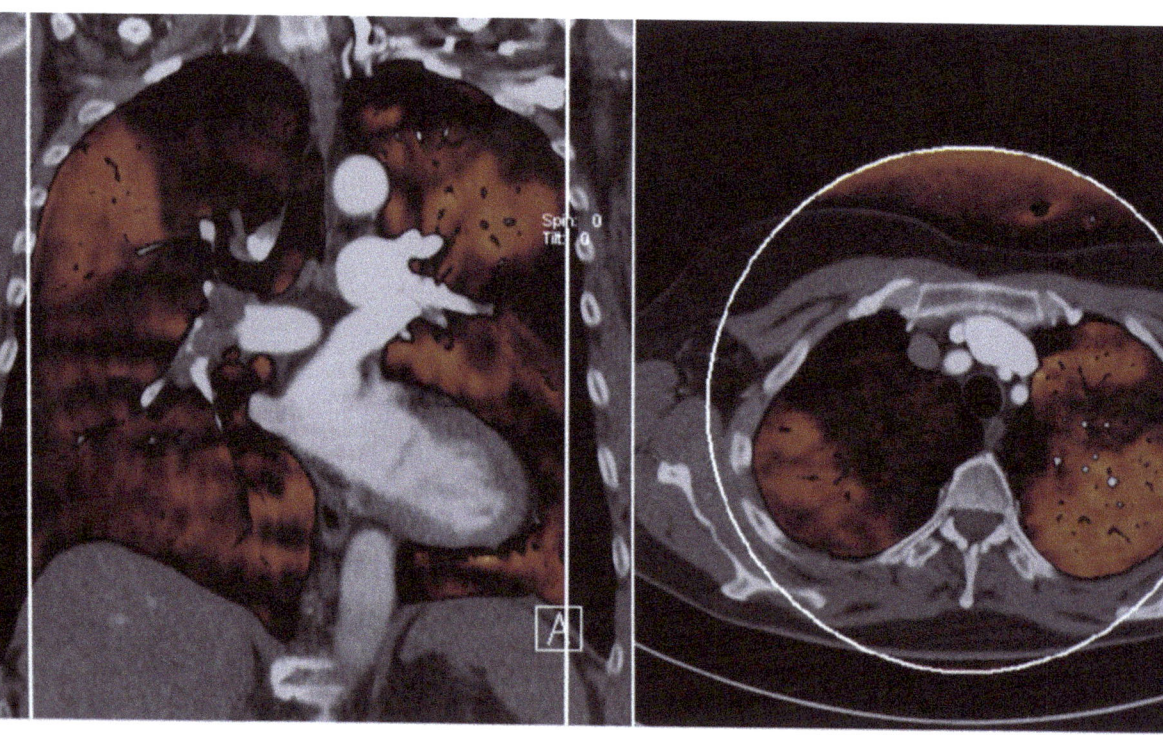

[1] Coronal view with presentation of a wedge shaped infarcted lung area in the right upper lobe.

[2] Axial view demonstrated perfusion deficits in the left and right upper lung due to infarction.

Findings

Thrombus clots are visualized in the right upper and right lower lobar pulmonary arteries. Only the clot formation in the right upper lobe leads to lung infarction, whereas the clots in the lower lobe arteries do not.

Take-home message

Spiral dual energy CT of the lung can display the perfusion defect or the infarcted territory of the lung independent of the direct visualization of thrombi in the pulmonary arteries. This provides a new functional aspect which makes a more comprehensive assessment possible, including the clinically more relevant effect of pulmonary emboli on peripheral perfusion.

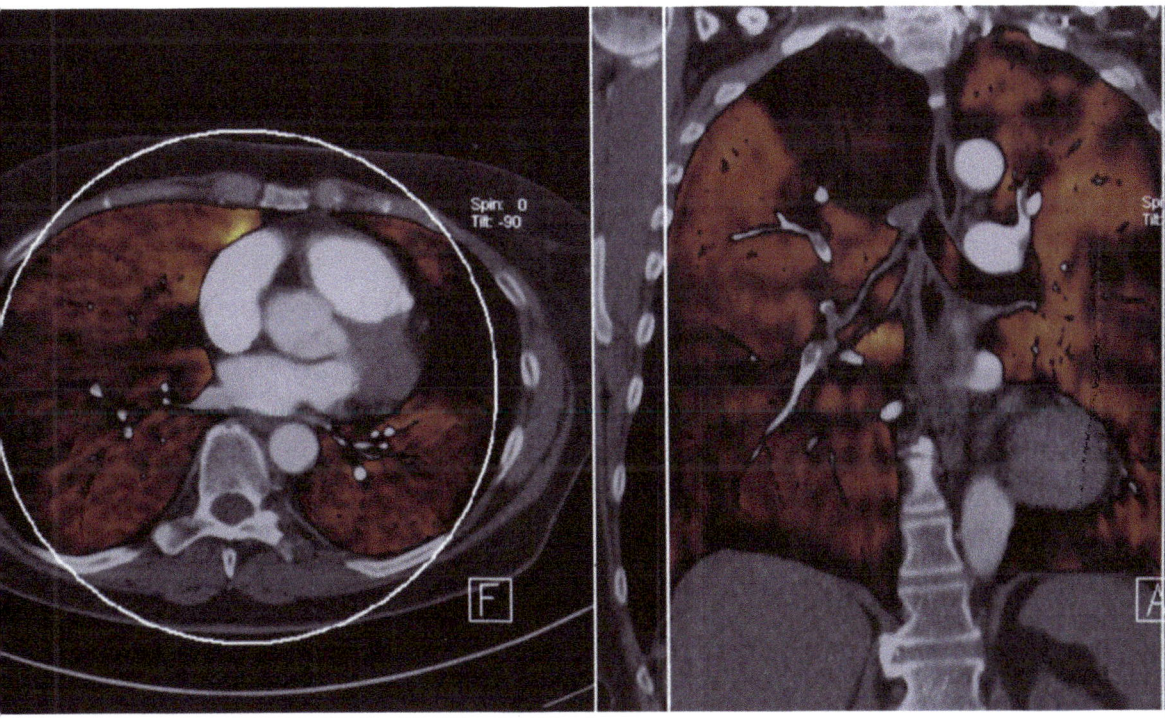

[3] Lower lobe of both lungs show normal perfusion, despite the fact that thrombus formation is present in the right lower lobe.

[4] Complete occluding clot in the right upper lobe and partially occluding clot in the right lower lobe.

Case 2 Pulmonary Hypertension Due to Chronic Recurrent Pulmonary Embolism

Case history

72-year-old female suffering from severe dyspnea is referred for pulmonary CT angiography to rule out pulmonary embolism.

Question

CT angiography is performed to rule out pulmonary embolism, right heart dilatation or pulmonary hypertension.

Diagnosis / Differential diagnosis

Apart from acute pulmonary embolism, differential diagnoses include primary right heart failure, secondary pulmonary hypertension, congestive heart failure, coronary artery disease, pneumonia and pneumothorax.

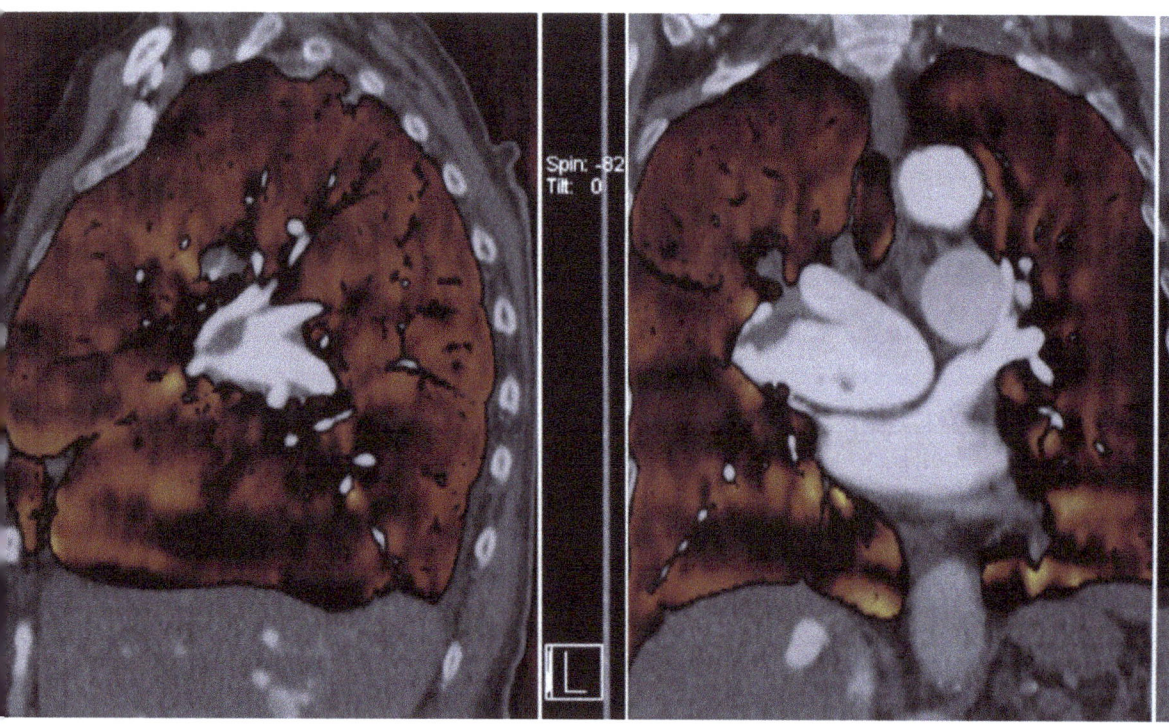

[1] Sagittal view of the lung with normal perfusion.

[2] Coronal view with normal lung perfusion and thrombus clot in the central pulmonary artery on the right side.

Findings

Clots of pulmonary emboli are displayed in the main pulmonary artery. However, there are no occlusive emboli shown in the lobar or segmental arteries. The peripheral parenchyma shows a normal perfusion without segmental defects.

Take-home message

Dual Energy CT can depict functional lung tissue in which both air and iodine are present and which can therefore be assumed to participate in blood oxygenation. In this patient, pulmonary embolism is present, but presumably older and it does not cause a perfusion defect, i.e. it is not impeding blood oxygenation.

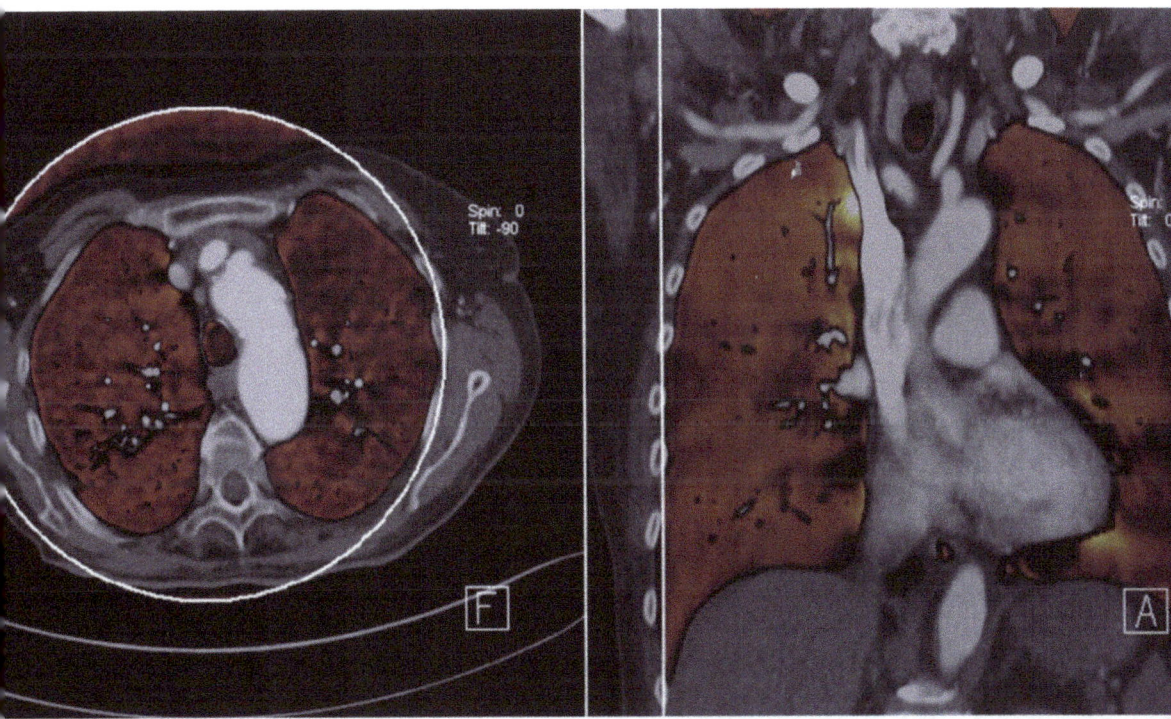

[3] Normal lung perfusion in the axial view of the upper lung.　　[4] Normal lung perfusion displayed in coronal view.

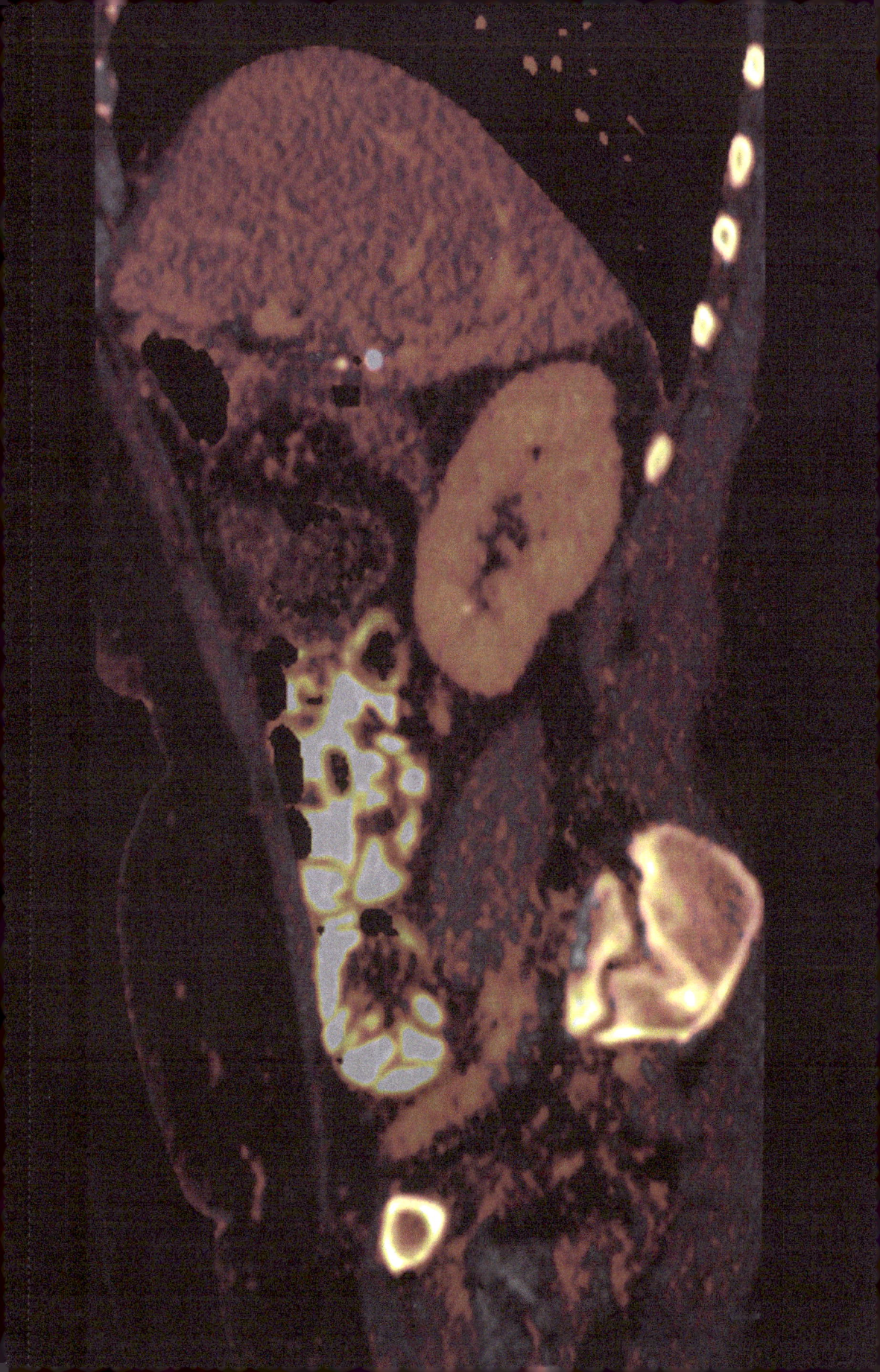

Dual Energy: Virtual Non-Contrast

Axel Kuettner · Katharina Anders · Michael Lell

Case 1: Scanning of a Small Polyp in Gallbladder

Case 2: Exclusion of Urolithiasis in the Presence of Contrast Media

The latest spiral dual energy scanning techniques facilitate easy derivation of "virtual non-enhanced" scans. Put simply, it gives us the possibility to derive non-contrast images from contrast scans without scanning the patient twice.

Background

The introduction of multi-detector row CT scanners has substantially broadened the spectrum of clinical applications and examination techniques in recent years. Thinner slices enable improved spatial resolution with a current minimal resolution of 0.3 mm. The true isotropic voxel has been realized since the 64-slice scanners and now the image quality of arbitrarily reconstructed planes is the same as the image quality of the scan plane. Faster scanning not only allows for the examination of long scan ranges such as the thoracoabdominal aorta or even the entire vascular tree, but also for studies in distinctively different contrast phases. This is very helpful for better discrimination of benign or malignant lesions especially in the highly vascularized organs such as the kidney or liver.[1, 2] In kidney exams, the different phases of contrast uptake can be differentiated using either the non-enhanced, arterial, cortico-medullary, nephrographic or excretory phase. In liver imaging, these phases include non-enhanced, early arterial, late arterial, portal venous and late. Even vascular studies such as the assessment of the aorta may require several phases to depict all possible pathologies.[3]

Despite these technical advances, the basic principle of image acquisition has remained virtually unchanged since the introduction of Computed Tomography in the 1970s. The x-ray attenuation of any scanned object or organ is measured and expressed in Hounsfield Units.[4] The scale was defined as follows: -1000 HU is air and 0 HU is water; the positive range of the scale has no limit. The variability of HU values found in a human body generally do not vary tremendously with the exception of bone (high HU values) and gas (air)-filled spaces. Soft organ tissue is generally iso-dense compared with the surrounding tissue, making the injection of contrast media necessary to better delineate individual organs or specific structures within the organ (e.g. focal liver lesions). However, sometimes the sought after pathology is only very subtly delineated, such as intramural hematomas when scanning on suspicion of aortic dissection. In these cases, contrast media should not be applied

Dual Energy: Virtual Non-Contrast

in order to avoid masking the pathology with highly dense contrast material inside the aorta. Another example is kidney stones. Since the kidneys actively secrete i.v. administered contrast agents, small calculi within the ureter or the renal pelvis may be masked by the surrounding contrast medium.

Clinical diagnostics not only involves detecting a given structure, but also its characterization. The detection of a "focal liver lesion" is clinically insufficient as the spectrum of a lesion can vary from a simple benign cyst to a hepatocellular carcinoma or a metastasis from a cancer of different origin. Thus the assessment of a lesion's behavior in the presence of contrast medium is a routinely used to characterize a lesion and thus calls for multiphase scanning. Considering all the scanning possibilities and requirements, multi-detector CT carries the risk of increased dose exposure to a given patient population due to thinner slice collimation and multiphase imaging. The simplest solution for this problem seems to be the use of strict scan indications, ensuring that only those patients that really need them are examined using multiphase protocols. However, the clinician ordering the scan typically does not know exactly what the underlying causes are despite an extensive and thorough clinical work up. This is precisely the strength of Computed Tomography in daily clinical routine, where CT is successfully used for patients with unclear thoracic pain ("triple rule out" concept) or patients with abdominal pain of unclear origin. The alternative could be to apply multiphase protocols to every patient scanned to allow for diagnosis of the full spectrum of diseases. This strategy on the other hand would dramatically increase the radiation dose applied to the population, result in longer scan times, lead to excessive amounts of images to read for one patient and, consequently, make CT considerably more expensive.

Virtual Non-Enhanced CT

Spiral dual energy CT may overcome this clinical problem in a unique way by being able to omit the non-contrast enhanced scan phase for all imaging studies.[5]

The two main mechanisms responsible for attenuation in the photon energy range used in CT are the Compton scatter and the photo effect, which have been extensively described in this book. Materials can be differentiated further by applying different x-ray spectra and analyzing the differences in attenuation. This works especially well in materials with large atomic numbers due to the photo effect. Iodine is one of these materials, and it is generally known to have stronger enhancement at low tube voltage settings. This effect makes it beneficial to use the spectral information to differentiate iodine from other materials that do not show this behavior. By applying dual energy, the iodine content of any object in the scan field can be "removed" without removing the object itself. The resulting image appears to have no contrast material in it at all; it is "virtually non-enhanced".[6] This technique allows for scanning any given contrast phase whether it is early arterial phase, portal venousphase or excretory phase and retrospectively generate non-enhanced images. the correct settings are used, the applied total dose to the patient should not be higher than using a standard 120 kV protocol setting.

As a result, the non-enhanced contrast phase could be spared in clinical routine for all imaging protocols, thereby reducing the applied dose and at the same time allowing clinicians to view non-enhanced images only when clinically required.[1] Omitting a scan phase may also gain time in emergencies, such as suspected aortic dissection. If no clear dissection is found in the arterial phase, an intramural hematoma could be looked for in the virtually non-enhanced images in a second step when time is no longer as critical.

Axel Kuettner · Katharina Anders · Michael Lell

University of Erlangen-Nuremberg

Department of Diagnostic Radiology

**Universitätsklinikum
Erlangen**

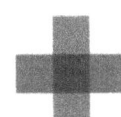

References

[1] Coppenrath EM, Mueller-Lisse UG. Multidetector CT of the kidney. Eur Radiol. 2006 Nov;16(11):2603-11

[2] Winterer JT, Kotter E, Ghanem N, Langer M. Detection and characterization of benign focal liver lesions with multislice CT. Eur Radiol. 2006 Nov;16(11):2427-43

[3] Rubin GD. MDCT imaging of the aorta and peripheral vessels. Eur J Radiol. 2003 Mar;45 Suppl 1:S42-9

[4] Ambrose J, Hounsfield G. Computerized transverse axial tomography. Br J Radiol. 1973 Feb;46(542):148-9

[5] Flohr TG, McCollough CH, Bruder H, Petersilka M, Gruber K, Süss C, Grasruck M, Stierstorfer K, Krauss B, Raupach R, Primak AN, Kuettner A, Achenbach S, Becker C, Kopp A, Ohnesorge BM. First performance evaluation of a dual-source CT system. Eur Radiol. 2006 Feb;16(2):256-68

[6] Johnson TR, Krauss B, Sedlmair M, Grasruck M, Bruder H, Morhard D, Fink C, Weckbach S, Lenhard M, Schmidt B, Flohr T, Reiser MF, Becker CR. Material differentiation by dual energy CT: initial experience. Eur Radiol. 2007 Jun;17(6):1510-7

Dual Energy: Virtual Non-Contrast

Basic considerations

The virtual non-enhanced imaging protocol is a technique applicable for many indications. Exams of parenchymal organs such as renal scans, liver scans or even scans of vasculature may require a non-enhanced image phase and thus accumulating radiation dose for any given patient. However, the non-enhanced scan seldom really contributes to the diagnosis. At the same time it is difficult to predict its necessity prior to the scan. Virtual non-enhanced imaging allows for obtaining non-enhanced scans out of any contrast enhanced scan at lower dose when compared with combined scanning protocols. This holds true for any contrast phase, since the protocol removes iodine from the image while maintaining all underlying structures.

Scan Parameters (exemplified for liver)

Scan mode	Spiral dual energy with Dual Source
Scan area	variable
Scan direction	cranio-caudal
Scan time	no special time
Tube voltage A/B	140 kV/80 kV
Tube current A/B	95 quality ref. mAs/404 quality ref. mAs
Dose modulation	CARE Dose4D
$CTDI_{vol}$	~19 mGy
Rotation time	1 s/0.5 s
Pitch	0.55
Slice collimation	1.2 mm
Acquisition	14 x 1.2 mm
Slice width	1.5 mm
Reconstruction increment	1 mm
Reconstruction kernel	D30s/D30f

Tricks

· In order to get full scan coverage of the liver, position the patient off-center. For other indications, the patient should be placed in the isocenter.

· Reduce the rotation time of the gantry to 1 s, if possible. For aortic scans the rotation time may be 0.5 s.

Pitfalls

This protocol is robust and only includes a few pitfalls. The only parameter to consider carefully is the patient's positioning. Problematic combinations are lateral liver segments VI/VII in combination with the left kidney, as not all organs are within the 26 cm field of view in most patients.

Contrast Injection Protocol

	Iodine concentration 300 mg I/ml	Iodine concentration 370 mg I/ml
Injection scheme	Monophasic	Monophasic
Iodine delivery rate	1.11 g/s–1.85 g/s	1.11 g/s–1.85 g/s
CM volume	100–148 ml	80–120 ml
CM flow rate	3.7–6.2 ml/s	3–5 ml/s
Body weight adaption	no	no
Bolus timing	–	–
Bolus tracking threshold	–	–
ROI position	–	–
Scan delay	–	–
Saline flush volume	50 ml	50 ml
Saline injection rate	3.7–6.2 ml/s	3–5 ml/s
Needle size	18 G	18 G
Injection site	antecubital vein	antecubital vein

Case 1 Scanning of a Small Polyp in Gallbladder

Case history

66-year-old male presents with gallbladder lesion. Multiple MRI scans and ultrasound scans were not able to definitively conclude the nature of the lesion.

Question

Can CT differentiate between cholesterol rich gallstone and polyp? Could the virtual non-enhanced technique possibly spare scanning sequences?

Diagnosis / Differential diagnosis

The ultrasound and MRI indicated that the lesion contained no calcium. No significant growth was documented, so that the major differential diagnosis for this entity was cholesterol rich gallstone vs. polyp.

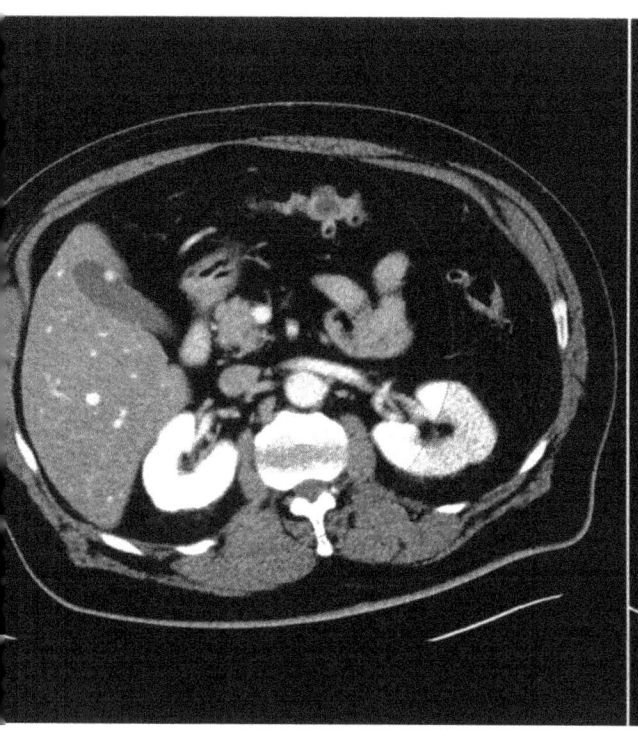 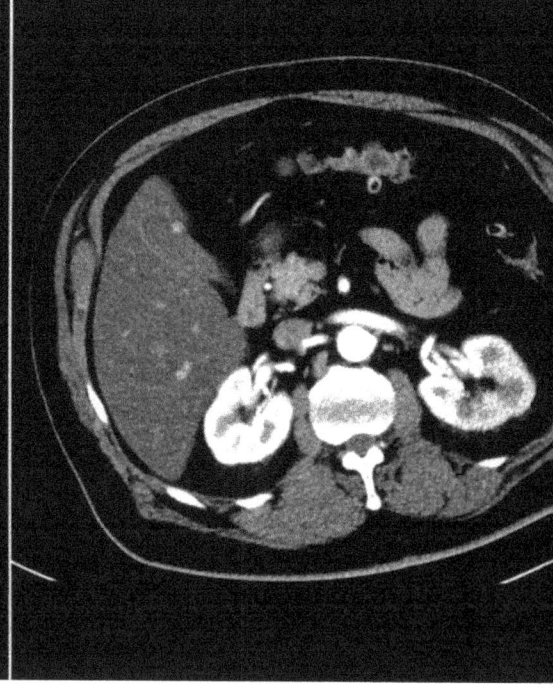

[1] Conventional non-enhanced scan of the liver and gallbladder. The gallbladder is without signs of radiopaque gallstones. Presence of cholesterol stones not excluded.

[2] Conventional early arterial scan. Same slice as image 1. Note the apparent contrast enhancing nodular lesion of the ventral aspect of the gallbladder.

Findings

In the portal venous phase, a lesion smaller than 1 cm and high attenuation is seen in the ventral aspect of the gallbladder. The lesion takes up contrast when comparing it to the non-enhanced and arterial phase scan. These finding make the presence of a small polyp very likely.

Take-home message

In the portal venous phase the ventral aspect of the gallbladder a lesion smaller than 1 cm and high attenuation is seen. The lesion takes up contrast when comparing it to the non-enhanced and arterial phase scan. These finding make the presence of a small polyp very likely. When comparing it with previous exams, the missing growth makes a malignant lesion such as gallbladder carcinoma very unlikely.

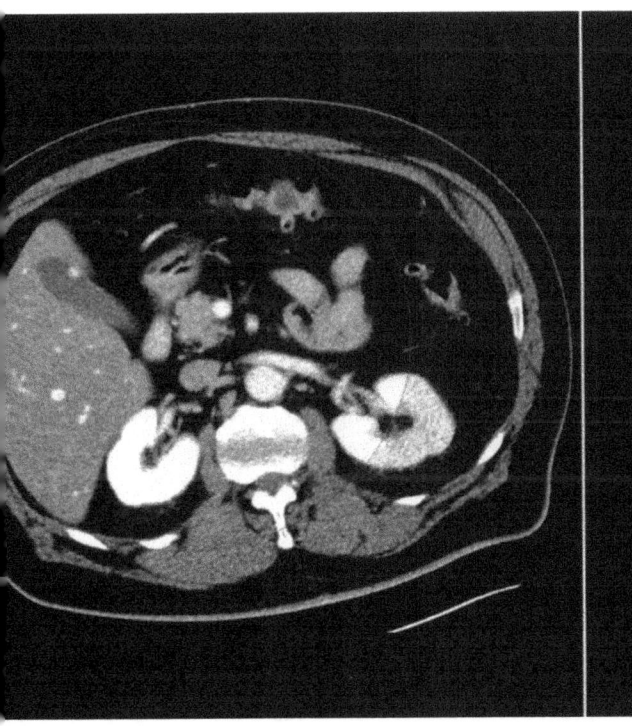

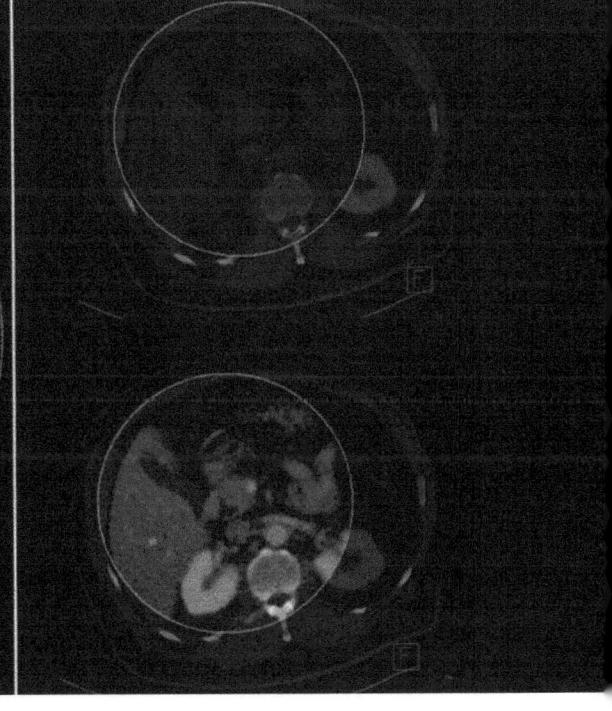

[3] Conventional portal venous phase scan. The lesion continuously takes up contrast media, confirming the presence of a polyp.

[4] Virtual non-enhanced analysis. The color coding confirms the iodine content of the polyp. The virtual non-enhanced image is not different from the conventional image.

Case 2 Exclusion of Urolithiasis in the Presence of Contrast Media

Case history

45-year-old female with cholangiocellular carcinoma and known peritoneal carcinosis presents for follow-up scan post surgery and post chemotherapy.

Question

Can virtual non-enhanced imaging confirm the presence of a small renal stone in the lower pole of the right kidney found incidentally?

Diagnosis / Differential diagnosis

The two major differential diagnoses of hyperenhancing areas in the collecting system of the kidneys after the administration of contrast medium can be renal calculi and excreted contrast media. If a non-enhanced scan is not present, the differential diagnosis is difficult to assess.

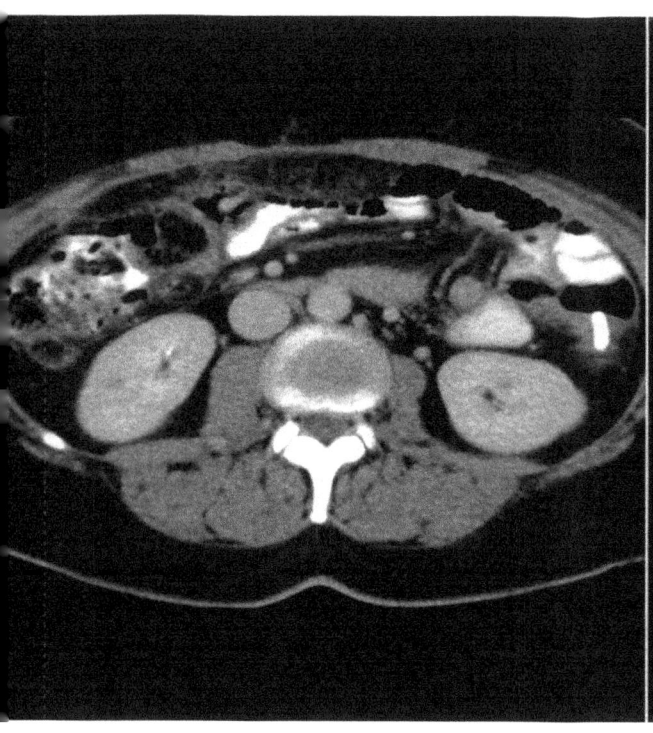

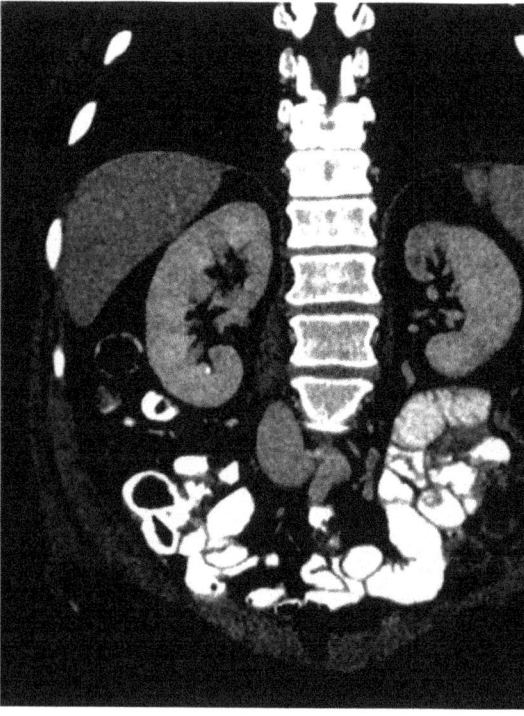

[1] Conventional 5 mm axial image of the lower pole of the kidneys. In the right kidney, the hyperenhancing area could be a calcified nodule.

[2] High resolution coronal reconstruction displays a nodular hyperenhancing nodule.

Findings

Singular scan in portal venous phase. A small hyperenhancing nodule was found in the right lower pole collecting system. No nephrolithiasis was known prior to the scan. Virtual non-enhanced analysis demonstrated an iodine containing nodule that was no longer present in the virtual non-enhanced image. Thus a renal calculi could be excluded and the diagnosis of excreted contrast media could be made.

Take-home message

This case demonstrates that the use of dual energy scanning may make any non-enhanced scan phase obsolete. The scan technique gives one the flexibility to reconstruct a non-enhanced image when needed. Especially in incidental findings or to save dose, the virtual non-enhanced imaging technique allows for full imaging capacities without compromising image quality.

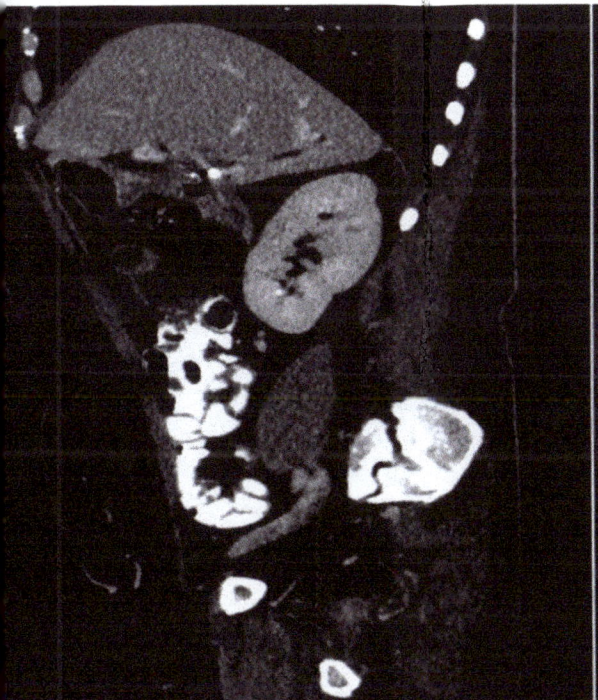

[3] High resolution sagittal reconstruction confirms the presence of a nodular hyperenhancing nodule, making the diagnosis of a renal calculus likely.

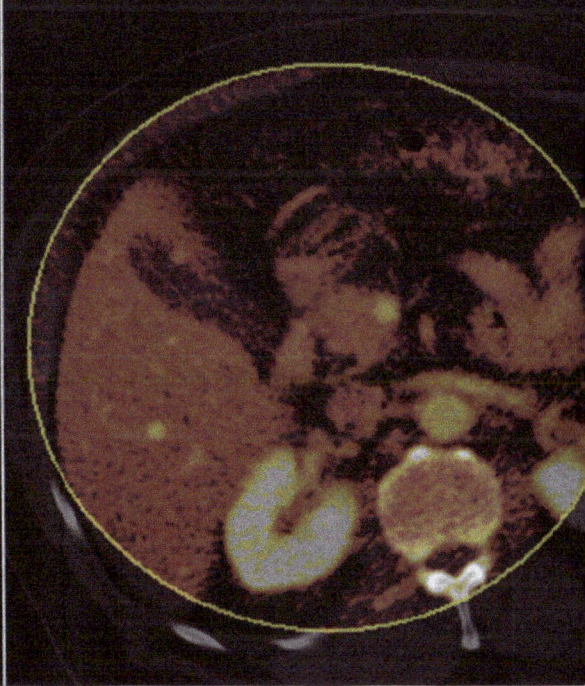

[4] Virtual non-enhanced analysis shows that the major component of the nodular formation is iodine, which is no longer present in the virtual non-enhanced image.

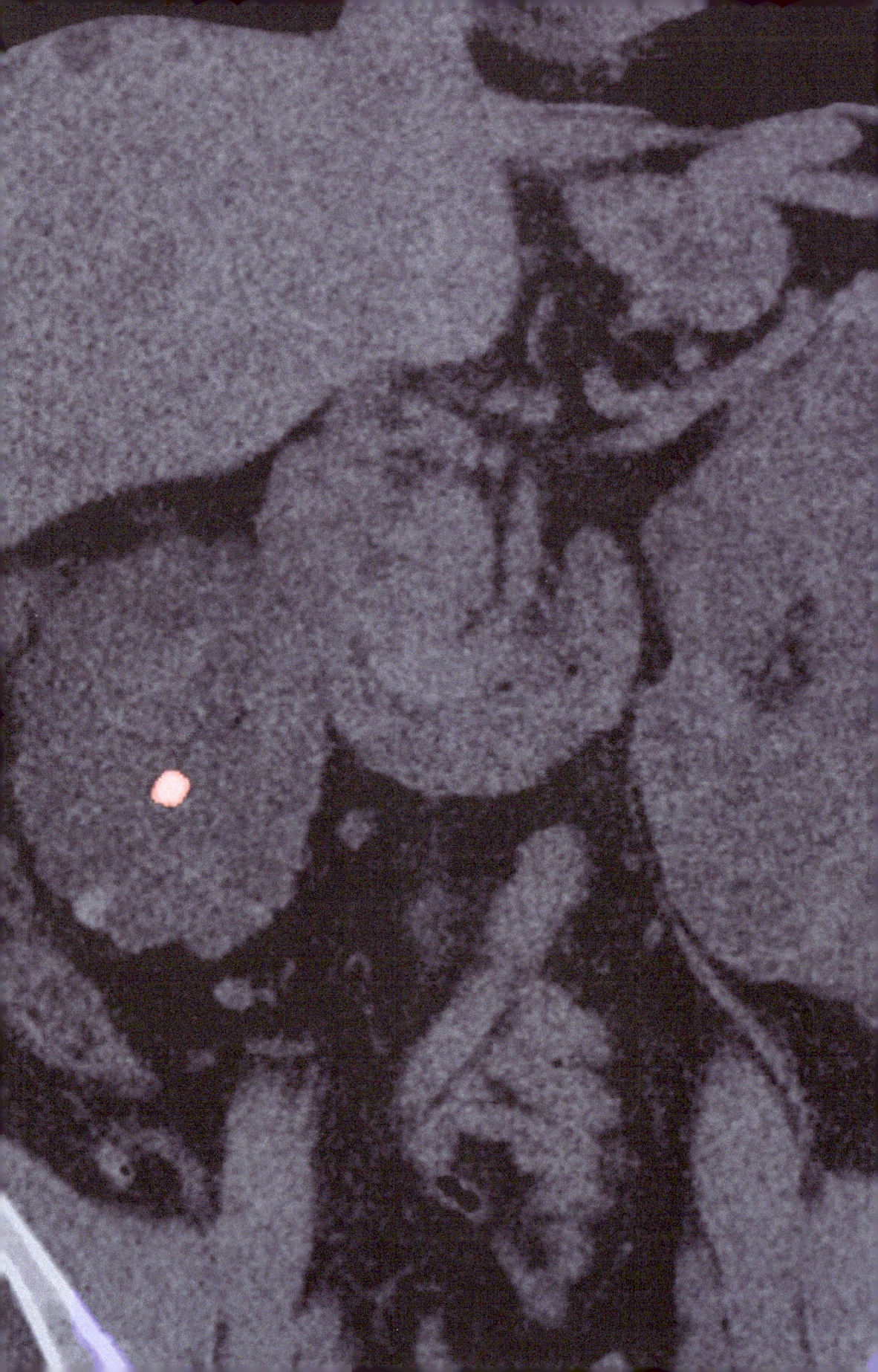

Dual Energy: Characterization of Kidney Stone Composition

Andrew Primak · Terri J. Vrtiska · Cynthia McCollough

Case 1: Ex Vivo Validation of Algorithm Accuracy

Case 2: In Vivo Characterization of Large Renal Stone

Symptomatic urinary stone disease affects approximately 900,000 people in the United States each year resulting in annual medical cost of $5.3 billion (National Kidney and Urological Diseases Advisory Board, 1990). Nephrolithiasis has traditionally been evaluated using radiographic techniques with intravenous (IV) contrast administration. In recent years, however, CT has supplanted these traditional techniques due to increased sensitivity, speed and lack of IV contrast. Furthermore, improved CT acquisition techniques can use less radiation dose than was required for a traditional excretory urogram.

Although modern state-of-the-art CT provides accurate submillimeter details of the size and location of renal stones, current routine clinical image analysis does not differentiate stone composition.[1,2] This is most important in the case of uric acid stones, which comprise approximately 10% of all stones, since urinary alkalinization is likely to dissolve uric acid stones and could be initiated at presentation rather than following lengthy metabolic work-up. Therefore, simple and reliable differentiation in terms of uric acid versus non-uric acid stone composition will allow patients with uric acid stones to avoid a typical shock wave lithotripsy procedure, which is expensive and sometimes results in renal hemorrhage, fibrosis and/or hypertension.

Previous attempts to predict stone composition using spiral CT were based on the analysis of CT attenuation values. Several in vitro and in vivo studies have shown that this approach has the ability to discriminate uric acid from non-uric acid stones. Combining the analysis of CT attenuation values with visual assessment of stone morphology using a wide window setting (e.g. bone window) substantially improves the accuracy of stone characterization.[3] Bellin et al. reported the prediction of stone composition in vitro with 64–81% accuracy, while Zarse et al. demonstrated that high resolution spiral CT yields unique attenuation values for common types of stones if proper window settings are used to localize homogeneous regions within the stones.[4,5]

Although the CT value approach to predict stone composition is feasible, it is not yet robust and reliable enough to be used as a routine clinical application. As an alternative, spiral dual energy CT appears to be a very promising tool for the uric acid vs. non-uric acid stone characterization. Since

Dual Energy: Characterization of Kidney Stone Composition

uric acid stones are composed only of light chemical elements (H, C, N, O), their x-ray attenuation properties at high and low kV are very different compared with those for other (non-uric acid) stone types (calcium oxalate, calcium hydroxyapatite, cystine), whose composition includes heavy elements (P, Ca, S). Consequently uric acid stones have higher CT numbers at higher kV than at lower kV, while non-uric acid stones, on the contrary, have higher CT numbers at lower kV than at higher kV. Some previous studies have already exploited this fact and used the difference between CT values at high and low kV as extra information to improve the prediction accuracy of the CT value approach.[4, 6]

Dual Source CT allows simultaneous dual energy acquisition with high spatial resolution and immediate post-scan image processing with a commercial material decomposition algorithm available on the system. We determined the accuracy of this approach using an ex vivo model. Forty human renal stones comprised of uric acid (n=16), hydroxyapatite (n=8), calcium oxalate (n=8) and cystine (n=8) were inserted into four porcine kidneys (10 each) and placed inside a 32 cm water tank above a cadaver spine. The stone sizes varied from approximately 2 to 7 mm, with 12 'small' stones being less than 2–3 mm. Spiral dual energy scans were obtained on a Dual Source CT system (Siemens SOMATOM Definition) using a clinical protocol with automatic exposure control (100 quality reference mAs at 80 kV, 425 quality reference mAs at 140 kV, pitch 0.7). Scanning was performed with two collimations (32 x 0.6 x 2 and 14 x 1.2) and three phantom sizes, half-full tank (medium), full tank (large) and full tank with extra attenuating material (extra-large). Images were reconstructed using a 1.0 mm slice thickness with 0.8 mm interval (32 x 0.6 x 2) and a 1.5 mm slice thickness with 1.0 mm interval (14 x 1.2) resulting in total of 6 image datasets. These datasets were analyzed using the commercial software tool (*syngo* Dual Energy Viewer, Siemens AG) available on the CT system and both accuracy (number of stones correctly classified as either uric acid or non-uric acid) and sensitivity (number of uric acid stones classified as uric acid) were determined.

After the spiral dual energy CT data acquisition, detailed stone characterization was performed using micro CT. For all stones, micro CT confirmed the major mineral compositions as determined by infrared spectroscopy. However, micro CT revealed visible content of other minerals in many of the stones; this is expected, as most stones contain more than one mineral component. In particular, micro CT revealed calcium salt content in 13 of the 16 uric acid stones. However, this content was quite minor (< 2% by volume) in all cases.

For the medium and large phantom sizes, the dual energy software tool demonstrated 100% accuracy, regardless of collimation. For the extra-large phantom size and the 0.6 mm collimation (the noisiest dataset); three (two cystine and one small uric acid) stones could not be classified (93% accuracy and 94% sensitivity). For the extra-large phantom size and the 1.2 mm collimation, the dual energy tool failed to identify two small uric acid stones (95% accuracy and 88% sensitivity). Thus, our work has demonstrated a high degree of accuracy for the spiral dual energy CT in differentiating between uric acid and non-uric acid stones.

Andrew Primak · Terri J. Vrtiska · Cynthia McCollough

Mayo Clinic College of Medicine

Department of Radiology

References

[1] Williams JC, Jr., Kim SC, Zarse CA, McAteer JA, Lingeman JE. Progress in the use of helical CT for imaging urinary calculi. J Endourol 2004; 18(10):937-941

[2] Vrtiska TJ. Quantitation of stone burden: imaging advances. Urol Res 2005; 33(5):398-402

[3] Williams JC, Jr., Paterson RF, Kopecky KK, Lingeman JE, McAteer JA. High resolution detection of internal structure of renal calculi by helical computerized tomography. J Urol 2002; 167(1):322-326

[4] Bellin MF, Renard-Penna R, Conort P, et al. Helical CT evaluation of the chemical composition of urinary tract calculi with a discriminant analysis of CT-attenuation values and density. Eur Radiol 2004; 14(11):2134-2140

[5] Zarse CA, McAteer JA, et al. Helical CT accurately reports urinary stone composition using attenuation values: in vitro verification using high-resolution micro-computed tomography calibrated to fourier transform infrared microspectroscopy. Urology 2004; 63(5):828-833

[6] Mostafavi MR, Ernst RD, Saltzman B. Accurate determination of chemical composition of urinary calculi by spiral computerized tomography. J Urol 1998; 159(3):673-675

Dual Energy: Characterization of Kidney Stone Composition

Basic considerations

Use of 14 x 1.2 mm collimation and 1.5 mm slice width is preferred in obese patients to reduce the impact of image noise. For average and small patients, use of 64 x 0.6 mm collimation is preferred, as it allows reconstruction of 1.0 mm images. Thinner images reduce partial volume averaging, hence improve accuracy for smaller stones.

In the case of very small stones (< 2.0 mm), the use of 20 x 0.6 mm collimation may yield to improved accuracy in stone differentiation due to better image quality.

Scan Parameters

Scan mode	Spiral dual energy with Dual Source
Scan area	kidney or region of known stones
Scan direction	cranio-caudal
Scan time	~6 s
Tube voltage A/B	140 kV / 80 kV
Tube current A/B	90 quality ref. mAs / 382 quality ref. mAs
Dose modulation	CARE Dose4D
$CTDI_{vol}$	~17 mGy
Rotation time	0.5 s
Pitch	0.6
Slice collimation	0.6 mm (1.2 mm)
Acquisition	64 x 0.6 mm (14 x 1.2 mm)
Slice width	1 mm (1.5 mm)
Reconstruction increment	0.8 mm (1 mm)
Reconstruction kernel	D20f

Tricks

· Centering the patient is very important. Make sure the region of interest is located within the central 26 cm FOV. For patients with known stones, a limited scan can be performed only over the stone region to reduce patient dose.

· Keep pitch below 0.7.

Pitfalls

· Some very small stones may not be able to be discriminated.

· High levels of image noise in obese patients may compromise accuracy of discrimination, especially for small stones.

Contrast Injection Protocol

CM volume	–
Iodine delivery rate	–
CM flow rate	–
Iodine concentration	–
Body weight adaption	–
Bolus timing	–
HU target	–
ROI position	–
Scan delay	–
Saline flush	·
Needle size	–
Injection site	–

Case 1 Ex Vivo Validation of Algorithm Accuracy

Case history

40 human renal stones of known composition were placed in explanted porcine kidneys immersed in water and scanned using clinical dual energy protocols.

Question

Determine the accuracy and sensitivity for the discrimination of uric acid vs. non-uric acid stones.

Diagnosis / Differential diagnosis

Not applicable.

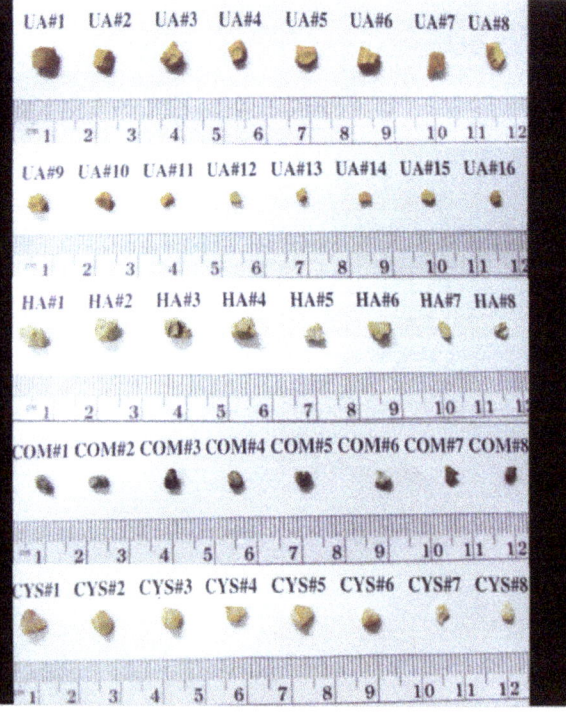

[1] Photographs of the 40 human stones used for ex vivo validation.

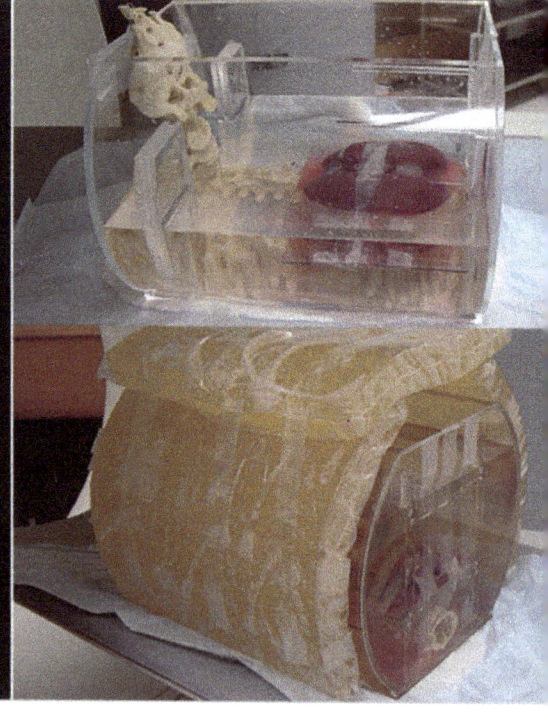

[2] Photographs of the water-filled cylinders used to simulate medium, large and extra-large patients. A spine was laid under the porcine kidneys.

Findings

100% accuracy was achieved when the attenuation simulated medium and large patients. For the simulation of extra-large patients, increased image noise decreased accuracy to 93–95%.

Take-home message

Spiral dual energy CT can accurately discriminate uric acid vs. non-uric acid stones. In obese patients, it is important to use wider collimation and slice width to decrease the influence of noise.

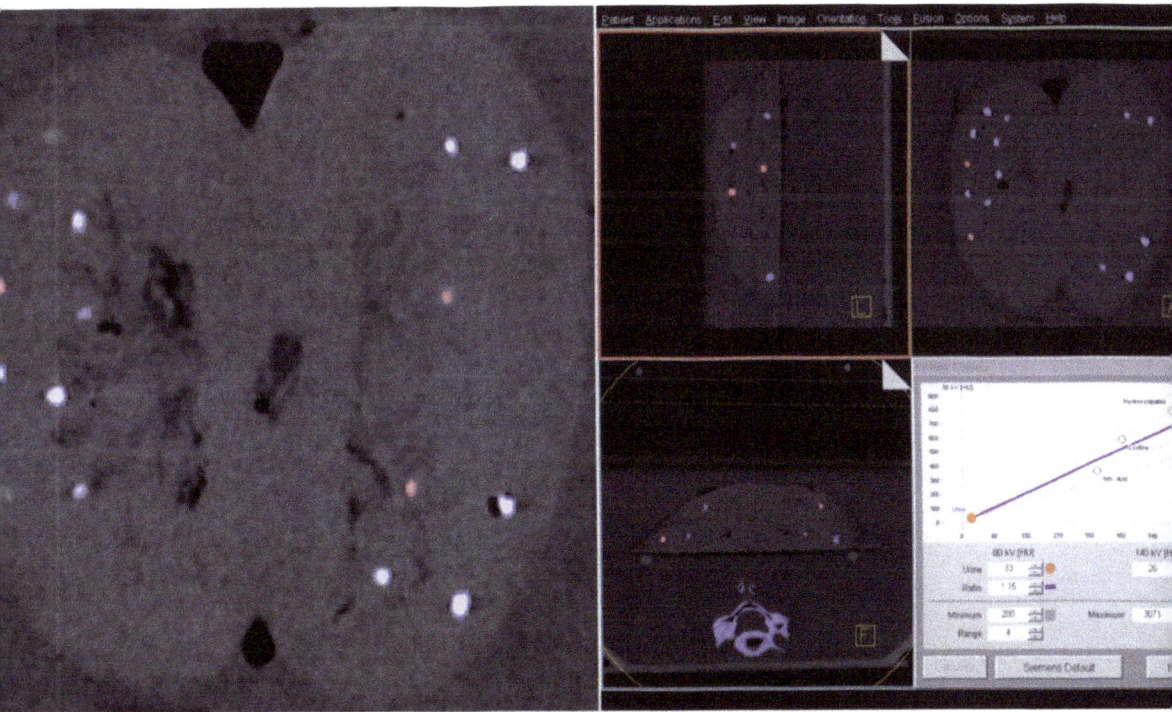

[3] Stones are color-coded according to composition. Results are independent of the absolute HU-value and only depend on the absorption difference between 140 kV and 80 kV.

[4] Color-coded display of uric acid (red) and non-uric-acid (blue) stones produced using the kidney stone workflow of the Syngo Dual Energy software tool.

Case 2 In Vivo Characterization of Large Renal Stone

Case history

43-year-old male with cystinuria managed by oral medications. He underwent CT evaluation for consideration of renal preservation percutaneous stone removal.

Question

What is the extent of the stone disease?
Are there any complications of stone disease?

Diagnosis / Differential diagnosis

· Right staghorn calculus.
· Small calyceal calculi in the lower pole of the left kidney.
· No ureteral calculi.
· No urinary tract obstruction.
· No renal masses.
· Moderate right renal parenchymal scarring.

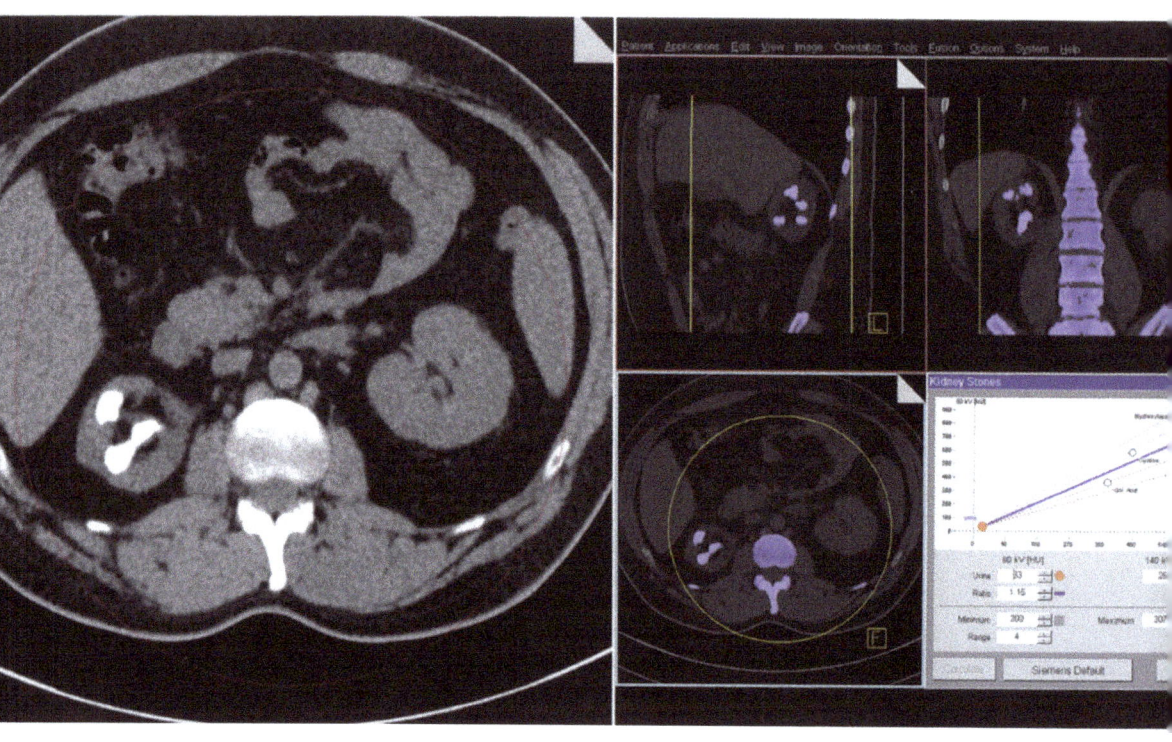

[1] Axial non-contrast image through the kidneys showing a large branching calculus in the right kidney. There is parenchymal scarring and atrophy of the right kidney.

[2] Stone composition processing; blue indicates non-uric acid stone types, such as this patient's large cystine stone. Advanced users may alter the processing parameters.

Findings

Large branching calculus filling the right intrarenal collecting system and renal pelvis. Moderate diffuse parenchymal loss involving the right kidney. A few small calculi in the lower pole calyces of the left kidney.

Take-home message

Currently renal stone CT is the optimal exam for stone disease, not only can symptomatic ureteral calculi be directly visualized using non-enhanced CT, but complications of stone disease can also be accurately visualized such as ureteral obstruction, intrarenal urinary tract dilatation, periureteral/perinephric edema and renal parenchymal scarring.

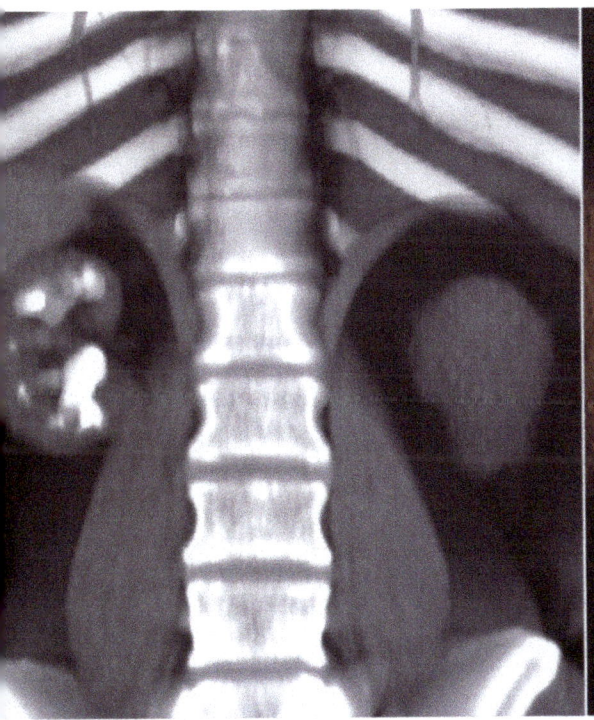

[3] Coronal 3D rendering demonstrates the branching calculus in the right kidney with parenchymal atrophy.

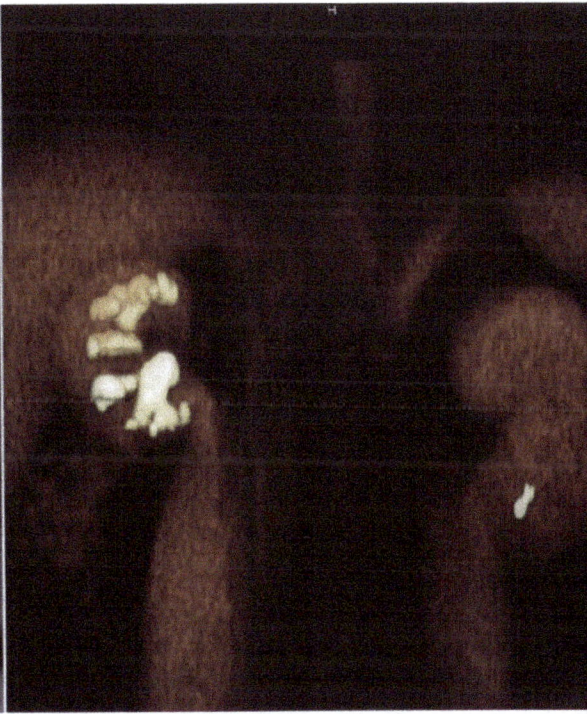

[4] Semi-transparent 3D rendering of the kidneys shows a staghorn calculus filling the intrarenal collecting system of the right kidney and a small stone in the left kidney.

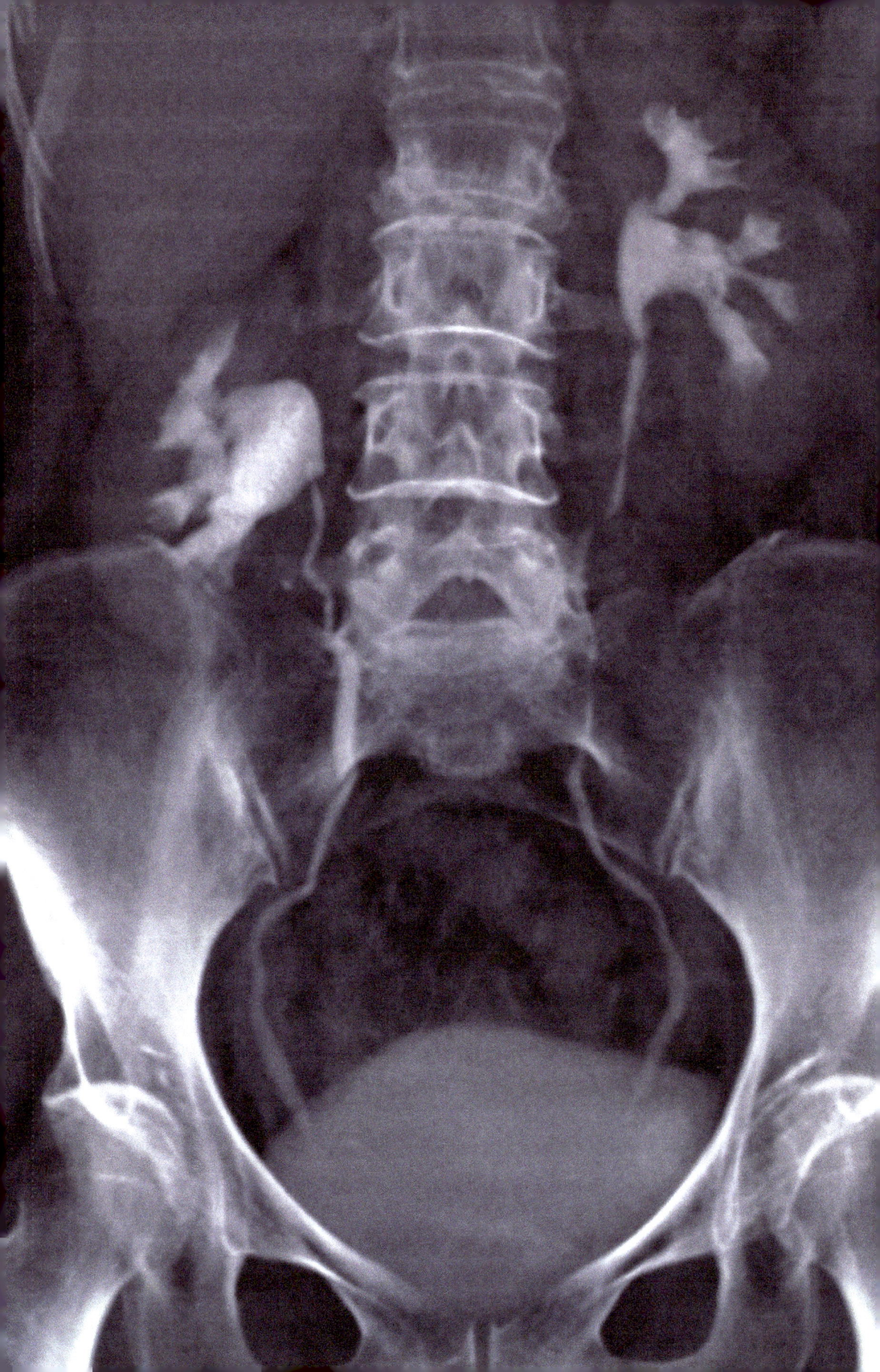

Dual Energy: Urography

Robert P. Hartman · Terri J. Vrtiska · Cynthia McCollough

Case 1: Virtual Non-Contrast CT for Identification of Stones from Contrast enhanced CT

Case 2: Dual Energy CT for the Differentiation of Renal Cyst vs. Mass

In recent years, developments in CT, especially the development of multi-detector CT (MDCT), have provided new and better tools for the evaluation of patients presenting with hematuria and flank pain. The ability of MDCT to provide rapid contiguous thin-slice imaging through the abdomen allowed for the development of CT urography (CTU) protocols for the detection of urolithiasis, renal masses and urothelial neoplasms such as transitional cell carcinoma.

Typically, CTU protocols include a non-contrast acquisition, a nephrographic phase of enhancement of the renal parenchyma and a delayed or excretory phase for distension and opacification of the urinary tract and bladder. A number of different CTU protocols have been developed at various institutions over the years. These protocols utilize variations in the timing of the scan relative to the contrast bolus, as well as single or split bolus contrast injections.

The detection of urolithiasis or calcification within renal lesions requires the use of a non-contrast scan. Smith et al. were the first to show the usefulness of CT in the detection of urolithiasis.[1] Advantages of CT over plain film radiography and IVU include the ability to localize the calculus within the intrarenal collecting system, ureter or bladder. This is particularly helpful in distinguishing pelvic phleboliths from distal ureteral stones. An additional benefit of spiral dual energy CT is the detection of particular stone compositions including uric acid stones, cystine stones, and xanthine stones which are known to be radiolucent on plain x-ray.

In many instances, the detection and characterization of renal masses require enhancement of the renal parenchyma. The nephrographic phase, when the cortex and medullary regions of the kidney have a homogeneous enhancement, is excellent for the detection of renal masses. The conspicuity of lesions in the kidney is greatest during this phase of enhancement as the lesions have a lower attenuation than the background of the enhanced renal parenchyma. However, studies have shown a similar detection rate with excretory phase imaging.[2]

Evaluation of the intrarenal collecting system and ureters requires a later phase following contrast injection, often termed an excretory phase. During this phase, the kidneys have filtered and excreted

Dual Energy: Urography

much of the iodinated contrast from the blood stream to opacify and distend the intrarenal collecting system and ureters. Given this background enhancement within the urinary tract, tiny lesions such as transitional cell carcinoma or other urothelial abnormalities are often depicted as a filling defect.

A non-contrast scan is of particular use in CTU for the detection of stones and calcifications. However, a secondary use for the non-contrast scans is in the characterization of renal masses. In many instances of renal cell carcinoma (RCC), discreet identifiable enhancement is visible on the post-contrast images without the need for comparison to the baseline non-contrast scan. However, there is a small percentage of lesions (including hemorrhagic cysts and occasionally hypo-perfusing malignancies such as papillary RCC) that can be difficult to confidently identify in the presence or absence of enhancement on the post-contrast acquisition without a non-contrast baseline for comparison. Investigators have identified thresholds for changes in the attenuation of lesions from baseline to post-contrast as they relate to benign or malignant etiologies. Lesions acquiring less than a 10 Hounsfield unit (HU) increase in attenuation on post-contrast images are benign, usually a renal cyst. Lesions acquiring greater than a 20 HU increase in attenuation on post-contrast images have been shown in most instances to be a solid lesion. In these instances, renal cell carcinoma is a likely diagnosis requiring surgical intervention. Those lesions obtaining an increased attenuation between 10 and 20 HU on the post-contrast images are often indeterminate in part due to a phenomenon known as pseudo-enhancement that has been described in CT evaluation of renal masses.[3]

With contemporary CTU, there may be variations in the protocol following the injection of contrast material, but all require a pre-contrast examination for the detection of stones and as a baseline for the evaluation of a renal mass. With the availability of spiral dual energy CT and its potential for delivering a virtual non-contrast image set, there is a potential for the elimination of the true non-contrast series.[4]

Differentiation of materials using dual energy CT was described in the late 1970s.[5] Given this ability of dual energy CT, it is possible to produce image sets where iodine from injected contrast media can be localized and subtracted, thereby producing a virtual non-contrast exam. In addition, an image set with a color overlay depicting particular locations where iodine is present can also be produced.[6] These spiral dual energy CT features are the basis by which the non-contrast acquisition may be rendered obsolete.

A virtual non-contrast image set can be produced from a CT acquisition performed during an excretory phase when the intrarenal collecting systems and ureters are opacified with iodinated contrast. With the iodine signal eliminated, the detection and localization of the urinary stones would be possible.

The iodine overlay image would provide the necessary information regarding enhancement of renal lesions. With dual energy CT's ability to identify iodine, the overlay would show iodine signal within the center of an enhancing solid mass. A renal cyst without blood flow would contain no iodine signal. Given the lack or presence of iodine signal within a particular lesion, the radiologist would have the ability to determine whether a mass was a cyst or solid lesion.

The capability to provide virtual non-contrast and iodine overlay images will allow spiral dual energy CT to provide an examination that is complete without a non-contrast acquisition. This could reduce the dose of radiation to all patients regardless of the particular protocol for CT urography. In the particular case of a split bolus technique, this would allow for a complete CT urogram to be performed during the single post-contrast, combined nephrographic and excretory phase, providing all required information during a single acquisition.

Robert P. Hartman · Terri J. Vrtiska · Cynthia McCollough
Mayo Clinic College of Medicine
Department of Radiology

References

[1] Smith RC, Verga M, McCarthy S, Rosenfield AT. Diagnosis of acute flank pain: value of unenhanced helical CT. AJR Am J Roentgenol 1996; 166:97-101

[2] Yuh BI, Cohan RH, Francis IR, Korobkin M, Ellis JH. Comparison of nephrographic with excretory phase helical computed tomography for detecting and characterizing renal masses. Can Assoc Radiol J 2000; 51:170-176

[3] Bae KT, Heiken JP, Siegel CL, Bennett HF. Renal cysts: is attenuation artifactually increased on contrast-enhanced CT images? Radiology 2000; 216:792-796

[4] Flohr TG, McCollough CH, Bruder H, et al. First performance evaluation of a dual-source CT (DSCT) system. Eur Radiol 2006; 16:256-268

[5] Millner MR, McDavid WD, Waggener RG, Dennis MJ, Payne WH, Sank VJ. Extraction of information from CT scans at different energies. Med Phys 1979; 6:70-71

[6] Johnson TRC, Krauss B, Sedlmair M et al. Material differentiation by dual energy CT: initial experience. Eur Radiol. 2007; 17(6):1510-7

Dual Energy: Urography

Basic considerations

The use of spiral dual energy CT can be incorporated into nearly any CT urography protocol. However, with current algorithms the iodine subtraction works best if the attenuation of the intrarenal collecting system and ureter is 1600 HU or less (measured at 120 kV). This value is seldom if ever approached using a split bolus contrast technique but can be achieved with single bolus techniques. In cases where this is exceeded, the iodine subtraction can be incomplete leading to non-visualization of stones or overestimation of stone size.

Scan Parameters

Scan mode	Spiral dual energy with Dual Source
Scan area	top of kidneys to symphysis
Scan direction	cranio-caudal
Scan time	~10–11 s
Tube voltage A/B	140 kV/80 kV
Tube current A/B	95 quality ref. mAs/403 quality ref. mAs
Dose modulation	CARE Dose4D
CTDI	~18 mGy
Rotation time	0.5 s
Pitch	0.55
Slice collimation	0.6 mm
Acquisition	64 x 0.6 mm
Slice width	3 mm
Reconstruction increment	2.5 mm
Reconstruction kernel	D30f

Tricks

Ensure that the kidneys are centered in the 26 cm FOV both, in the left/right and a.p. patient plane. Use a compression belt and remove it directly before the 70 second abdomen/pelvis scan begins.

Pitfalls

Current subtraction algorithms can occasionally subtract some of the volume of urinary stones. This can lead to complete subtraction and non-visualization of tiny stones (<2 mm) or to underestimation of true stone size in larger stones that are identifiable on virtual non-contrast.

Contrast Injection Protocol

	Iodine concentration 300 mg I/ml	Iodine concentration 370 mg I/ml
Injection scheme	Biphasic	Biphasic
Iodine delivery rate	1.2 g/s	1.2 g/s
CM volume	140 ml (split dose 70 ml/70 ml)	120 ml (split dose 60 ml/60 ml)
CM flow rate	4 ml/s	3.2 ml/s
Body weight adaption	no	no
Bolus timing	70 ml/4 ml/s, saline flush, 7 min delay, 70 ml/4 ml/s, 60 s delay	60 ml/3.2 ml/s, saline flush, 7 min delay, 60 ml/3.2 ml/s, 60 s delay
Bolus tracking threshold	n.a.	n.a.
ROI position	n.a.	n.a.
Scan delay	70 s after second injection	70 s after second injection
Saline flush volume	150 ml	150 ml
Saline injection rate	4 ml/s	3.2 ml/s
Needle size	18 G	18 G
Injection site	antecubital vein	antecubital vein

Case 1 Virtual Non-Contrast CT for Identification of Stones from Contrast Enhanced CT

Case history

66-year-old male presenting for follow-up exam of known nephrolithiasis and prior history of bladder transitional cell carcinoma.

Question

Evaluate the kidneys and ureters for presence of calculi and any associated complications.

Diagnosis / Differential diagnosis

· There are two renal calculi present.

· No other abnormalities of the kidneys, ureters or bladder are identified.

· The stones lie within the intrarenal collecting system and were slightly larger than on previous exams.

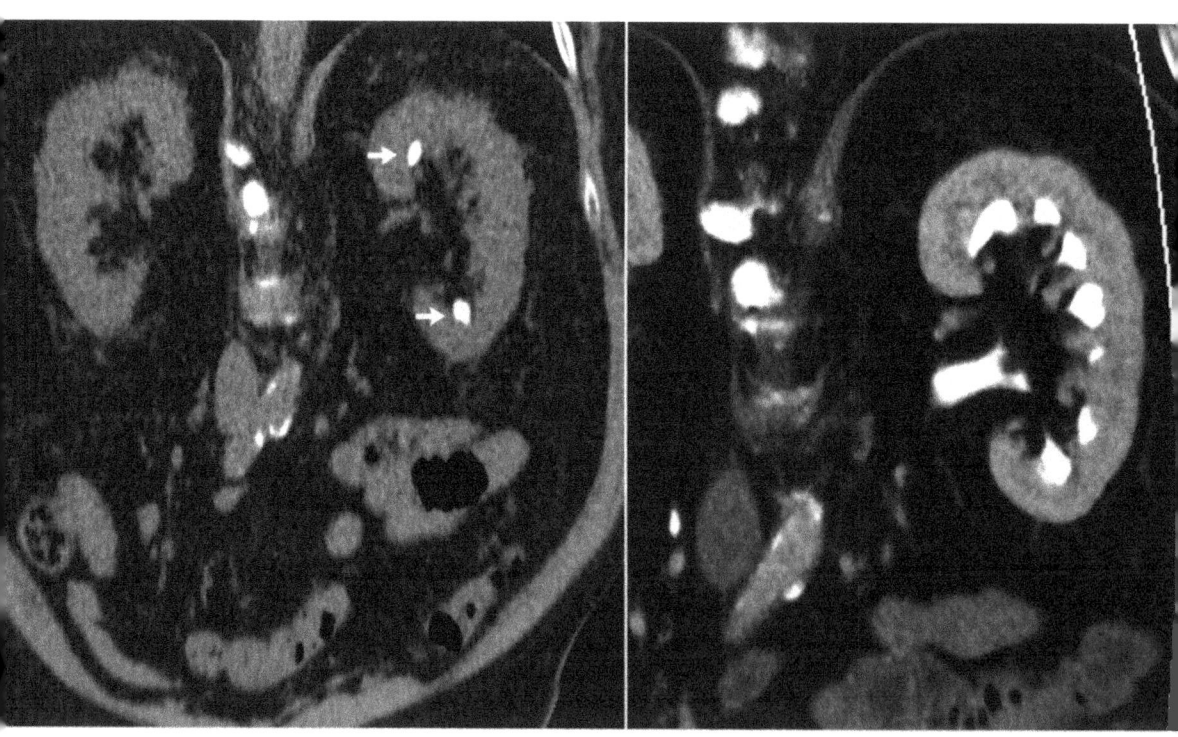

[1] Coronal MPR image from a non-contrast CT acquisition demonstrates stones in the upper and lower poles of the left kidney (arrows).

[2] Coronal MPR from the dual energy mixed images acquired during the excretory phase. The stones shown on the non-contrast acquisitions are now obscured.

Findings

Two renal calculi are present in the left kidney. The stone in the upper pole measures 5 mm and the stone in the lower pole measures 8 mm. No other urinary calculi or signs of obstruction. No recurrent transitional cell carcinoma is identified.

Take-home message

The virtual non-contrast images produced from the excretory phase of the CT urogram were capable of detecting the stones that were evident on the true non-contrast acquisition. Given this capability of spiral dual energy CT, a separate non-contrast acquisition may not be needed, which would reduce the radiation dose to the patient.

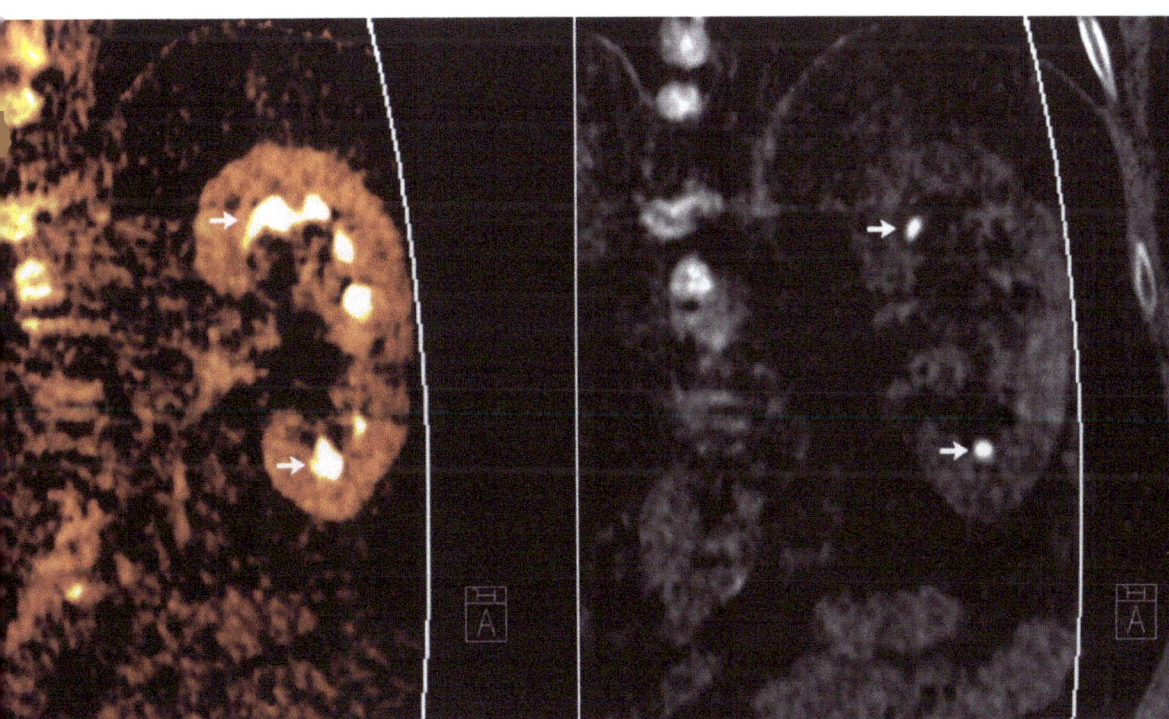

[3] Coronal MPR from dual energy data acquired in the excretory phase. The areas determined to be iodine are depicted with color. The stones are not visible (arrows).

[4] Coronal MPR image after iodine subtraction from the excretory phase. The stones previously obscured by the surrounding iodinated contrast are now easily visible (arrows).

Case 2 Dual Energy CT for the Differentiation of Renal Cyst vs. Mass

Case history

70-year-old female presents for follow-up of a suspected solid mass in the lower pole of the left kidney.

Question

Is the mass in the lower pole of the left kidney in fact solid or some complex renal cyst?

Diagnosis/Differential diagnosis

Given the presence of iodine signal exhibited on the iodine overlay images, this appears to be a solid renal mass. This was also established based on an increase in attenuation from true non-contrast to post-contrast images of 70 HU. This should be considered worrisome for a renal cell carcinoma, but an oncocytoma could have an identical appearance.

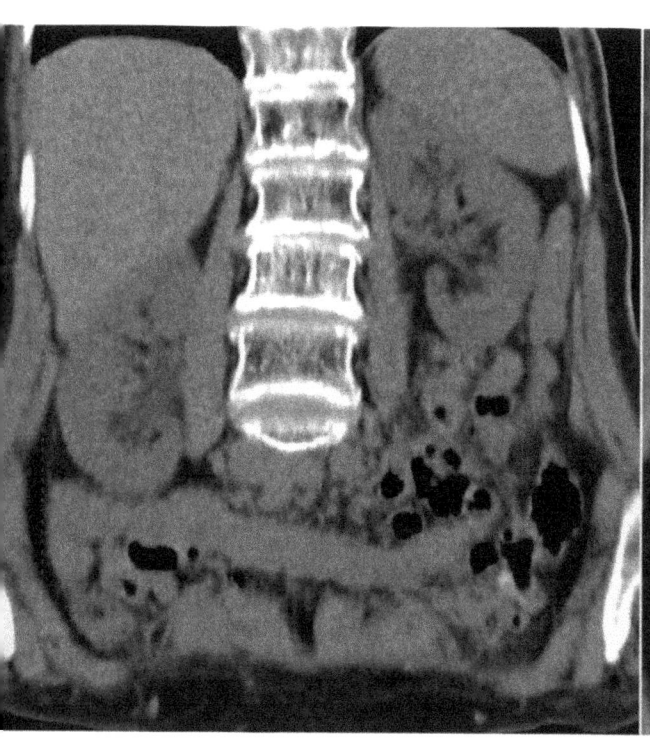

[1] Non-contrast coronal MPR. No stones were identified in either kidney.

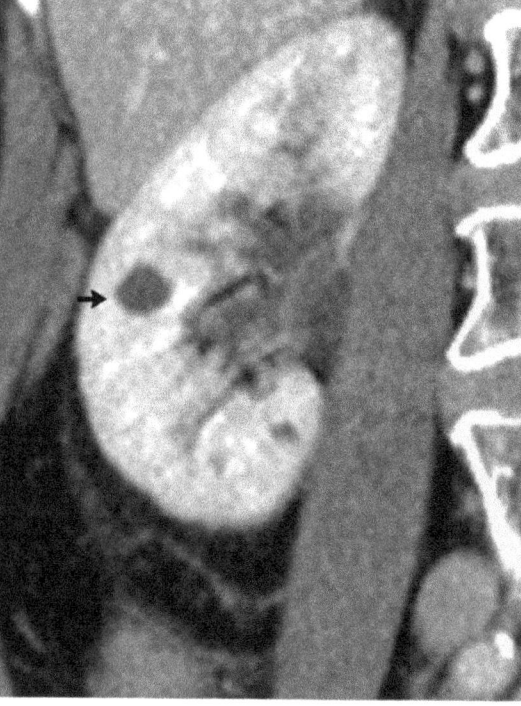

[2] Coronal image of the right kidney with a low attenuation mass in the mid portion (arrow) that has a typical appearance of a renal cyst.

Findings

1.2 cm mass in the lower pole of the left kidney is solid based on the presence of iodine signal centrally. A second lesion in the mid portion of the right kidney does not have iodine signal and is considered to be a benign cyst.

Take-home message

The use of the iodine overlay image that can be produced from a dual energy acquisition allows for the differentiation of a renal cyst from a solid mass. This capability may allow for the elimination of a dedicated non-contrast acquisition and reduce patient radiation dose.

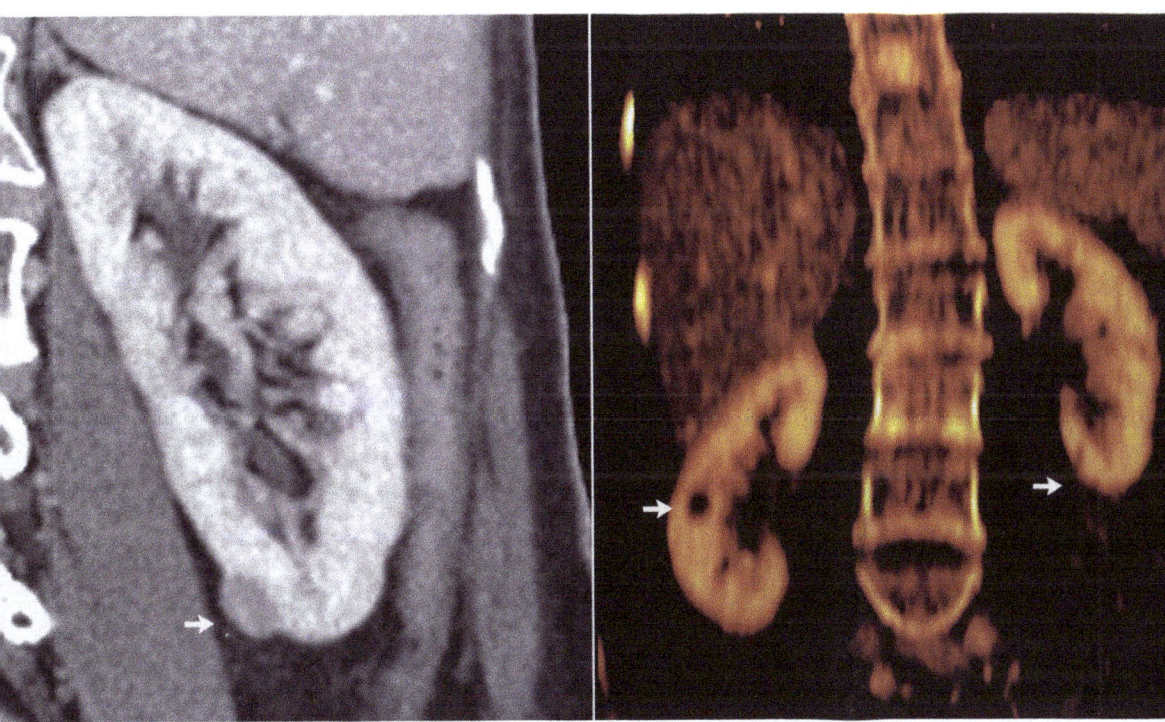

[3] Coronal image of the left kidney with an indeterminate lesion along the medial lower pole (arrow).

[4] Coronal iodine overlay image depicting both lesions (cyst in right kidney with signal void and mass in left kidney) identified on average weighted series (arrows).

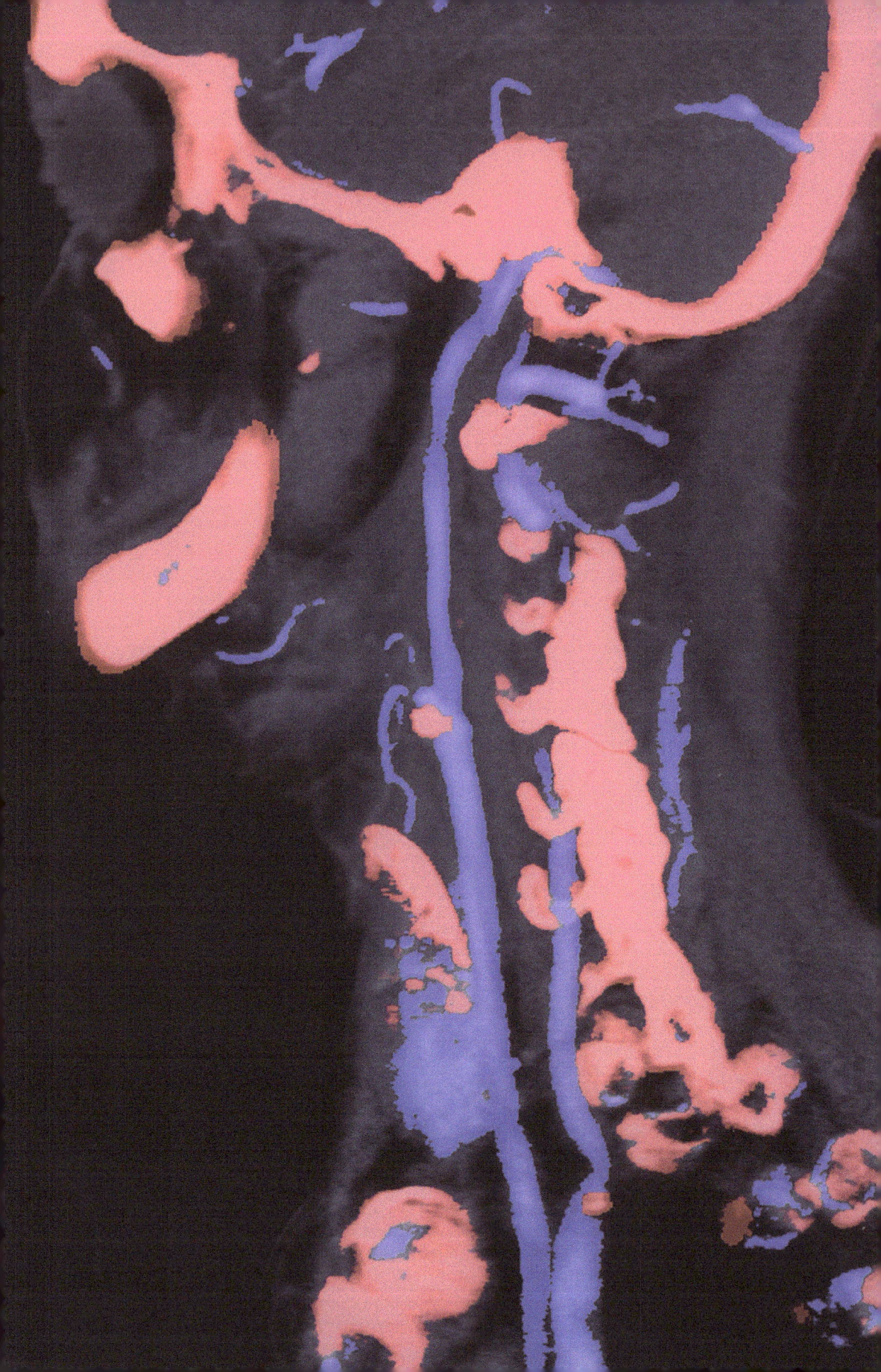

Dual Energy: Vascular Plaque Removal/Detection

Christoph Thomas · Harald Brodoefel · Martin Heuschmid · Andreas F. Kopp

Case 1: Calcification of the Carotid Artery

Case 2: Calcification of the Renal Artery

Manifestations of arteriosclerosis such as cardiovascular and arterial occlusive disease are among the major causes of death in the western world. Besides age, sex and genetic disposition, other common risk factors for arterial occlusive disease include diabetes, nicotine, high blood pressure and lipid metabolic disturbances.[1]

Challenges for imaging arteriosclerosis and its major complication, arterial occlusive disease, include an accurate quantification of stenosis, preoperative planning and monitoring disease progression or remission as well as plaque characterization. Intra-arterial digital subtraction angiography (IA-DSA) is considered the standard reference used to assess arterial occlusive disease. However, as DSA is an invasive modality, it may cause complications during examination, and it may be limited by overlaying of other vessels and the dependence of lumen measurements on the imaging angle due to its two-dimensional nature.[2]

The introduction of multislice CT (MS CT) systems has opened up the field of CT angiography (CTA) in recent years. CTA facilitates fast and robust data collection relating to the arterial vascular system within a single spiral acquisition. In clinical routine, CTA is used for the assessment of the whole aorta, cerebral and carotid arteries, pulmonary and coronary arteries, mesenteric, renal and iliac arteries as well as the vessels of the lower limb.[3] The axial source images can be used to grade the severity of stenosis and to visualize the arterial lumen and surrounding tissues. Furthermore, there are several post-processing techniques available to facilitate the evaluation of the images, such as shaded surface display (SSD) reconstructions or maximum intensity projections (MIP). However, because they depend on thresholds, these techniques are limited by osseous structures and calcified plaques. Consequently, an accurate quantification of stenosis often has to be performed manually, which is time-consuming and also user-dependent. Being able to further automate the post-processing workflow by applying automated plaque detection has the potential to further improve the accuracy and the acceptance of CTA.

Calcium and iodine are chemical elements with high atomic numbers (calcium: 20; iodine: 52). Their x-ray attenuations differ at different photon energy spectra such as generated by tube

Dual Energy: Vascular Plaque Removal/Detection

voltages of 80 and 140 kV$_p$.[4] Therefore, by using attenuation information from a dual energy scan and applying dedicated algorithms, calcium and iodine can be discriminated from each other.[5]

Currently, there is only one Dual Source CT scanner on the market that allows simultaneous dual energy scanning – the SOMATOM Definition (Siemens Medical Solutions). It is equipped with two x-ray tubes and two detectors mounted perpendicular within the gantry.[6] The *syngo* Dual Energy software package (Siemens AG) includes a module designed for the decomposition of calcium and iodine called "hard plaque": Applying a dedicated algorithm to the low- and high-kV$_p$ series, it creates a virtual image stack containing only calcium and iodine information, assigning positive numbers to all pixels containing iodine, and negative numbers to all pixels with calcium. All other image information is deleted. For visualization, this calcium/iodine map is fused with the original image. Depending on the choice of the color map for the overlay, the presence of calcium and iodine can be indicated by different colors.

Plaque removal is possible using the "Bone removal" module, which sets all voxels containing calcium to zero. As a result, bones and calcified plaques are removed from the images. The resulting image stack can be used to create 3D-images unimpaired by calcifications.

There are certain possible benefits in automated dual energy plaque detection. Since a sensitive calcium detection and delineation now seems to be possible in contrast enhanced scans, an additional non-enhanced scan, which is frequently performed prior to the enhanced scan, might be spared. This could lead to a relevant reduction in patient dose performing CTA. By using the dual energy bone removal tool, calcified hard plaques can now be automatically removed from the images, which might have a significant impact on the interobserver variability in the grading of stenosis. This is because the grading of stenosis partly depends on the window setting in single-energy scans and is, therefore, observer dependent. With an ability to automatically define calcified plaque, this variability might be reduced. Furthermore the ability to automatically color-code vessel calcifications has the potential to significantly reduce the post-processing and reading time and to simplify the presentation of radiological findings to the clinical referrers and especially to our patients.

Altogether, dual energy plaque detection is a promising and evolving technique that yields very interesting possible applications. Especially an automatic and precise quantification of calcium burden and the grading of arterial stenosis may improve vascular evaluations and image reading for routine applications.

Christoph Thomas · Harald Brodoefel

Martin Heuschmid · Andreas F. Kopp

Eberhard-Karls-University Tübingen

Department of Diagnostic and Interventional Radiology

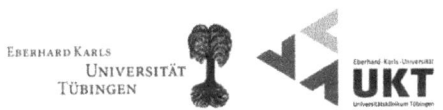

References

[1] Wilson PW, D'Agostino RB, Levy D, et al. Prediction of coronary heart disease using risk factor categories. Circulation 1998; 97(18):1837-47

[2] Elgersma OE, Wust AF, Buijs PC, et al. Multidirectional depiction of internal carotid arterial stenosis: three-dimensional time-of-flight MR angiography versus rotational and conventional digital subtraction angiography. Radiology 2000; 216:511-516

[3] Napoli A, Fleischmann D, Chan FP, et al. Computed tomography angiography: state-of-the-art imaging using multidetector-row technology. J Comput Assist Tomogr 2004; 28 Suppl 1:S32-45

[4] Huda W, Scalzetti EM, Levin G. Technique factors and image quality as functions of patient weight at abdominal CT. Radiology 2000; 217:430-435

[5] Johnson TR, Krauss B, Sedlmair M, et al. Material differentiation by dual energy CT: initial experience. Eur Radiol 2007; 17:1510-1517

[6] Flohr TG, McCollough CH, Bruder H, et al. First performance evaluation of a dual-source CT (DSCT) system. Eur Radiol 2006; 16:256-268

Dual Energy: Vascular Plaque Removal/Detection

Basic considerations

Because dual energy plaque detection/removal can be performed in any part of the body, the examination protocol design is variable, depending on the body region examined. Apart from choosing a different scan mode (dual energy), the procedure resembles conventional CTA with the iodine delivery rate as the decisive factor determining contrast attenuation.

A CTDIvol comparable to conventional CTA should be delivered. In order to achieve an optimal arterial phase, different scan directions should be chosen (e.g. cranio-caudal for abdomen and caudo-cranial for neck).

Scan Parameters (exemplified for the neck region)

Scan mode	Spiral dual energy with Dual Source
Scan area	aortic arch to circle of Willis
Scan direction	caudo-cranial
Scan time	~4 s
Tube voltage A/B	140 kV/80 kV
Tube current A/B	55 quality ref. mAs/234 quality ref. mAs
Dose modulation	CARE Dose4D
CTDI$_{vol}$	~9 mGy
Rotation time	0.5 s
Pitch	0.7
Slice collimation	0.6 mm
Acquisition	64 x 0.6 mm
Slice width	1 mm
Reconstruction increment	0.7 mm
Reconstruction kernel	D30f

Tricks

Tube current modulation (CARE Dose4D) should be switched on to smoothen the image noise profile of the scan for an efficient dual energy analysis. Scanning should be performed in an early arterial phase.

Pitfalls

· Spiral dual energy evaluation is only possible within the inner field of view of 26 cm in the center of the gantry, therefore the patient has to be positioned carefully.

· In obese patients or in anatomical regions with irregular attenuation profiles such as the shoulders, image quality might be degraded if scan parameters are not adjusted accordingly.

Contrast Injection Protocol

	Iodine concentration 300 mg I/ml	Iodine concentration 370 mg I/ml
Injection scheme	Monophasic	Monophasic
Iodine delivery rate	1.85 g/s	1.85 g/s
CM volume	100 ml	80 ml
CM flow rate	6.2 ml/s	5 ml/s
Body weight adaption	no	no
Bolus timing	bolus tracking*	bolus tracking*
Bolus tracking threshold	130 HU	130 HU
ROI position	aortic arch	aortic arch
Scan delay	2 s	2 s
Saline flush volume	60 ml	60 ml
Saline injection rate	6.2 ml/s	5 ml/s
Needle size	18 G	18 G
Injection site	antecubital vein	antecubital vein

* Depending on the preference of the individual site, test bolus can be used as an alternative

Case 1 Calcification of the Carotid Artery

Case history

63-year-old hypertensive patient presenting with transient amaurosis fugax and aphasia for 8 hours. MRI angiography was not possible because a cardiac pacemaker is present.

Question

Abnormal anatomy of the carotid vessels? Severe carotid artery stenosis? Plaques of the carotid arteries?

Diagnosis / Differential diagnosis

· Arteriosclerosis of the internal carotid artery.
· Occlusion of carotid artery due to thrombosis / embolism.
· Soft or calcified plaque of the carotid artery.
· Vascular abnormalities.

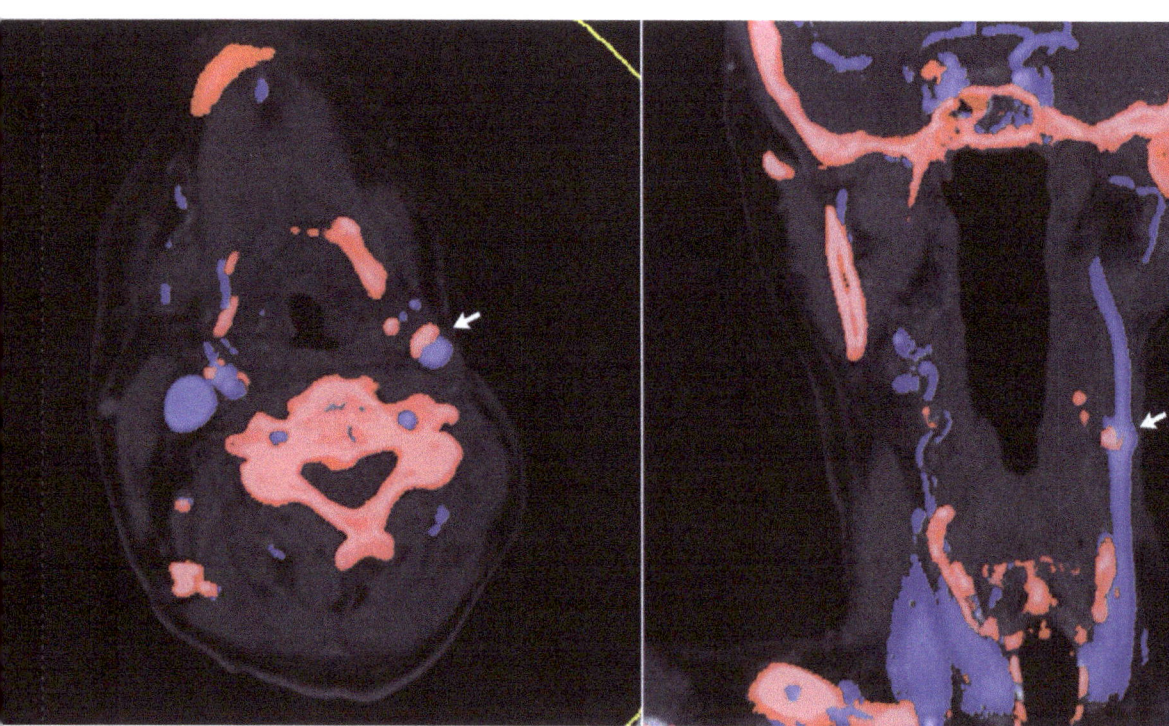

[1] Axial dual energy image of a calcified plaque at the bifurcation of the left carotid artery (arrow). Note the differentiation of iodine (blue) and calcium (red).

[2] Coronary dual energy image (MPR) of the same plaque (arrow).

Findings

Abnormal anatomic findings of the carotid arteries could be excluded. Fused dual energy images show calcified plaques at both carotid bifurcations. Severe vascular stenosis due to calcified or soft plaque was not found.

Take-home message

Dual energy CTA enables a differentiation of iodine-filled vessel lumina from calcified vessel plaques, making a more accurate quantification of carotid stenosis possible. Color-coded visualization further simplifies diagnosis and presentation.

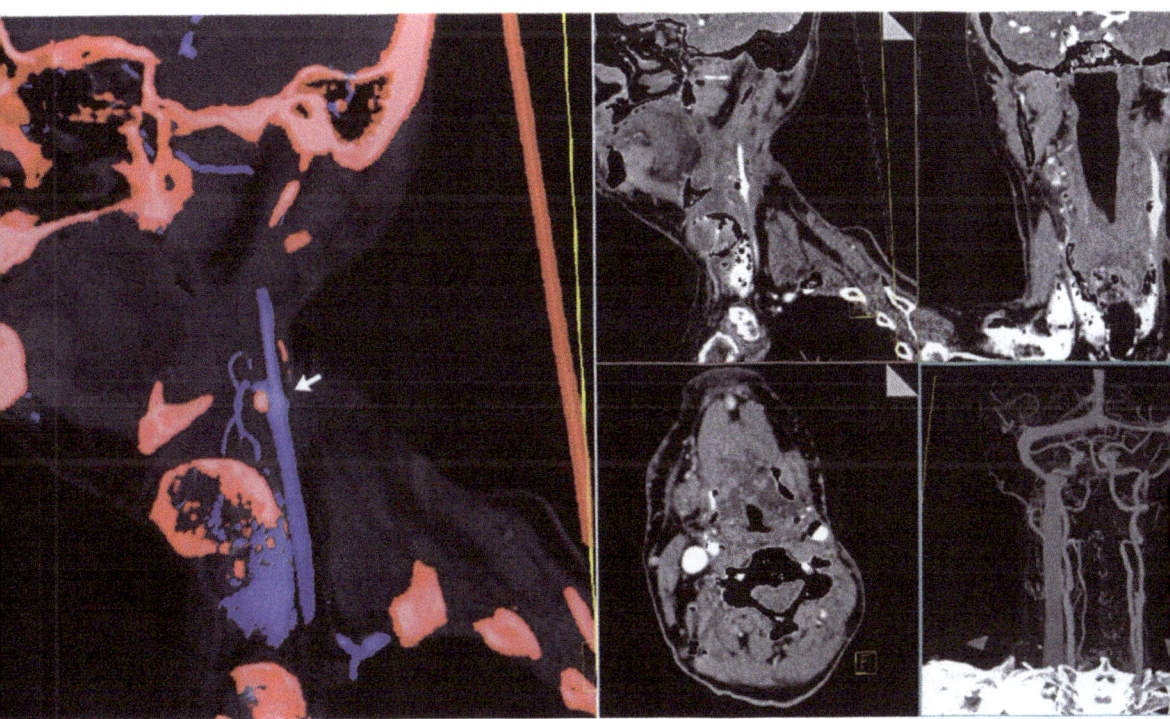

[3] Sagittal dual energy image (MPR) of the same plaque (arrow).

[4] Application of dual energy bone / plaque removal: All voxels containing calcium (hard plaques and bones) have automatically been removed from the images.

Case 2 Calcification of the Renal Artery

Case history

62-year-old female presenting with hypertension. She had undergone right nephrectomy 12 years prior. Since she is severely claustrophobic, an MRI cannot be performed.

Question

Anatomical abnormalities? Calcified or soft plaque lesions? Stenosis of the left renal artery?

Diagnosis / Differential diagnosis

· Arteriosclerosis of the left renal artery.
· Stenosis of the left renal artery.
· Soft or hard plaque.
· Fibromuscular dysplasia.
· Other pathologies.

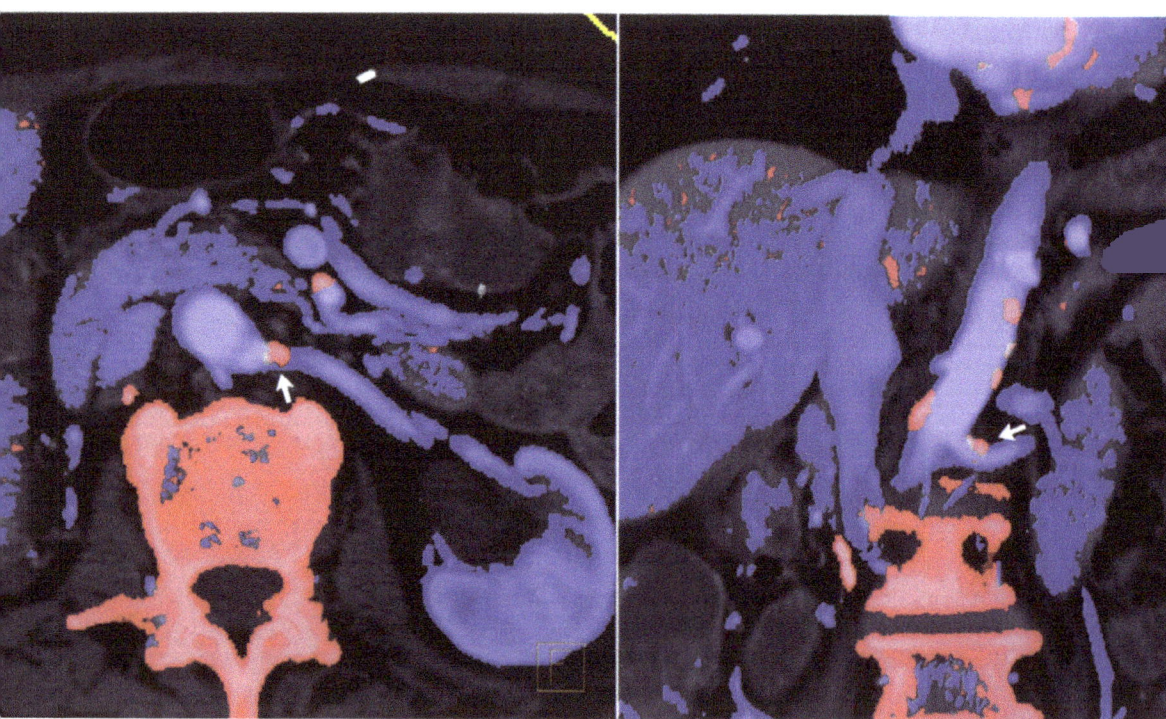

[1] Axial post-processed image from a dual energy abdominal scan. Note a calcified plaque at the outlet of the left renal artery (arrow).

[2] Coronary reformatted image of the same plaque (arrow).

Findings

Abnormal anatomic findings were excluded. Fused dual energy images show a mixed plaque at the ostium of the left renal artery as well as several calcified plaques at the aortic wall. No severe vascular stenosis could be found.

Take-home message

Detection of calcified plaques with dual energy CTA is feasible also in abdominal scans. Even small calcified plaques are detected and color-coded. With the bone removal tools, plaques can be removed from the images, making an unimpaired view onto the vessel lumen possible.

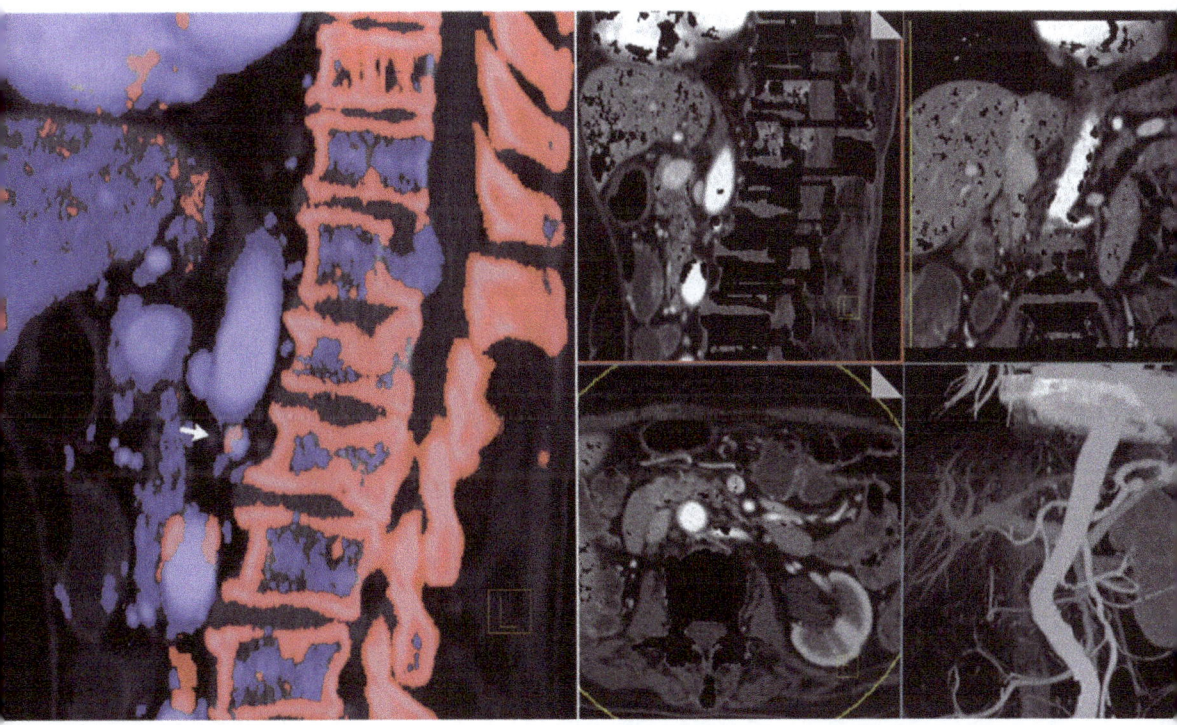

[3] Sagittal image of the same plaque (arrow).

[4] Images after the application of dual energy bone removal. Bones and plaques have been removed from the images.

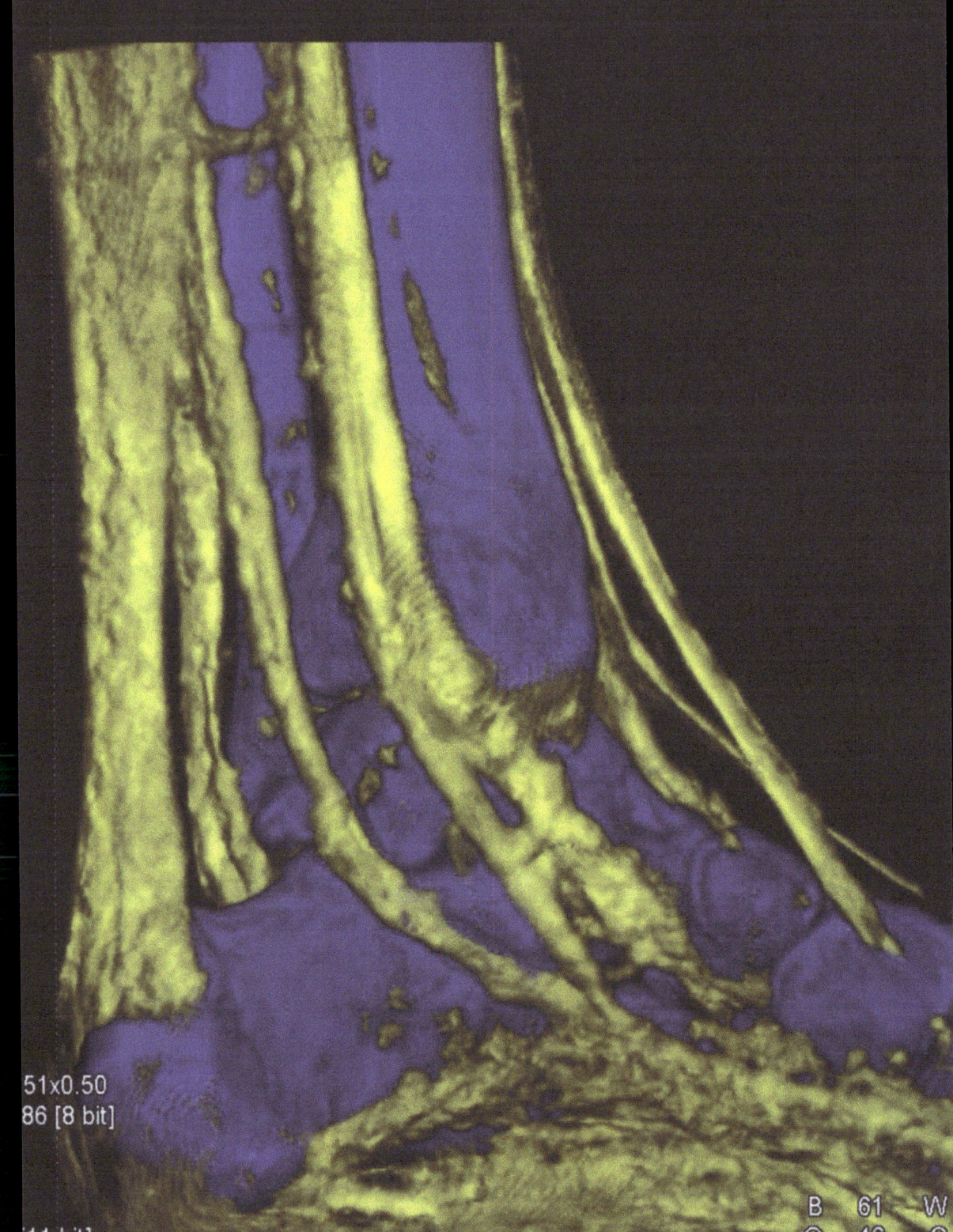

51x0.50
86 [8 bit]

B   61   W

Dual Energy: Tendons and Cartilage

Stefan G. Ruehm · Derek Lohan · Christoph Panknin

Case 1: Suspected Tear of Achilles Tendon

Case 2: Suspicion of Intraarticular Free Body

The introduction of multi-detector row computed tomography (MDCT) has lead to remarkable advances in the field of musculoskeletal imaging. MDCT enables the acquisition of isotropic data sets in high-spatial-resolution, from which multiplanar reformatted images can be calculated in any desired plane. Magnetic resonance imaging (MRI), based on its good low contrast resolution, remains the gold standard for musculoskeletal imaging. However, there is a wide range of situations when MRI cannot be performed, for example, when MRI is contraindicated as in patients with pacemakers or claustrophobia, or in emergency situations where access to the patient is critical. In general, MRI is still less widely available and more costly than CT.

In postoperative situations, susceptibility artifacts caused by metallic implants can render an MRI study non-diagnostic. CT may still yield diagnostic results, particularly when a volume-rendering algorithm is employed, which offers the potential to minimize the impact of streak artifacts caused by metallic hardware. Therefore, MDCT is commonly used for the evaluation of hardware complications and for monitoring of the healing process of fractures in the presence of post-surgical hardware.[1] In the setting of trauma, CT generally allows the precise assessment of the extent of fractures by providing a three-dimensional (3D) display of fracture lines and fragments. If the data is acquired with isotropic resolution, accurate positioning of the extremity prior to the scan is not crucial. When the peripheral skeleton is imaged, the x-ray dose can be significantly reduced because of the small volume of the examined structures, particularly distal to elbow and knee.[2] In contrast to MRI, CT provides the ability to detect and characterize calcifications. Material differentiation capabilities of dual energy CT may even be able to further characterize soft tissue calcification. Initial studies have shown that dual energy CT may actually allow the differentiation of uric acid deposits in gout from other calcifications. CT provides advantages when a large anatomic area needs to be covered, for example, in patients with skeletal dysplasias or thoracic deformities, or when structures not easily assessed by MRI, such as ribs, need to be visualized.

MDCT in combination with 3D image reconstruction has shown to be useful for the evaluation of a variety of tendon abnormalities. MDCT may serve as a valuable alternative imaging tool for the assessment of soft tissues when Ultrasound or MRI cannot be used, for example, in the presence of

Dual Energy: Tendons and Cartilage

large open wounds or when there is post surgical metallic hardware close to the anatomical area of interest. MDCT has been evaluated for imaging of tendons in foot, ankle and hand.[3,4] Promising results have been reported for the diagnosis of peroneal tendon dislocations in patients with a fractured calcaneus or for the delineation of ruptured tendons in the hand.[3,4]

In the knee, MDCT may visualize the intact anterior and posterior cruciate ligaments with high accuracy. However, the precise diagnostic evaluation of torn ligaments still appears challenging.[5]

While MRI is still widely accepted as the primary imaging technique for the evaluation of articular cartilage, CT arthrography may be used as an alternative imaging modality. Based on the ability to reconstruct thin overlapping slices with multiplanar reformations in any desired plane, the introduction of MDCT has actually prompted a revival of CT arthrography for the assessment of intraarticular structures, including the evaluation of articular cartilage. Common causes for articular pathology are osteoarthritis, acute or chronic inflammatory disease, chondrocalcinosis and posttraumatic osteochondral fractures (osteochondrosis dissecans). Often clinical symptoms are non-specific and imaging is mandatory for diagnosis and therapeutic strategy.

CT characterization of body tissue is generally based on differences in x-ray attenuation measured in Hounsfield units (HU). Different attenuation values are displayed as different shades of grey on reconstructed CT images. CT attenuation of a specific material varies with the energy of the x-ray photons applied, and this variation is depending on the material. This effect makes material differentiation with dual energy feasible. Early experiments with dual energy CT applications have been performed in the late 1970s. However, limited spatial resolution, long data acquisition times, and misregistration between the two separate acquisitions at different energy levels prevented the widespread application of dual energy techniques for material characterization. Furthermore, the tube technology available at that time was unable to deliver sufficient tube current to achieve the necessary dose at low voltage. Material differentiation works particularly well in materials with large atomic numbers. This allows for the reliable differentiation of iodine from other dense structures such as bone, a technique currently used for bone removal algorithms. The ability to differentiate soft tissue structures, such as muscle, tendons, ligaments and cartilage is limited, since these tissues mainly contain atoms with small atomic numbers, which show similar x-ray attenuation values at different energy levels. Nevertheless, initial studies have shown that the differentiation of collagen may be possible, probably due to densely packed hydroxylysine and hydroxyproline in side chains of the collagen macromolecule.[6]

In summary, due to its superior contrast resolution, MRI remains the imaging modality of choice for the evaluation of the musculoskeletal system. However, MRI cannot be used in a variety of situations, either because it is contraindicated, impractical or not available. High resolution MDCT may then play an increasing role in addition to its current value for the work-up of trauma patients when imaging of complex skeletal injuries is the primary requirement. Dual energy techniques, employing the simultaneous operation of two x-ray sources at different kVp levels, hold promise to offer additional diagnostic information regarding the integrity of ligaments, tendons and potentially cartilage. Further studies are required to evaluate the diagnostic value of dual energy MDCT for musculoskeletal applications.

Stefan G. Ruehm · Derek Lohan · Christoph Panknin
David Geffen School of Medicine at UCLA
Department of Radiology

References

[1] Ohashi K, El-Khoury GY, Bennett DL, Restrepo JM, Berbaum KS. Orthopedic hardware complications diagnosed with multi-detector row CT. Radiology 2005; 237:570-577

[2] Dalrymple NC, Prasad SR, Freckleton MW, Chintapalli KN: Informatics in radiology (infoRAD): introduction to the language of three-dimensional imaging with multidetector CT. Radiographics 2005, 25:1409-1428

[3] Sunagawa T, Ochi M, Ishida O, Ono C, Ikuta Y. Three-dimensional CT imaging of flexor tendon ruptures in the hand and wrist. J Comput Assist Tomogr 2003; 27:169-174

[4] Ohashi K, El-Khoury GY, Bennett DL. MDCT of tendon abnormalities using volume-rendered images. AJR Am J Roentgenol 2004; 182:161-165

[5] Mustonen AO, Koivikko MP, Haapamaki VV, Kiuru MJ, Lamminen AE, Koskinen SK. Multidetector computed tomography in acute knee injuries: assessment of cruciate ligaments with magnetic resonance imaging correlation. Acta Radiol 2007; 48:104-111

[6] Johnson TR, Krauss B, Sedlmair M, et al. Material differentiation by dual energy CT: initial experience. Eur Radiol 2007; 17:1510-1517

Dual Energy: Tendons and Cartilage

Basic considerations

For muskuloskeletal applications the acquisition of data sets with maximized spatial resolution is generally recommended (collimation: 0.6 mm). A volumetric 3D data set with thin overlapping slices (increment: 0.3 to 0.4 mm) and isotropic spatial resolution is then reconstructed. It allows the calculation of multiplanar reconstructions in any plane or volume rendered displays.

Volume rendered displays are particularly helpful for 3D visualization of tendons and ligaments. The administration of contrast agent is generally not required for standard musculoskeletal protocols, but may be required for oncologic applications and for the evaluation of inflammatory disease.

Scan Parameters

Scan mode	Spiral dual energy with Dual Source
Scan area	any; depending on indication
Scan direction	cranio-caudal
Scan time	~15–45 s
Tube voltage A/B	140 kV/80 kV
Tube current A/B	45 eff. mAs/190 eff. mAs
Dose modulation	no
CTDI$_{vol}$	~8 mGy
Rotation time	0.5 s
Pitch	~0.55–0.75
Slice collimation	0.6 mm
Acquisition	64 x 0.6 mm
Slice width	0.75 mm
Reconstruction increment	0.5 mm
Reconstruction kernel	D30f/B60f

Tricks

The tube current needs to be adjusted to the anatomical region and size of the patient to achieve the desired low contrast resolution. CARE Dose4D should be used to compensate for changes in attenuation (eg. from shin to foot). 3D reconstructions can greatly aid visualization of ligaments and tendons. Despite promising early results for DE imaging of intraarticular cartilage arthrography may still be needed.

Pitfalls

Potential of increased image noise with improper adjustment of tube current settings. Off-center positioning of the area of interest needs to be avoided to achieve maximum in-plane resolution and to allow optimal post processing.

Contrast Injection Protocol

CM Volume	–
Iodine delivery rate	–
CM flow rate	–
Iodine concentration	–
Body weight adaption	–
Bolus timing	–
HU target	–
ROI position	–
Scan delay	–
Saline flush	–
Needle size	–
Injection site	–

Case 1 Suspected Tear of Achilles Tendon

Case history

31-year-old recreational soccer player. Direct trauma to back of ankle during soccer. History of Achilles tendon tear on the contralateral side.

Question

The patient is referred to rule out an acute tear of the Achilles tendon. In addition, the bony structures should be assessed.

Diagnosis / Differential diagnosis

Non contrast enhanced Dual Energy MDCT of ankle shows no evidence of Achilles tendon tear. There is no evidence of bone lesions or larger hematoma. Peroneal and flexor tibial tendons are intact.

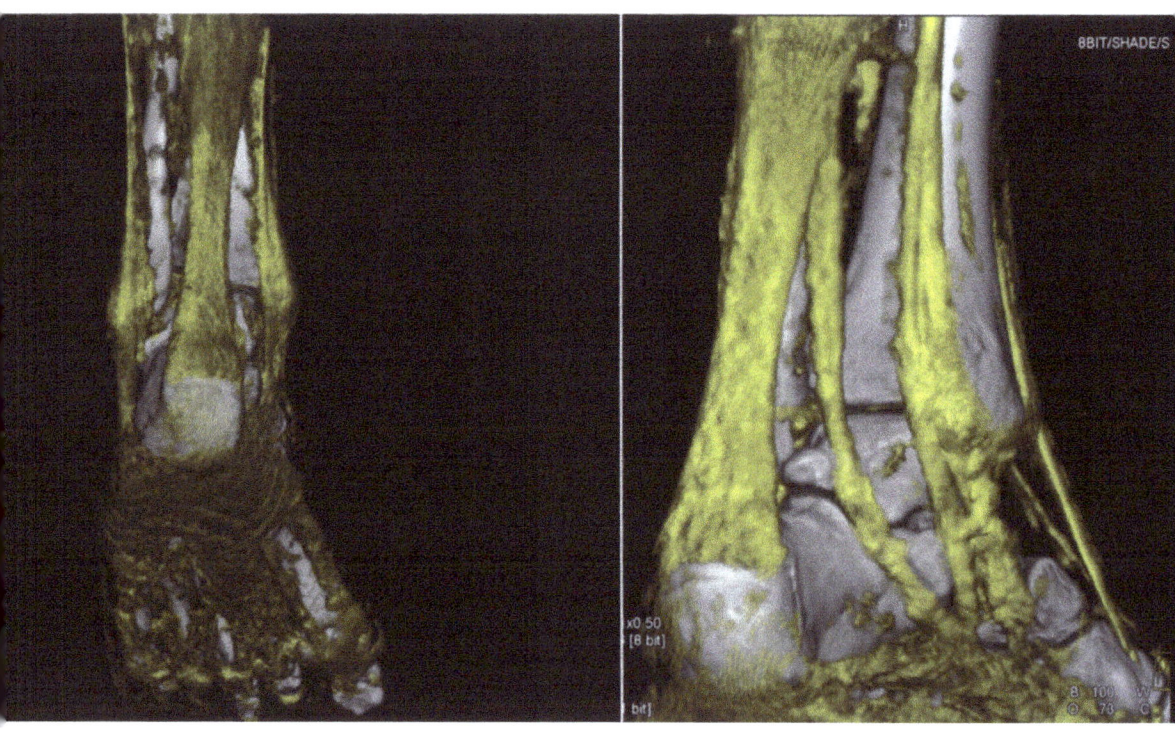

[1] 3D volume rendered image of ankle tendons; posterior view.

[2] 3D volume rendered image of ankle tendons; medial oblique view.

Findings

Dual energy MDCT of ankle shows continuity of tendons in the ankle with no evidence of tendon rupture. Peroneus longus, peroneus brevis, achilles and tibial tendons are clearly demarcated. The bony structures are unremarkable.

Take-home message

Dual energy MDCT imaging of tendons is feasible. Isotropic high spatial resolution allows three dimensional visualization of tendons in combination with display of bony structures. Contrast administration is not necessary for imaging of the ankle to rule out tendon rupture.

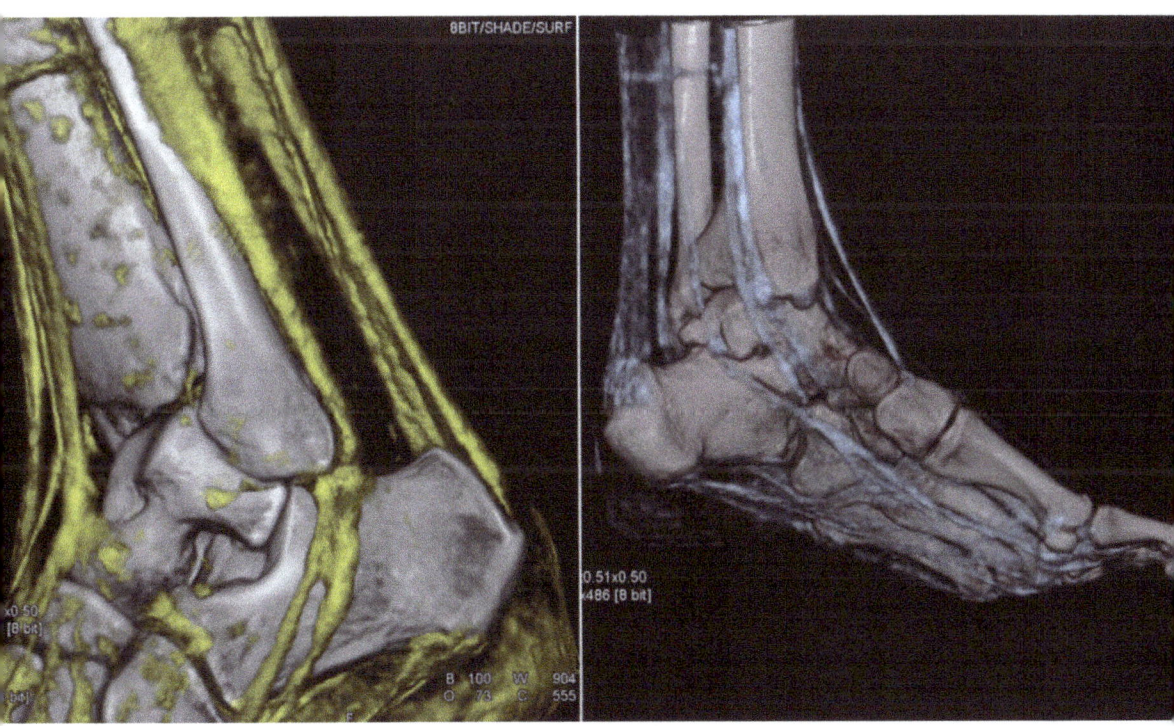

[3] 3D volume rendered image of ankle tendons; lateral oblique view.

[4] 3D volume rendered image of foot; normal display of ankle tendons.

Case 2 Suspicion of Intraarticular Free Body

Case history

40-year-old athlete with recurrent episodes of knee joint blockades. Minor trauma due to bicycle accident 2 years ago. Recurrent episodes of swelling of left knee.

Question

Derangement of meniscus? Intraarticular free body? Normal size and shape of menisci?

Diagnosis / Differential diagnosis

Normal dual energy MDCT study of left knee joint. There is no evidence of a free intraarticular body. There is no evidence of a mensiscal dislocation or larger tear. There is no intraarticular free fluid.

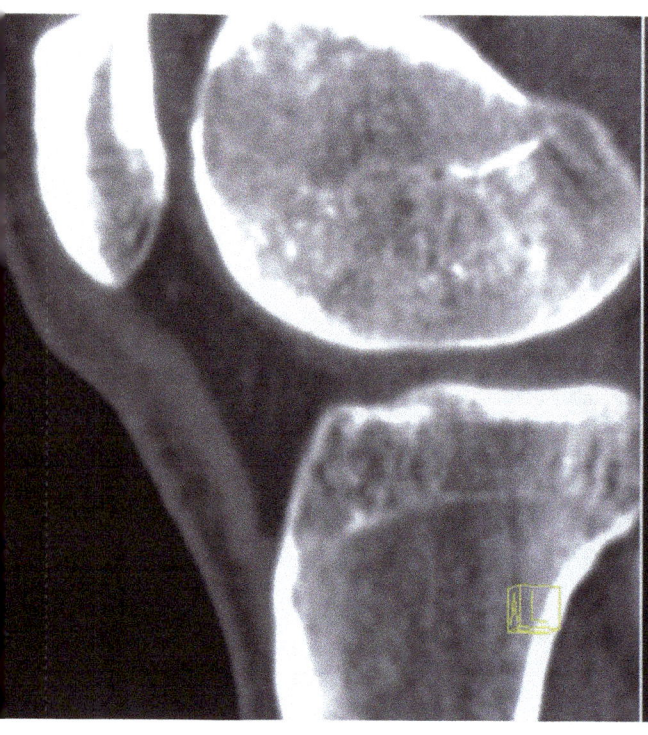
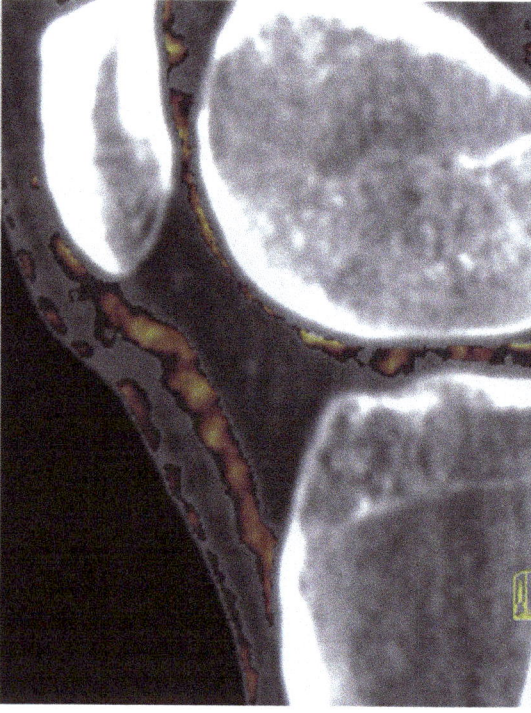

[1] Sagittal reformatted image of left knee with no evidence of joint effusion or fracture.

[2] Spiral dual energy MDCT display of left knee visualizes normal infrapatellar tendon.

Findings

Dual energy MDCT study of left knee nicely delineates medial and lateral meniscus with normal shape and in normal location. There is no evidence of a larger meniscal tear extending to the surface of the meniscus. The bony structures are unremarkable. There is no evidence of an osteochondral fragment.

Take-home message

Dual energy MDCT allows visualization of medial and lateral meniscus of knee joint. In addition, bony structures as well as ligaments can be clearly delineated. Dual energy MDCT appears well suited to rule out osteochondral fragments, and to assess teh size and location of the menisci in the knee joint.

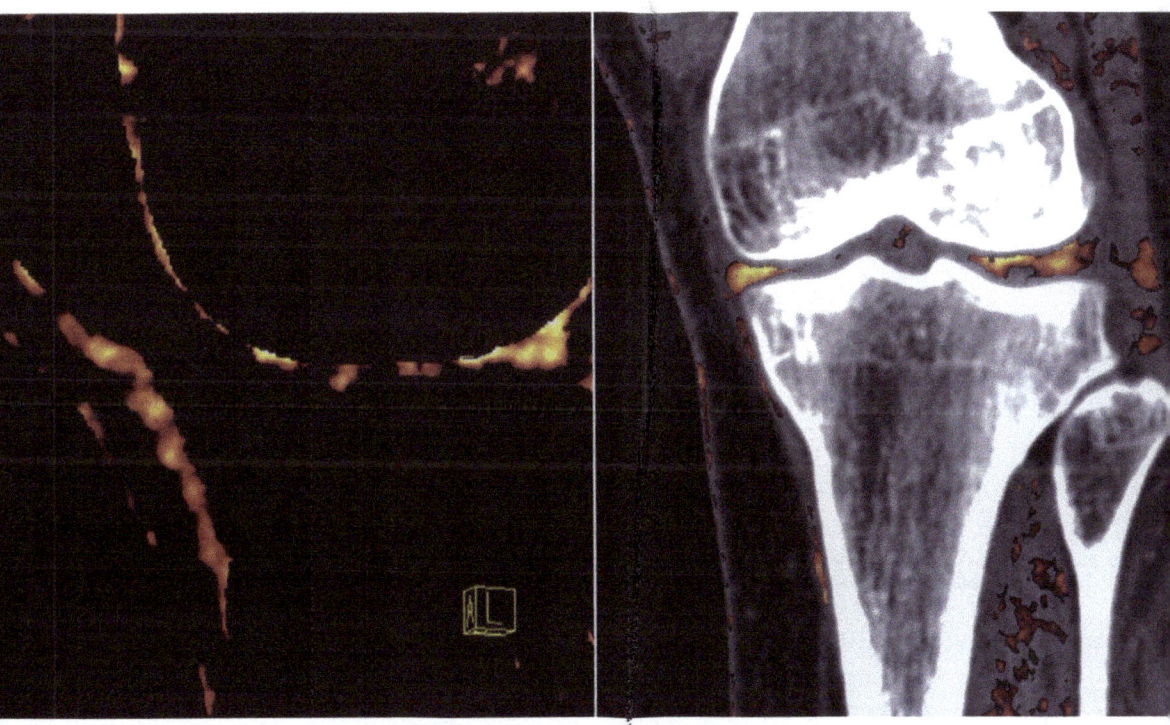

[3] Spiral dual energy MDCT display of left knee aimed at the visualization of hyaline femoral cartilage shows normal articular thickness at femoral condyle.

[4] Coronal reformatted spiral dual energy MDCT display of left knee shows normal position of medial and lateral meniscus.

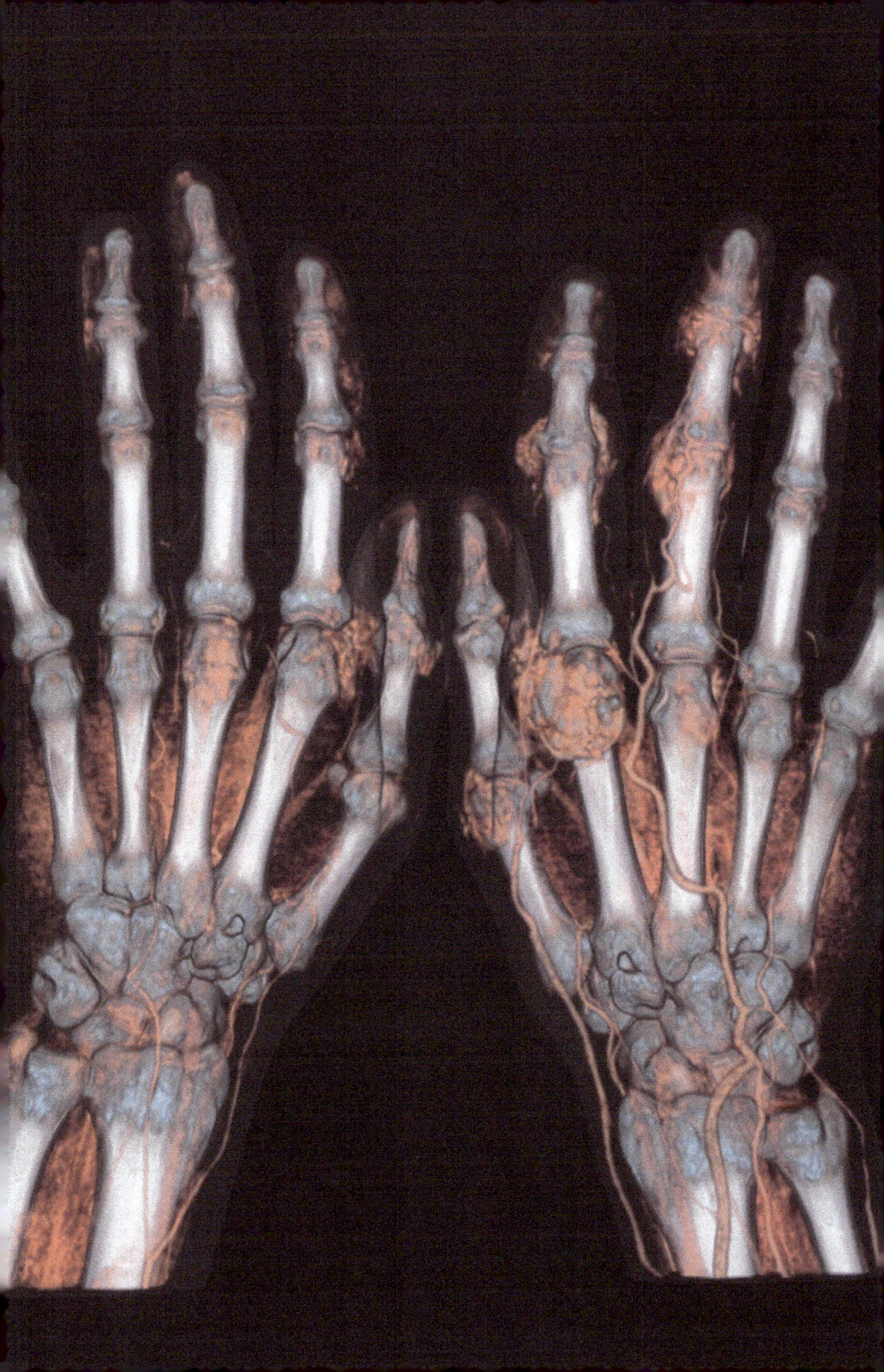

Dual Energy: Gout

Thorsten R. C. Johnson · Sabine Weckbach · Christoph R. Becker

Case 1: Adult Male with Soft Tissue Swelling of Right Middle Finger

Gout is caused by genetic disposition and alimentary factors. It comprises a heterogeneous group of disorders characterized by deposition of monosodium urate crystals in the joints and tendons. Asymptomatic hyperuricemia is common and should not ordinarily be treated. Gout progresses through four clinical phases: asymptomatic hyperuricemia, acute gouty arthritis, intercritical gout (intervals between acute attacks) and chronic tophaceous gout. A combination of increased production of uric acid and insufficient excretion causes the disease to become clinically evident. The causes are deposits of uric acid that can be found in the distal extremities, especially adjacent to joints, primarily in the toes but also in the fingers. The foot, heel, ankle, knee, hands, wrists and elbows are the other joints that are frequently involved (i.e. rather peripheral joints). A familial pattern is observed in up to 15% of cases. Obesity, high blood pressure and atherosclerotic heart disease are often associated.

Gout occurs acutely as intermittent attacks of inflammatory arthritis with severe joint pain, swelling, redness and warmth of affected joint. In 90% of initial episodes, a single joint is involved, especially the joint at the base of the hallux. Severe attacks of joint pain can occur at any age, but the first attack often affects men between the ages of 40 and 50. Gout occurs 20 times more frequently in men than in women. Attacks can be triggered by alcohol, high purine food (meat, seafood, kidney), diuretic drugs or anti-cancer chemotherapy.[1, 2]

Although hyperuricemia predisposes patients to gout and nephrolithiasis, it does not need to be treated in the asymptomatic patient. However, efforts should be made to modify or correct underlying causes.

Colchicine, an antimitotic drug derived from the roots of the herb Colchicum autumnale, is one of the oldest treatments for gout. Although colchicine is effective in treating acute gout, 80 percent of patients experience gastrointestinal side effects, including nausea, vomiting and diarrhea, at therapeutic dosages.

Therefore, nonsteroidal anti-inflammatory drugs are the treatment of choice for acute attacks of gout in most patients, but should be used sparingly in elderly patients and avoided in patients with renal disease and peptic ulcer disease. Corticosteroids are a valuable treatment option for patients in whom non-steroidal anti-inflammatory drugs are contraindicated. Acute gouty arthritis and chronic gout

Dual Energy: Gout

require different treatment strategies. After the acute gouty attack is treated and prophylactic therapy is initiated, the issue of ongoing urate deposition should be addressed. A common practice is not to initiate drug therapy aimed at lowering urate levels after the initial attack. Rather, most clinicians prefer to aggressively correct or reverse sources of hyperuricemia in hopes of lowering the serum urate level without the use of medication.

Demonstration of intra-articular monosodium urate crystals is necessary to establish a definitive diagnosis of gouty arthritis. Thus, a definitive diagnosis usually requires aspiration and examination of synovial fluid to confirm the presence of monosodium urate crystals. The crystals are identified by their characteristic birefringence under polarized light microscopy.

In cases of unclear soft tissue swelling, elevated serum levels of uric acid and response to treatment with colchicine can support the diagnosis. Plain film radiography shows soft tissue affections and calcium deposits in earlier stages, and chronic gout leads to asymmetrical forms of osseous destruction.[3]

Spiral dual energy CT provides the unique opportunity to directly show the presence of uric acid crystals in the tophi. Moreover, inflammation can be assessed by administering contrast material, and areas of enhancement can also be identified by spiral dual energy CT due to the dual energy properties of iodine. Thus, a more specific and reliable diagnosis can be made within a few minutes, including high-resolution morphology of the affected joint, depiction of inflammatory changes and visualization of uric acid deposits in the tophi.[4]

As described in a recent case report, a 46-year-old male was referred for imaging of his hands to clarify an acute inflammation with hyperemia, swelling and tenderness of his right middle finger.[1] There were several areas of painless soft tissue swelling on both hands. Known hyperuricemia was suggestive of gout, but the inflammation of the palmar soft tissue of the right middle finger without relation to a joint was considered less characteristic, and imaging was to rule out other causes.

Spiral dual energy CT was performed on the SOMATOM Definition at 140 and 80 kV$_p$ tube potential after intravenous injection of iodinated contrast material (Ultravist® 370, Bayer Schering Pharma). The three material differentiation shows a spectral behavior characteristic for uric acid in the area of inflammation and multiple other areas of painless soft tissue swelling (encoded blue in the image). The differentiation of iodine clearly shows the contrast enhancement in the area of inflammation (encoded red). Thus, the inflammatory changes could be attributed to acute gout. The diagnosis was confirmed by response to treatment with Colchicine. The patient received appropriate medication and dietary advice and is now scheduled for surgical resection of the gout tophi.

This case shows the ability of spiral dual energy CT to enhance the diagnostic value of computed tomography, not mainly by increasing its spatial resolution or its soft tissue contrast but by adding a higher specificity to the obtained information. Depending on the further development of the technique and ongoing research, it is conceivable that other substances which represent markers for a certain diseases can be differentiated and detected due to their spectral properties. Then, other dual energy protocols can offer more specific diagnostic information as well as a direct and precise assessment of the disease with diagnostic certainty and high resolution morphology, replacing the current, merely morphology-based diagnostic reading in CT.

Thorsten R. C. Johnson · Sabine Weckbach · Christoph R. Becker
University of Munich-Grosshadern
Department of Clinical Radiology

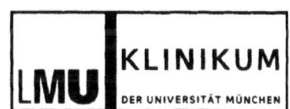

References

[1] Tausche AK, Unger S, Richter K, Wunderlich C, Grassler J, Roch B, Schroder HE Hyperuricemia and gout: diagnosis and therapy. Internist 2006. May;47(5):509-20

[2] Muller-Fassbender H, Bach GL. Radiologic findings in gout. Wien Med Wochenschr. 1997;147(16):377-81

[3] Perez-Ruiz F, Naredo E. Imaging modalities and monitoring measures of gout. Curr Opin Rheumatol. 2007.19(2):128-33

[4] Johnson TR, Weckbach S, Kellner H, Reiser MF Becker C. Dual-energy computed tomographic molecular imaging of gout. Arthritis Rheum. 2007 Jul 30;56(8):2809

Dual Energy: Gout

Basic considerations

As uric acid has spectral properties that can be exploited for dual energy imaging, unenhanced images are sufficient to detect uric acid and to confirm gout. Contrast material can additionally show hyperenhancement in areas of inflammation at the same time to assess disease activity and diagnose acute gout as the cause of current symptoms. The thinnest slice thickness and low image noise are desirable in order to detect small uric acid particles. Both hands should be positioned flat next to each other on the scanner table. If the hands are extended over the head, a very low radiation exposure for the body can be achieved.

Scan Parameters

Scan mode	Spiral dual energy with Dual Source
Scan area	hands or feet
Scan direction	proximal to distal
Scan time	~15 s
Tube voltage A/B	140 kV / 80 kV
Tube current A/B	70 quality ref. mAs / 300 quality ref. mAs
Dose modulation	CARE Dose4D
CTDI$_{vol}$	~12 mGy
Rotation time	0.5 s
Pitch	0.7
Slice collimation	0.6 mm
Acquisition	64 x 0.6 mm
Slice width	1 mm
Reconstruction increment	0.7 mm
Reconstruction kernel	D30f

Tricks

Hands should be extended above the head in prone position as it is usually easier for the patient to hold his hands still for the exam. Dual topograms in anterior-posterior and lateral projection can help positioning. Consider examining hands including wrists and feet including the ankles to cover the most commonly affected areas.

Pitfalls

· High image noise can hinder the detection of small uric acid cristals.
· Make sure that both hands are placed in the isocenter.

Contrast Injection Protocol

	Iodine concentration 300 mg I/ml	Iodine concentration 370 mg I/ml
Injection scheme	Monophasic	Monophasic
Iodine delivery rate	0.75 g/s	0.75 g/s
CM volume	100 ml	80 ml
CM flow rate	2.5 ml/s	2 ml/s
Body weight adaption	no	no
Bolus timing	–	–
Bolus tracking threshold	–	–
ROI position	–	–
Scan delay	70 s	70 s
Saline flush volume	50 ml	50 ml
Saline injection rate	2.5 ml/s	2 ml/s
Needle size	20 G	20 G
Injection site	antecubital vein	antecubital vein

Case 1 Adult Male with Soft Tissue Swelling of Right Middle Finger

Case history

A middle-aged male presents with unclear painful soft tissue swelling of his right middle finger.

Question

Although the patient has gout tophi, the new swelling is not considered typical. CT is performed to confirm gout or rule out other causes.

Diagnosis / Differential diagnosis

For soft tissue swelling of the hands or feet, differential diagnoses include other forms of arthritis, e.g. rheumatoid arthritis, or hallux valgus, or bacterial inflammation. Spiral dual energy CT offers the unique potential to identify deposits of uric acid in the tophi and thus confirm gout. Acute gout can be diagnosed if additional contrast enhancement is observed in the tophi.

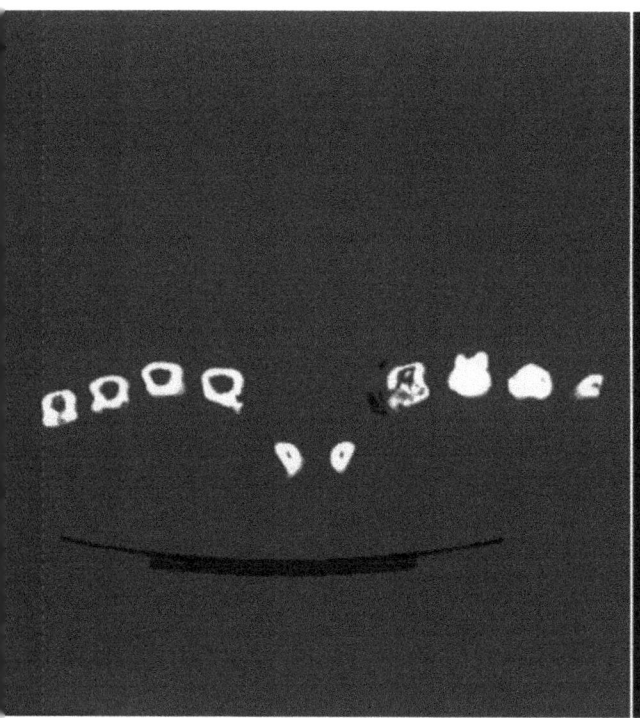

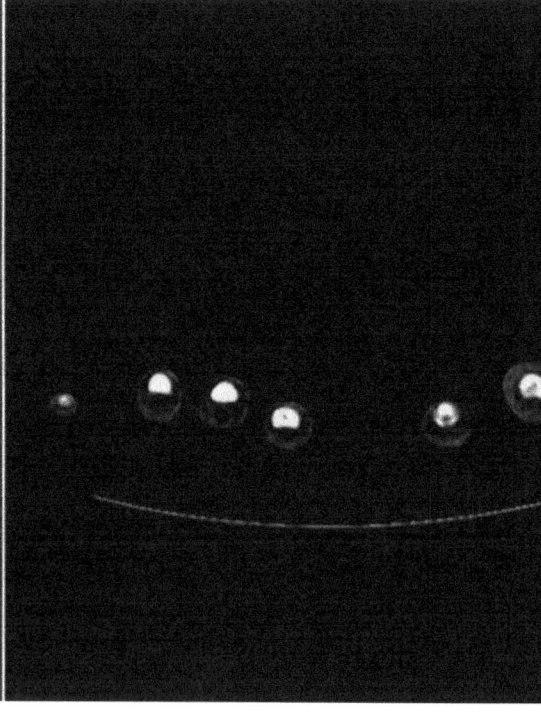

[1] Dual Energy material decomposition shows deposits of uric acid, e.g. in a tophus on the left index finger.

[2] Additional analysis for iodine shows contrast enhancement of the left middle finger, showing active inflammation.

Findings

Multiple areas of soft tissue swelling are found on both hands, preferentially around the metacarpophalangeal joints. The presence of uric acid can be confirmed in those areas due to its typical spectral dual energy properties. Additionally, contrast enhancement can be shown in the area of acute inflammation due to the spectral behaviour of iodine.

Take-home message

Spiral dual energy CT offers the unique possibility to directly visualize uric acid in gout tophi and thus to detect the specific substance causing the disease. With this information, the diagnosis of gout is much more specific than the mere description of arthritis, possibly with destruction of the joint, which would otherwise be the most precise information obtainable by CT or MRI.

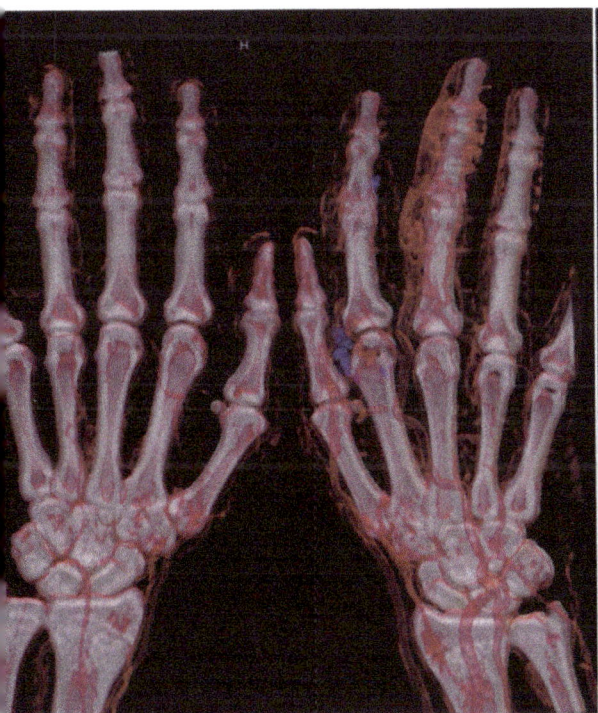

[3] The volume rendered image combines all information with the uric acid color-coded in blue and iodine-encoded in red.

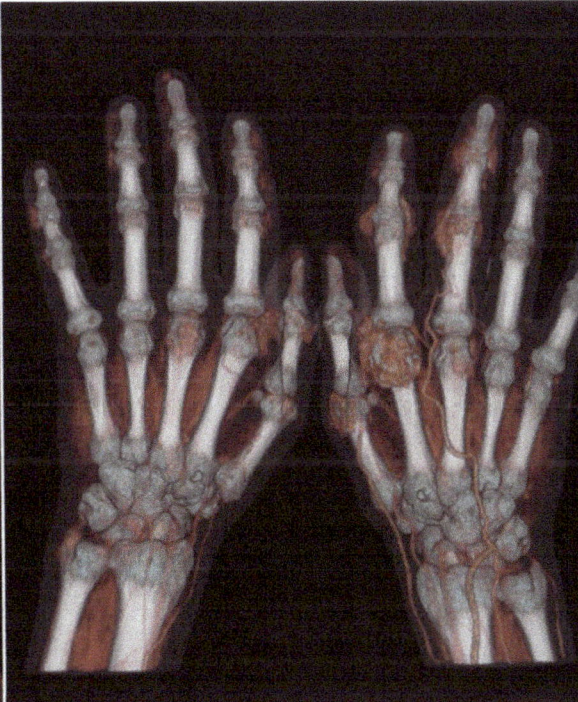

[4] This volume rendered image shows multiple tophi on both hands of the same patient.

Abbreviations

AAA	abdominal aortic aneurysm		p.a.	posteroantierior
AF	arterial fibrillation		PAOD	peripheral arterial occlusive disease
ARVCM	arrhythmogenic right-ventricular cardiac morphology		PBV	perfused blood volume
			PCI	percutaneous coronary intervention
BMI	body mass index		PCT	perfusion CT
bpm	beats per minute		RAS	renal artery stenosis
CABG	cardiac artery bypass graft		RCA	right coronary artery
CAD	coronary artery disease		RCC	renal cell carcinoma
CBF	cerebral blood flow		RCX	circumflex artery
CBV	cerebral blood volume		RFCA	radio-frequency catheter ablation
CCTA	coronary CT angiography		ROA	regurgitant orifice area
CM	contrast media		ROI	region of interest
CRT	cardiac resynchronization therapy		RVOT	right-ventricular outflow tract
CTA	CT angiography		SAH	subarachnoid hemorrhage
$CTDI_{vol}$	computed tomography dose index		SPECT	single-photon emission CT
CTO	total coronary artery occlusion		SSD	shaded surface display
CTP	CT perfusion (scan)		s/p	status post
CTU	CT urography		SVC	superior vena cava
DSA	digital subtraction angiography, dual source angiography		trot	rotation time
			TTP	time to peak enhancement
DSCT	Dual-Source computed tomography		VRT	volume-rendering technique
DWI	diffusion-weighted imaging		VSD	ventricular septal defect
EBCT	electron beam CT			
ECG	electrocardiogram			
EDV	end-diastolic volume			
EF	ejection fraction			
ESV	end-systolic volume			
EVAR	endovascular aortic repair			
FMD	fibromuscular dysplasia			
FoV	field of view			
Gd-DTPA	gadolinium diethylene triaminopenta-acetic acid			
HU	Hounsfield units			
ICD	implantable cardioverter defibrillator			
IMA	internal mammary arteries			
LAD	left anterior descending artery			
LVH	left-ventricular hypertrophy			
MCA	middle cerebral artery			
MDCT	multi-detector row CT			
MI	myocardial infarction			
MIP	maximum intensity projection(s)			
MPR	multiplanar reformations			
MRA	magnetic resonance angiography			
MRI	magnetic resonance imaging			
MSCT	multislice spiral CT			
MTT	mean transit time			
NECT	non-enhanced CT			

Editors

Peter R. Seidensticker, radiologist, was born on April 25, 1970, in Hamburg, Germany. After a year of economic IT studies at the PTL Wedel, Hamburg, he started studying medicine at the Ruprecht-Karls-University in Heidelberg, Germany, in 1992. Accomplishing most of his radiological residency in the Department of Diagnostic Radiology at Heidelberg University, he finalized his dissertation on the histological background of TIPSS stenoses in 2004. Completing his radiological training at the Charité Clinic, University of Berlin, Germany, he joined the Diagnostic Imaging unit of Bayer Schering Pharma AG, Berlin, Germany, as a medical expert in 2004. At present, he is responsible for the field of x-ray imaging in the Department of Global Medical Affairs.

Lars K. Hofmann, MD, was born on March 7, 1974, in Landau/Pfalz, Germany. In 1995, he began studying medicine at the Philips-University Marburg, Germany, and wrote his medical dissertation on breast cancer genomics at the Lombardi Cancer Center, Georgetown University, Washington D.C. A research fellowship in thoracic radiology at the Brigham & Women's Hospital, Harvard Medical School in Boston, sparked his interest in cardiac CT imaging. Dedicated to become a cardiac surgeon, he started his residency at the Heart Center of the University of Leipzig, Germany. In 2004, he decided to join Siemens Medical Solutions and was responsible for the global clinical marketing of cardiac and acute care CT. At present, Lars Hofmann runs the Siemens Med Learning Academy, an institution providing medical and clinical workflow knowledge to employees.